Breathing: Violence In, Peace Out

New Approaches To Peace And Conflict

Ivana Milojević

16

EasyRead Large

RHYW

Copyright Page from the Original Book

First published 2013 by University of Queensland Press
PO Box 6042, St Lucia, Queensland 4067 Australia

www.uqp.com.au
uqp@uqp.uq.edu.au

Cover concept by i2i design
Cover design by Kate Barry
Typeset in Adobe Garamond Pro 11.5/15pt by Post Pre-press Group, Brisbane
Printed in Australia by McPherson's Printing Group

National Library of Australia Cataloging-in-Publication Data
http://catalogue.nla.gov.au

978 0 7022 4969 3 (pbk)
978 0 7022 5113 9 (pdf)
978 0 7022 5114 6 (epub)
978 0 7022 5115 3 (kindle)

University of Queensland Press uses papers that are natural, renewable and recyclable products made from wood grown in sustainable forests. The logging and manufacturing processes conform to the environmental regulations of the country of origin.

TABLE OF CONTENTS

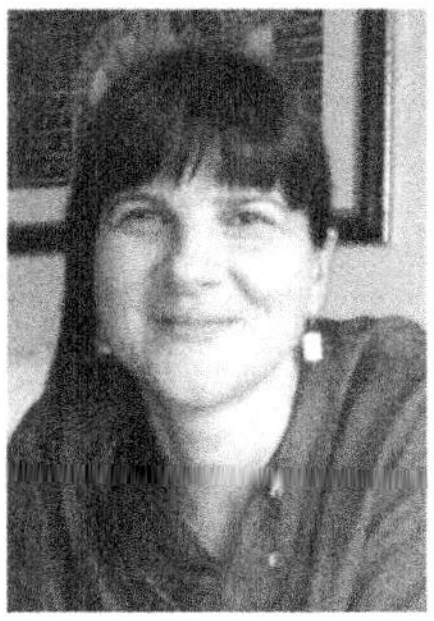

Professor Ivana Milojević is a researcher, writer and educator with a professional background in the fields of sociology, education, gender, peace and futures studies. Born in the former-Yugoslavia, she currently resides at the Sunshine Coast, Australia, where she is an Adjunct Professor (University of the Sunshine Coast, Faculty of Arts and Business). Since 2008, Dr Milojević has also been Visiting Professor at the Association of Centres for Interdisciplinary and Multidisciplinary Studies and Research, University of Novi Sad, Serbia.

She is the author of over sixty journal articles and book chapters, as well as the author, co-author and/or co-editor of: *Ko se boji vuka još? [Who Is Afraid of the Big, Bad Wolf?],* a peace education guidebook (2012); *Uvod u rodne teorije [Introduction to Gender Theories]* (2011); *Alternative Educational Futures: Pedagogies for an Emergent World* (2008); a special issue of *Futures* on Feminism/Gender (2008); *Neohumanist Educational Futures: Liberating the Pedagogical Intellect* (2006); *Educational Futures: Dominant and Contesting Visions* (2005, reprinted in

2011); and *Moving Forward: Teachers and Students Against Racism* (2001).

www.meta-future.org and www.breathinginout.weebly.com

Other titles in UQP's New Approaches to Peace and Conflict series

Reporting Conflict: New directions in peace journalism
by Jake Lynch & Johan Galtung

When Blood and Bones Cry Out: Journeys through the soundscape of healing and reconciliation
by John Paul Lederach & Angela Jill Lederach

Peacemaking and the Imagination: Papua New Guinea perspectives
by Andrew Strathern and Pamela J Stewart

Peace and Security: Implications for women
by Elisabeth Porter and Anuradha Mundkur

Ending Holy Wars: Religion and conflict resolution in civil wars
by Isak Svensson

Note from Series Editor

UQP's New Approaches to Peace and Conflict series builds on the wisdom of the first wave of peace researchers while addressing important 21st century challenges to peace, human rights and sustainable development.

The series publishes new theory, new research and new strategies for effective peacebuilding and the transformation of violent conflict. It challenges orthodox perspectives on development, conflict transformation and peacebuilding within an ethical framework of doing no harm while doing good.

Professor Kevin P Clements
Chair in Peace and Conflict Studies
Director of The National Centre for Peace and Conflict Studies
University of Otago, New Zealand

Introduction

In: To breathe or not to breathe?

> I have intentionally made extensive use of my own story, for a number of reasons. For one thing, my own stories are the ones I know best. As Thoreau said in *Walden:* 'I should not talk so much about myself if there was anybody else whom I knew as well.' Another thing. When I read a book ... of healing, I'm engaged with the author in a personal way and want to know: How did she come to believe this? What in her life made her understand this subject in this particular way? I know I'm not alone in my nosiness. Most engaged readers of books on subjects like this one are voyeurs like me. The stories from my own life that you will read here will give you a sense of the ground from which this book sprouted (Greenspan 2004, pp.6–7).

When I began writing this book some years ago I had serious troubles breathing. My symptoms included an inability to breathe freely, breathlessness, a crushing sensation and sharp pain in the chest, frequent sighing, yawning and gasping, and a rising terror, a fear that something terrible was about to happen. The experience was frightening and deeply unsettling. The more I tried to control my breathing, the more uncontrollable it became. Trying to not think about it, paradoxically, made it the only thing to think about. Distraction was futile. Several months and doctor's appointments passed and I did not have a proper medical diagnosis or any treatment to minimise the symptoms. Appointments with a psychologist to ascertain if there was any underlying psychological cause also did not help. In fact, they somehow, albeit temporarily, managed to increase the symptoms. And so I started conducting my own research into the matter.

As I found out, the literature on the subject is abundant, and various causes and cures of my condition have been proposed. According to self-help author Louise L Hay, for example, the symptoms represent 'a fear or refusal to take in life fully' as well as 'not feeling the right to take up space or even exist'. In addition to her diagnosis of the main underlying causes of my symptoms she recommends a solution: create a 'new thought pattern' in your mind, along the lines of, 'it is my birthright to live fully and freely,' 'I am safe everywhere in the Universe. I trust the process of life' (1999, pp.184, 201). One of my friends, though, thought I was simply hyperventilating and brought me a piece of paper describing some of the symptoms that closely matched my own. But there was nothing on that sheet about how I could stop them to get on with my life. So I resorted to an analysis of yet another self-help author, Ann Gadd, who writes, 'When we make a habit of hyperventilating it is an indication that we often assume ourselves to be in "fight or flight" mode, where our security is in jeopardy.' And if we are 'constantly finding ourselves in situations that make us afraid, it is an indication that we have deep-rooted expectations that things will go wrong rather than right.' Her solution? 'Find the source of your fear' (2006, pp.40–45).

Not having much to lose, I sat down in front of an empty computer screen with one goal in mind. Can I find out what is behind my symptoms – my disturbed breathing and the feeling I might suffocate? Surprisingly, stories started pouring out of me. As they did, they astounded me. I wanted to know about *my* condition and I was thus utterly surprised that the first story took place in Slovenia and then in the Soviet Union in the 1930s, decades before I was even born. It was family history, and I was aware of scepticism towards historical narratives. For example, Brian Simon summarises this scepticism well: 'Why study history ... at all? After all, it's all dead, gone, finished – what is important lies in the future ... History ... is boring, arid, defunct. Such as it is, it were better forgotten' (1983, p.65). Mehni Khan Nakosteen, on the other hand, proposes that history is 'always a study of ourselves, our problems, our hopes and dreams, our failures and successes, our joys and anxieties.' Therefore, 'so conceived, history becomes in a wider context the study of [hu]man[s] in the present sense and in the present tense' (1965, p.13). Joseph Voros, too, suggests a rationale for reconciling past, present and future: '...historians, sociologists and futurists are all involved in pretty much the same work. The main difference [between them] is in the direction they look: historians look back, futurists look forwards, and sociologists look around' (2008).

My narratives, though, looked simultaneously back, forward and around, adding even more confusion to my already perplexed mind. They also oscillated between deeply personal narration and highly theoretical analysis, between local and global issues, and between historical, present and future times and various geographical spaces, making for a strange mix indeed. Furthermore, I was astonished to discover all these things that I never even *knew* I knew. At times it felt as if I was possessed by the spirit of my own and my family's past; as if the fractals of my ancestors' stories had to be depicted and announced to the world.

Writing my stories and their stories made me suffer, made me cry and made me struggle with how much I was allowed to reveal. It made me ask tough questions about authenticity and ethics, self-serving attributional biases and the politics of victimhood,[1] as well as whether I was a traitor or a truth seeker. At other times I wondered how much my ancestors were speaking directly to me. Did they perhaps speak through me? Did they project their fears on to me, or did I project mine on to them? What were these sentences describing events of the past that came out of me without much effort on my part? How did I know all these things? Where were the stories really coming from? Why am I writing in English? Who am I writing all this for? And, most importantly, can all these bits and pieces make for a coherent narrative?

Out: History, present, future

> Not only is another world possible, she is on her way. On a quiet day, I can hear her breathing (Roy 2003).

Breathing: Violence In, Peace Out investigates the long-term impact of transgenerational trauma and of personal and collective experiences with violence. As well, it looks at the possibilities for the emergence of more peaceful futures, including the individual/social practices necessary to bring them about. The text oscillates between a deeply personal and an academic tone of voice. The personal narratives, which I organised within the 'in' sections, are mostly employed for describing violent events and follow the loosely chronological order and thematic context around which the chapters are organised. The academic voice, the 'out' section, is used mostly for reflection, analysis of events and for making sense of the various experiences.

I have used the rhythm created by inhaling and exhaling as it symbolically reflects not only how we 'take in' life and the world but also what we 'give out' to the people around us. This in–out pace models efforts to understand the links between violence–peace, self–other, individual–world history, personal–political, trauma–healing, experience–sense making, stability–change, safety–threat, oppressing–freeing, perception of reality– reality and past–future. To make it easier for readers I have used different fonts for personal narratives/stories and the academic analysis of those events. At times, as is so often the case in life, the in and out narratives overlap. This becomes more so towards the end of the book, which focuses mostly on psychological processes.

Breathing: Violence In, Peace Out is therefore a result of an inquiry into my own condition of feelings of impending suffocation as well as into the possibility of changing the inner landscape of our collective thinking amid so much pain and suffering in the world now and in recent history. Up until the beginning of the actual writing of this book I was unaware how important the stories of the past and the stories of my ancestors had been in my life. Once I was engaged in the task of peeling away the metaphoric onion layers for the purposes of writing a reasonably coherent storyline, I discovered all sorts of memories that existed within the inner layers of my psyche. Like most other children and grandchildren of traumatised people I remember those memories in 'bits and pieces' (Danieli 1998, p.5). Like many other children and grandchildren of traumatised people I did not realise nor appreciate the burden they carried. I would like to acknowledge their resilience in the face of trauma by dedicating this book to them, to the three generations of people that came before me, people who are still alive in my mind, and people who, for better or worse, help(ed) make me the person I am today.

Neither those who came before me nor I exist(ed) in a vacuum, so the following chapters are also an inquiry into the links between my own and our collective personal histories and world events – how they shape and are shaped by each other. Large sections of the book analyse various ideologies and worldviews that have marked the twentieth century, the century when the events in the stories took place and which still influence the landscape of our thinking around issues of peace, conflict and violence. Lastly, this book is also an inquiry into alternative futures – a range of personal and global future possibilities.

Chapter 1, 'Communism, utopia: The personal is political', starts with a story of my great-grandfather who left Slovenia for the Soviet Union to avoid prosecution and to build a better future for him and his family. Events take place mostly in the Union of Soviet Socialist Republics (USSR) and, towards the end of the chapter, in the Socialist Federal Republic of Yugoslavia (SFRY or former Yugoslavia). This chapter deals with a totalitarian state and society's oppression–terror and seeks alternative understandings behind such oppression as well as for the ingredients that may prevent it in the future. The out section starts analysing the ways in which politics is not an abstract concept but 'a real and very powerful force influencing people's everyday lives' (Drakulić 1991, p. xv), which is a theme that runs throughout the book. Chapter 1 also starts an inquiry into another central theme: the ways our individual and collective images and views about the future impact on our actions that, in turn, help manifest particular preferred futures. Other topics discussed in this chapter include the raising of children, worldviews and 'othering' – all crucially important to understand the events described in this chapter as well as the practices of waging terror, or alternatively, of building positive peace.

Chapter 2, 'War, dystopia: The holy trinity of militarism, imperialism and nationalism', describes the impact of the Spanish Civil War and Second World War on my grandfathers as well as on one of my grandmothers. It gives context to my indirect dealings with these massive events of collective violence, the impact they had on me as a child, and on my family as well as our society. While the Second World War experiences are also touched on in Chapter 1, there I focus more on totalitarianism and repression by the state. Chapter 2 continues with these topics while predominantly focusing on wars and inter-ethnic conflict. Chapter 2 introduces yet another major theme within this book: the analysis of some of the mechanisms behind acts of collective violence and the devastating, long-term impact they have on the fabric of a society. As is apparent from the subtitle of this chapter, the three themes given most attention here are those of (social) militarism, imperialism (including the issue of 'balkanism') and nationalism.

Chapter 3, 'Feminism, eutopia: Challenging patriarchy and androcratic masculinities',[2] discusses the role gender identities play in the waging of war and other acts of collective violence. Some long-lasting debates on the gendered division of life-giver and life-taker roles are reflected upon, introducing the latest concepts from gender studies that are relevant for rethinking of gender–war/violence–peace connections and describing alternative nonviolent ways to conceptualise gender roles and identities. This chapter connects the social practice of androcratic–hegemonic masculinity with the doing of war, arguing that the 'doing of gender' remains one among several key variables in the doing of war/violence. The in stories are the personal experience of some members of my family, providing links between the personal and the political and showing again ways in which themes discussed in this chapter manifest in the lived experiences of concrete individuals.

Chapter 4, 'Living trauma, eupsychia: The political is personal',[3] deals with the long-term and ripple effects of violence and includes an investigation into the ways in which previous unhealed traumas impact political events. In addition to showing the depth and width of destruction of a society through war and violence, the question of the long-term impact of trauma on people's mental and physical health is also raised. As with all previous chapters, the analysis is followed by an inquiry into alternative futures – the range of nonviolent future possibilities, including for healing and post-traumatic growth. Again, events in the former Yugoslavia are provided as case studies. Some experiences of (post-)Yugoslav refugees, displaced persons and migrants are also brought into the discussion. The last in section of the book takes place in Australia. The analysis, however, is broader and global, linked to the specific theme and the current research that best explains the violence–peace dynamics behind these events.

Despite the many heavy and dark stories presented, it is my hope that *Breathing: Violence In, Peace Out* will help bring a little more light into the world and into the lives of its readers. Perhaps life is simply a balance of inhaling and exhaling, taking and giving, and receiving and releasing. If there is but one thing I would inhale, take and receive more of, it would be more inner and outer peace. If there is but one thing I could exhale, give and release, it would be sharing that inner and outer peace with others. May we all make better and more informed choices – including chosing the right thought patterns – to get us closer to more peaceful present– future realities.

Ivana Milojević

CHAPTER 1

Communism, utopia: The personal is political

> Growing up in Eastern Europe you learn very young that politics is not an abstract concept, but a powerful force influencing people's everyday lives (Drakulić 1991, p. xvi).

In: Mirko

Some time between 1937 and 1939, Mirko Weinberger was assassinated. Earlier, he had 'disappeared' in the middle of the night, naturally, for the cover of night is often needed when shameful and unjust deeds are performed. He left behind his wife and two children, who all went on to survive Stalin's Great Purge and the Second World War. When the family left Slovenia, which was then a constitutive part of the Kingdom of Yugoslavia, they left behind their culture, extended family and community in the hope that a better life awaited them. The Soviet Union held the promise of an advanced, stateless, classless society where workers were valued rather than exploited. It held the promise of a utopia in which the proletariat of the world united, each giving according to their abilities and receiving according to their needs. The family was not only escaping poverty in Slovenia, the rise in Italian fascism, the earlier Italian invasion of the Austro–Hungarian Empire and the Slovene-populated part of it but also, perhaps most importantly, the records that detailed Mirko had been arrested three times for political activities and wounded once by the police.

Towards the end of the First World War, Mirko had been mobilised into the Austrian army. Shortly after his discharge in 1920, he joined the Yugoslav communist party, which promised, among other things, to provide a viable alternative to the tradition of the proletariat forced to fight war after war for the bourgeoisie. In the 1920s, Mirko was an activist and member of the Zagorje miners' trade union and one of the founders of the Independent Workers' Party of Yugoslavia, as well as of an organisation called Vesna, the Union of Workers' Youth of Yugoslavia. As a member of these organisations he was accused, as the bill of indictment at the court case in Celje in November 1924 stated, of 'propagating communism and revolutionary ideas, which represent a disturbance of public law and order, and peace ... in addition to propagating communism, the intention of these organisations is to propagate anarchism, terrorism and commit murder in order to achieve such goals.' While the court eventually acquitted him of the charges, the threat of a fourth imprisonment still lurked.

Mirko thought that the communist police in the Soviet Union, on the other hand, would be on his side – initially, before and just after his migration to the Soviet Union, it was. New papers were arranged, work assignments given and accommodation provided. His successful completion of communist studies at the Communist University for Minorities (KUMPS) should have meant a stamp of approval, the achievement of a desirable skill set needed in a new society. Instead, years later a number of those who had studied together at the communist school came under suspicion. First, Yugoslav expatriates and successful KUMPS graduates were arrested and taken away to unknown places, then Mirko was also 'removed'.

We will never know what exactly happened on that fateful night when 40-year-old Mirko disappeared for good. Nothing was said. No one informed the family, mentioned a trial or issued a death certificate. It took nearly 20 years for Mirko's name to be uttered by the Soviet government's officials and bureaucracy. During Khrushchev's Thaw (1956–64), exactly a year after Khrushchev denounced Stalin in his speech 'On the Personality Cult and Its Consequences' (1956) while simultaneously squashing the anti-Soviet revolution in Hungary (for which the Soviet–Russian state apologised in 1991 and 1992), Mirko was quietly pardoned. Unlike the first one, this second pardon did not arrive in time. Twenty years late, it prevented Mirko from joining millions of Soviet political prisoners who were finally released from the Gulag labour camps during the Thaw.

Instead, decades after his disappearance, when the old files were finally opened, it was confirmed that Mirko was on the list of 'foreign suspects' killed in the spirit of the times, which demanded all potential sources of opposition to the government be removed. Neither Stalin nor the Politburo actually pulled the trigger, yet the collective madness that they helped create normalised killings for which no one was ever held accountable. What the files also showed was that, ironically for a Marxist-socialist revolutionary, Mirko was killed in front of a church and buried in an unmarked mass grave behind this sacred building.

Out: Salvation

Perhaps it was not ironic, but fitting, that Mirko died in front of a church. Like the story of Christianity, Marxist communism was also about salvation. The former promises to save us from the devil, from our inherited sin, from oblivion, from our carnal bodies, and sometimes even from ourselves. The latter promised salvation from exploiters, elites, social and economic injustices, and sometimes even from our own selfish desires. Both assure glorious times in some distant future, for which you must either repent and die or arduously work at changing yourself and society.

Utopian sentiments, religious and secular – heavens in the sky or havens on the Earth, or 'the human capacity to visualize The Other as different and better than the experienced present' – are found in all civilisational and cultural traditions. Utopia, 'at once a vision, a way of life, and a tool' (Boulding 1986, pp.345–46, 365), has been and remains a major force in picturing more peaceable and socially just ways of living, individually and collectively. Whatever their inspiration, their social and historical context, their understanding of peace and violence, or the degree of their rejection of violence, most pacifists and peace activists envision present/future societies in which conflicts are resolved (more) peacefully and where there is a 'moral commitment to cooperative personal, social, and international conduct based on agreement rather than force' (Cady 2010, p.313). It is hoped that such nonviolent arrangements – based on a rejection of the use of violence in personal life and in social, national and international affairs, affirming the moral principle of 'thou shalt not kill', and coupled with socially just arrangements – would result in 'harmony among individuals, justice in society, and peace in the world' (Woito 2010, p.308). Various debates within radical and reformist, principled and pragmatic pacifisms and pacificisms aside, some degree of implicit utopianism is always present within them. This is so in both its positive meaning (how things could and should be, the preferred, more peaceful states of collective and/or individual being) as well as in its negative function (critique of society as it exists, critique of war and various other forms of violence). As the utopian dreamers of Paxtopia explicitly state:

> In a Paxtopian World, nations and the people of the Earth will strive to live in peaceful coexistence. The world will share a common goal – to make life better for ourselves and those we care about, while respecting each other and the planet we share (Utopian Dreamer 2012).

At the beginning of the twenty-first century, however, we are generally expected to give up thoughts of utopia because it has failed us in the past. Even though some utopias have succeeded, and even though new utopias usually learn from the failures of the past, utopianism has become a 'sentiment' non grata. To a large degree, this is due to disappointment over the failures of twentieth-century progressivist politics, of which communism was, once upon a time, a shining example. The blame for a general scepticism towards utopia is also attributed to the other previously 'failed' utopian efforts, including many 'communitarian peace experiments' (Rigby 2010, Boulding 1986). The scepticism is also explained in terms of the socio-historical context of twentieth-century Europe, wherein the general dampening of optimism is connected to a collective reaction towards the carnage of two world wars and the emergence of several totalitarian societies. Sometimes, it is assigned to a 'reflective realism', given the condition in which '85% of people in today's world live physically and perhaps 98% psychically' (Suvin 2000). Suvin connects this situation with 'present day capitalism without a human face', or a capitalism that is perhaps showing its real face 'now that it fears communism no longer' (2000). Many other theorists of utopia make a connection between 'the regimes and subsequent collapse of communist Eastern Europe' and 'the failure not only of Marxism, socialism, or communism but also of utopian idealism' (Breton 2010, p.286).

Putting aside historical overviews of utopian thinking that have 'a predictable story line', often ending with 'a coda which proclaims or laments the death of utopia in our own century' (Kumar 1987, p. vii), the dominant and popular discourse on utopia does not share in this lament. Rather, it generally understands utopia 'as a perfect place or condition of existence' (Breton 2010, p.284) and as such considers it 'imaginary, dangerous, and misleading' (Polak 1973, p.162). In other words, 'of the many aspects hidden under the one concept of a utopia, one aspect – its imaginary quality, has stamped its mark on the whole and thus distorted it' (1973). Further:

> Although the critique of utopia is as old as the first utopias, most contemporary critiques owe something to ... liberalist arguments [which assert] ... that utopians fail to understand the diversity of human values and goals and that the desire for utopia exposes a naive faith in the benevolence of organizations, regulations, routines, disciplines, and unanimity (Breton 2010, p.284).

In line with such interpretation, utopia is then also understood as a tendency towards uniformity and sameness, which inevitably leads to tyranny. Accordingly, utopia is necessarily about failure (Hughes 2000, p.84) because its subjects are 'the fallacies and delusions of human hope':

> ...utopia means conformity, a surrender of the individual will to the collective or the divine [and, as such, utopia is] basically for authoritarians and weaklings (2000, p.84) ... while some might think that to be deprived of a life in utopia may be a loss, a sad failure of human potential [this can be the case only until they] consider how unspeakably awful the alternative would be (2000, p.85).

Most utopian experiments, of which communism is but one example, end up in mass killings, argues John Carey. This is because the aim:

> ...of all utopias, to a greater or lesser extent, is to eliminate real people. Even if it is not a conscious aim, it is an inevitable result of their good intentions. In a utopia real people cannot exist, for the very obvious reason that real people are what constitute the world that we know, and it is that world that every utopia is designed to replace. Though this fact is obvious, it is one that many writers of utopias are reluctant to acknowledge. For if real people cannot live in utopias, then the utopian effort to design an ideal commonwealth in which human beings can lead

> happier lives is evidently imperilled (Carey 1999, p. xii).

Consequently, continues Carey, proponents of various utopian experiments aim to eliminate real people by various means, whether by invasive methods such as punishment, eugenics, genocide or purges; subtle methods such as education, alternative social arrangements, including transforming the family organisation, or the justice system; or requests for reforming one's self. Such inclinations may be connected to another key aspect of utopian thought, 'the rage for order' (Boulding 1986, p.347), which Boulding defines as 'the powerful drive to impose rational, efficient, just and peaceful behavioural protocols and structures on irrational, inefficient, untidy and impulsively aggressive human beings'. Coupled with the fact that utopia is always 'the other – something totally different from existing society, and implying a radical restructuring of the existing order', this rage for order too often results in revolutionary violence, 'even when there is a commitment to peaceableness' (1986).

So was it utopia, or more specifically a communist utopia that killed my great-grandfather Mirko? In the meaning-making quest I have embarked upon in writing this book, should I be adamant that all utopian dreaming, including those of big and small pacotopias,[1] therefore be abandoned? Should I simply accept the world as it is, including that large-scale violence is unavoidable? Should I argue against communism and socialism in all its forms and manifestations?

Perhaps some answers to these questions could come from further investigation into twentieth-century political utopias, including the communist ones, as well as into utopian sentiment in general. This is important, as (communist) utopia has been accused of many evils, including of murderous outcomes resulting from their insistence on sameness and (totalitarian) order. However, not all utopias show a tendency towards the rage for order and sameness wherein both change and difference are undesirable; indeed, 'many utopias are libertarian ... and allow for a great deal of variety (more, perhaps, than what is truly offered in the modern world), change, development, and fluctuating desire' (Breton 2010, p.285). Contemporary ecotopias, for example, argue for greater biodiversity as well as against 'monocultures of the mind' (Shiva, 1993). Feminist and multicultural utopias envision greater gender and cultural diversity than is currently allowed expression in most present-day societies. And contemporary paxtopias or pacotopias envision a *multitude* of peaceful and nonviolent ways of resolving conflict and negotiating differences.

Utopias always have 'roots in the real world, reflecting the values of the time and place in which they were composed or created, even as they express desire to change the world that produced them' (Breton 2010, p.286). Utopias in the sixteenth and seventeenth centuries were thus 'dominated by an emphasis on authority and religion', eighteenth-century utopias were 'marked by an emphasis on the importance of reason', and those of the nineteenth century mostly depicted 'the emergence of peaceful societies in concert with universal economic cooperation and equality, as well as reflecting the rise of socialist and anarchist thought' (2010). The rage for order, sameness, uniformity and abandonment of individual differences are thus as much a feature of a modernist industrial civilisation relying on standardisation as they are of utopias of those eras.

Even though the 'standard critique of utopia' may recognise that 'there are different kinds of utopias' (Hughes 2000, p.84), it still maintains that '[a]ll utopians err in preferring the fulfilment of ideal representation to the mundane improvements which are possible in their time. It also faults utopians for opting for maximal value orientations' (2000). Grand designs for social reconstruction, the argument continues:

> ...are nearly always disasters. While contemporary social institutions may be far from perfect, they are generally serviceable. At least, it is argued [generally by conservatives], they provide the minimal conditions for social order and stable interactions. These institutions have evolved through a process of slow, incremental modification as people adapt social rules and practices to

> changing circumstances. The process is driven by trial and error much more than by conscious design, and by and large those institutions which have endured have done so because they have enduring virtues. This does not preclude institutional change, even deliberate institutional change, but it means that such change should be piecemeal, not whole scale ruptures with existing arrangements (Wright 2010).

By this logic, the global international system – wherein national security is paramount and the theory of 'just war' acceptable – is only a result of trial and error and of incremental modifications over many centuries, which have been proven to ensure more lasting peace. Consequently, if the current system is radically changed, even by global 'cultures of peace' dreamers, chaotic wholescale ruptures will be imminent, potentially bringing chaos and unforeseen dangers. This also implies that grand utopia, such as pacotopia may be, is not only unrealistic and impractical but also outright dangerous (Hudson 2003, p.16). This is because any grand utopia has the capacity to encourage human beings to 'give vent to totalist adolescent psychological states' and provide 'an illusory basis for human action'. Therefore:

> According to this critique, utopia is a form of subjectivism which ignores the fact that we cannot reshape the world in our own image. It is irrational in its refusal to acknowledge objective

> reality, immature in its inability to realise the limited nature of the possible, and irresponsible in its failure to understand the role of fallibility in the realisation of the good (2003).

Despite good intentions, the utopian dream of peace may inevitably result in, as some critics of pacifism argue, the 'dismemberment of your country as well as murder of innocents, political oppression, social injustice, and appeasement of terrorist' (Woito 2010, p.308). It is by a lack of a particular 'action' – meaning reluctance to use violence to prevent further potentially more massive and harmful use of violence – by 'good men' that the triumph of evil is assured. As such, pacifism remains the luxury, even the pathology, of the privileged.

Such warnings about the dangers of utopia within our current sociohistorical context make it imperative that paxtopian or pacotopian sentiments be restrained, for fear of such sentiments being labelled unrealistic, naive, or worse. As a consequence it has by now become critically important to tread carefully on utopian grounds. Not so long ago and all over the world, as a factsheet on the 'Cultures of Peace' by the United Nations Association of Canada states, war was 'considered as inevitable and peace was only a vague utopian dream' (UNAC 2010). But with the development of necessary instruments to establish peace, such as, for example, modern-day peacekeepers:

> The UN established several programs intended to reduce, as much as possible, all the factors leading to outbreaks in [violent] conflicts. These programs did not only focus on peace keepers, who intervene after a conflict has erupted, but also on economic and social development, human rights, and the struggle to end world poverty and hunger. Indeed, all of these United Nations programs contribute directly or indirectly to the prevention of conflicts and thus to peace on earth. It is certainly true that, in the last 50 years, not everyone in the world has known peace, but it is gradually gaining ground. The dream of peace in the world is becoming less and less utopian and more and more attainable (2010).

Parallel to the request to refrain from dreaming and to focus on practicality, there is an imperative to demonstrate workable strategies that may close the gap between utopian dreaming (for example, peace on Earth) and the current world (ridden with violent conflict). This means that salvation from violence, individually and collectively, for us and others, lies not so much in the construction of an idealised peaceful world, but in the practice of devising nonviolent approaches that deliver more peaceful outcomes. Perhaps then, the argument goes, unlike previous failed utopian experiments, a *strategic utopianism* or the *practical utopia* of more peaceable societies in the future has a solid chance of becoming reality. This is because the main problem with earlier unsuccessful utopias was that their proponents were 'rarely able to devise political strategies to achieve their utopia which [did] ... not destroy the very goals described' (Boulding 1986, p.345). Consequently, this means that the strategies and methods must match the vision, as in the general motto, 'there is no way to peace – peace is the way'. In other words, what is absolutely necessary is the use of specific and concrete peacemaking, peacekeeping and peace-building approaches, all of which are continuously invented, trialled and evaluated. If this is achieved, it can be concluded that the gap between utopian peace promoting goals and new realities will remain minimal, if not obliterated altogether. At the end, however, we are still left with the following problem: how is one to travel if one knows not where s/he wants to go?

In: Zinka

Zinka (Terezija) Martelanc was born in 1899 in the village of Šempeter, near the northeastern Italian town of Gorizia. After her father Alojz Martelanc, a worker in a factory, died when she was 12 years old, she left home to become an apprentice housemaid for Austrian nobles. Her mother, a seamstress, died six years later, when Zinka was 18. With little family support, Zinka relied on her labour to make ends meet. She followed work opportunities and left the region of Šempeter when heavy fighting broke out in the area during the First World War. She moved to

Ljubljana and worked in a storage facility and then in a messroom for soldiers, which Mirko frequented.

The period when they met was a turbulent one. Their country had recently proclaimed independence from the Austro-Hungarian Empire and joined other southern Slavs to create a new state (the internationally initially unrecognised State of Slovenes, Croats and Serbs). In that context, both Zinka and Mirko became connected with groups and organisations that spoke for them. After the war and the birth of their firstborn, a daughter, they moved to Mirko's hometown Zagorje on the river Sava, where Mirko found work as a highly qualified glasscutter. At the same time, he was also working in the illegal communist party. By the time Zinka and Mirko had three young children under the age of five, he was arrested for the third time and consequently lost his job. The family's survival depended on the generosity of their fellow party members and others in the glasscutters' union. In return for their generosity, Zinka became the first women in Zagorje to join the Communist Party of Yugoslavia, actively participating in its work.

In 1927 the party sent Mirko to summer school at the International Lenin School. When it was over, Zinka asked her colleagues from *Kominterna* (Comintern or the Third International) when he was coming back. They told her he wasn't. He was not allowed to return because he was now apparently a Trotskyist. With their two surviving children, Zinka decided to join him in Moscow and succeeded in doing so in 1930.

When Zinka first arrived in Moscow she also studied at the KUMPS (Communist University for Minorities). She found the classes difficult, as she had to learn in both Russian and Serbo-Croatian, rather than in her native Slovene. After the successful completion of her communist studies she started working in a factory producing airplane engines. Her hard work paid off and she became a *brigadirka,* the leader of a work group, and an *udarnica,* 'outstanding worker'. Her reward for these efforts was '100 grams of sugar and half a kilogram of flour'. This may not seem much but this was during the period when four million Soviet peasants died from starvation. Ironically, while her husband became an 'enemy of the state', she was earning the trust of Soviet society.

Between 1942 and 1945 Zinka also belonged to a group that organised and led the Moscow radio station Free Yugoslavia, which focused on 'promoting anti-fascist uprising in Yugoslavia and lobbied for the international recognition of a new, democratic Yugoslavia' (*Vojna enciklopedija* 1974). In 1945, after communism came to power in her country of origin, she returned with her now adult children to Belgrade. She found employment in the library where she was put in charge of 'bourgeois print', a post given only to tried and tested communists due to the potential 'dangers' of such genre. In 1954 she took early retirement from her role as manager of the Central

Belgrade library and moved back to Ljubljana. She died there in 1985 but not before being awarded prestigious communist awards: the *Spomenica* 1941 (Partisan Medal), the Order of Brotherhood and Unity with the Golden Wreath (1969) and the Order of People's Merit with the Golden Star (1974).

Paradoxically for a Slovenian anti-fascist, she is buried but 40 easy steps from the *Cimitero Militare Italiano,* a memorial site containing the graves of hundreds of Italian soldiers who fell fighting for the supremacy of those lands during the First World War.

Out: Progress and regress

Perhaps it was only fitting Zinka was buried there, at Ljubljana's Žale Central Cemetery, which became the final resting place for fallen soldiers from all sides. Enemies in life, they lay side by side in death. Death, as they say, is the great equaliser. The communist utopia, on the other hand, imagined a society where such equality would exist for the living.

Even if 'Marx himself would have been horrified to have the Russian socialist experiment called utopian' (Boulding 1986, p.353), communism was indeed a utopian experiment par excellence. The nineteenth-century founders of 'modern' and 'scientific' communism and socialism, Karl Marx and Friedrich Engels, envisioned a society in which the 'abundance of resources would replace scarcity, individual freedom would be guaranteed, and historical cycles would disappear since discontent would no longer drive change' (Hollis 1998, p.145). Other shared key elements that gave the various socialist and communist utopias their recognisable features could also perhaps be deduced to include no large differentiation and power imbalance between towns and villages or mental and manual labour, no differentiation and hierarchical arrangements between social classes, no private property but more a communal ownership of goods and services, all goods distributed according to need, self-governance, demonetisation of finances, universal education and healthcare, international cooperation, and equality of sexes and peoples.

This communist promise of 'universal emancipation [was] supported by three centuries of critical, international and secular philosophy that exploited the resources of science and mobilized, at the very heart of the industrial metropolises, the enthusiasm of both workers and intellectuals' (Badiou 2010, p.3). Furthermore, this promise was an expression of a larger human desire for social unity, harmony and equality that at times also manifested in the formation of communes and utopian communities. Intentional political and social communes, often marked by features such as self-determination, sharing of resources (including property, finances and income), common interests, non-hierarchical structure and consensual decision-making, formed many times in history – any time when groups of people 'banded together in communities to bring about the fulfilment of their own utopian aspirations' (Kanter 1972, p.2). Thousands of experiments followed, all aimed at creating a new reality where society reflects 'humankind's deepest yearnings, noblest dreams, and highest aspirations ... [and] where all physical, social and spiritual forces work together, in harmony, to permit the attainment of everything [founding] people ... [considered] necessary and desirable' (1972, p.1).

Despite these shared elements there were also many differences between the subsequent socialist and communist utopian (preferred futures) visions of various theorists and practitioners. It is only logical that, among generations of communists and socialists spread across the globe, huge differences in viewpoint on a whole range of issues existed. Contrary to some later interpretations, the communist utopia was never monolithic; rather, it was fluid and flexible, a result of many debates and differences of opinion, even though at times certain utopian discourses became the most dominant. Utopian socialists, for example, wanted to 'replace ruinous competition with cooperation' but did not propose the abolition of private property as 'the later scientific socialists and anarchists' (Hollis 1998, p.256) had. They believed capitalism was flawed, not that it was irredeemable (1998). Some socialist thinkers were keen on revolutions. Others preferred to focus on reforms. In fact, prominent socialist (including social democrats) and communist thinkers often disagreed on almost everything. Mikhail Bakunin argued with Karl Marx ('not all revolutions need to be violent' verus 'dictatorship of the proletariat'), Leon Trotsky with Joseph Stalin (over the role of bureaucracy in the Soviet Union and whether socialism could exist in one country alone), and Eduard Bernstein with August Bebel and Karl Kautsky (gradual peaceful reforms within capitalism or its revolutionary overthrow) (Kolakovski 1980).

While the majority of socialists and communists believed in the necessity of gruelling work in order to change the old society, as early as 1883 Paul Lafargue wrote his best-known work, *The Right to Be Lazy,* arguing against a clerical–bourgeois conspiracy that lifts work to the level of a cult, creating all the personal and social suffering. He also proposed an antidote – refusal to work for more than three hours per day – that would see the 'earth, the old earth, trembling with joy ... feel[ing] a new universe leaping within her' (Lafargue 1883). Amusingly, his essay concludes with an ode to laziness: 'O Laziness, have pity on our long misery! O Laziness, mother of the arts and noble virtues, be thou the balm of human anguish!' (1883). For her part, fellow activist Clara Zetkin took issue with what she saw as the nationalistic and warmongering attitude of some of her colleagues. Rosa Luxemburg went as far as to critique the despotic forms of behaviour by Bolsheviks and the complete liquidation of democratic freedoms under their rule. Zetkin and Luxemburg defended, again and again, internationalism, before some of their more chauvinistic male colleagues. Another Marxist–socialist, Ber Borochov, published '*Poalei Tziyon* [the Jewish Socialist Labor Confederation] Peace Manifesto' in 1917 in which he wrote:

> We see the main purpose of the impending deliberations to be: to oppose the war aims of the various states by the will to peace and the conditions of peace of a reunited world proletariat, and to organize the struggle for peace. The imperialist governments, which have on their consciences the horrible, universal slaughter, are unable to control the unchained elements of destruction: they have neither the power to consummate their war purposes nor the courage to relinquish them. The bleeding human race awaits its deliverer. The international proletariat must become conscious of its historical mission to take into its hands the destiny of nations, to establish a peace that will preclude the danger of future wars by the strength of its union and to pave the way for the social emancipation of mankind (Borochov 1917).

Not all socialists and communists bought into the dominant discourse on the necessity of violent social change normative in violent societies – socialist/communist and non-socialist/communist alike. Indeed, an important element of mainstream communist ideology was a detrimental view that justified organised violence as 'the best means to end class violence and social oppression' (Barash & Webel 2002, p.21). And yet, parallel to this dominant strand of 'realist' politics that promoted revolutionary violence, a rich antimilitarist, socialist–communist–pacifist tradition also always existed (Burke 2010; Young 2010a). Even though it was marginalised within communism and socialism – just as peace movements and pacifism are marginalised within contemporary global society – it nonetheless provided an influential critique of wars that were, according to their interpretation, waged due to imperialism and the expansionist character of capitalist economies, to the detriment of working classes everywhere.

This Marxist and communist argument – that war efforts may be misplaced, that structural inequalities should be addressed with a 'war on poverty' and on other similar grievances related to socially unjust arrangements by the wealthy and powerful – remains important. It is especially so during the post-communist era, which is marked by a general consensus on reverting to 'capitalism and non-egalitarian dogma' (Badiou 2010, p.3). We are only now starting to realise on a mass scale the dangers of such a reversal; that is, the dangers of moving back to capitalist omnipresence without balancing such a change (and the consequent excesses) with the critique coming from some (powerful) alternative discourses.[2]

Pacifist alternatives are and have always been critical for balancing the excesses of bellicose societies and civilisations. However, due to the negative connotations that both utopianism and pacifism have often had, many pro-pacifist socialists went to great pains to distinguish themselves from these traditions. The difference between the 'bourgeois peace enthusiasts' and socialists, argued Rosa Luxemburg, lies 'in the fact that the bourgeois apostles of peace are relying on the influence of fine words, while we do not depend on words alone'. In fact:

> Our very points of departure are diametrically opposed: the friends of peace in bourgeois circles believe that world peace and disarmament can be realised within the frame-work of the present social order, whereas we, who base ourselves on the materialistic conception of history and on scientific socialism, are convinced that militarism can only be abolished from the world with the destruction of the capitalist class state. From this follows the mutual opposition of our tactics in propagating the idea of peace. The bourgeois friends of peace are endeavouring – and from their point of view this is perfectly logical and explicable – to invent all sorts of 'practical' projects for gradually restraining militarism ... The Social Democrats, on the other hand, must consider it their duty in this matter, just as in all matters of social criticism, to expose the bourgeois attempts to restrain militarism as pitiful half-measures (Luxemburg 1911).

In the 1930s, the American James Burnham, then a socialist, argued that it is 'the duty of socialists to attack pacifism sharply and uncompromisingly' (Bennett 2003, p.62). Similarly, Italian Marxist Coletti, 'paraphrasing Lenin's work *State and Revolution*' (Sullivan 2002, p.30) wrote, 'It is impossible to be a Communist ... if your aim is not a violent seizure of power.' Coletti denounced the pacifist tendencies of German social democrats, criticising them as 'accommodation with capitalism', whilst Bolsheviks subsumed them under derogatory rubrics such as 'social chauvinism', 'social pacifism', 'centrism', and 'power sharing with the burgouise' (2002). This reaction, at the very least, testifies to the existence of and the necessity for engagement with pacifism, if not to the strength and prominence of pacifistic minority views, both within and outside the ranks of socialists and communists. In other words, there were always pacifist alternatives within socialist and communist discourses, even though it was their opposite that, by and large, became more popular and accepted.

Sadly, it was precisely such attacks on pacifism and utopianism, rather than socialist–communist utopia per se, that were instrumental in creating the 'pragmatic' policies of Stalin's era. Violence is rarely promoted as an ideal; rather, it is usually justified on the counts of being 'the only realistic and workable strategy'. In other words, we do not engage in violence because we want to, we use it because we must. Unlike utopians and idealists, who provided positive elements of preferred/utopian visions, it was predominantly the 'realists' and 'pragmatists' within communist ranks that argued for ways out of various (and continual) crises via military means and revolutionary violence. Furthermore, the idealism and the violent end of the first socialist government in history, or the first government of the proletariat, the Paris Commune of 1871, were not forgotten. Despite its many successes, the majority of socialist–communist theorists and leaders, including Marx, Lenin and Stalin, focused on the violent ending of the Commune, the brutal reprisal by which conservative repression saw tens of thousands of Communards slaughtered. Among Communards' mistakes, Marx (1871) and Lenin (1917b) later concluded, was their generosity towards the enemy. In other words, the compromising and idealism of the Communards did not work, and this overshadowed what did.

Large-scale violence always leaves behind a trail of (individual and collective) traumas, and such trauma often skews survivors' views of the past in a way that selective remembering of violence becomes paramount. Partially due to this, cultures of peace, or peaceful change and transformation, remain history's hidden side (Boulding 2000). It then takes conscious and concentrated effort to recover and remember such hidden history. For example, during the 72 days the Paris Commune existed it introduced many social measures, such as the regulation of work and pay to the benefit of the workers, the separation of church and state, and electoral and educational reforms (including the introduction of free education). The intent was to help create a more democratic and progressive society. The Commune's violent end informed the views of many prominent socialist–communist thinkers, but so did its peaceful attempts to better society. Subsequent generations of socialists and communists were inspired by these attempts, even though the Commune failed within a few months. Later generations consequently went ahead and, via social and political activism, helped create policies benefiting many worker-class families who gained from the increase in higher education and other opportunities.

This was not limited only to the influence of the Paris Commune. Likewise, in some historical phases and countries, many of the utopian goals of early socialist–communist visions were achieved – universal health and education, higher literacy rates, affordable housing, nearly full employment, more opportunities for women to get paid work and an increase in overall living standards for the majority of the population. Unfortunately, these achievements, which mostly took place in the more liberal socialist countries and historical periods, were overshadowed by the brutality of the more totalitarian countries and historical periods. Some inner contradictions also helped with the eventual collapse of socialist–communist societies almost everywhere. These collapses – and their often-violent endings – overshadowed the more peaceful and just periods that are also part of socialist–communist history, achievements and traditions. But, in the end, the feeling of security, sense of community and equality, idealism and concern for exploited classes that existed as a consequence of progressivist socialist policies were eventually replaced by the overwhelming sense of dissatisfaction about the lack of democracy and individual liberties, such as freedom of speech and thought, as well as economic stagnation and poor material standards (in comparison with Western capitalist and democratic nations). Too much focus on wealth distribution and too little on wealth creation, coupled with issues around communal property (such as resentment over differing input and degrees of care by various communal co-owners, the controlling behaviour of petty tyrants) were some of the inner contradictions that helped bring down communist systems.

In addition to economic stagnation, perhaps most damaging was the reproduction of hierarchies and inequalities by the socialist–communist elite vanguard in all socialist–communist countries. This situation helped to 'spread [an] atmosphere of bribery and dishonesty throughout the whole society ... [leaving] deep wounds inside and [hampering] normal relations between people' (Svoboda 2004). A number of socialist systems, including the Soviet Union, eventually collapsed because in reality they were not following their own utopian principles. Rather, they became *absurd* societies, 'with an intolerable disjunction between myth and reality' (Galtung 2008, p.34). In the end, it was the discrepancy between utopian goals (such as equality) and the reality on the ground (such as reproducing inequalities) that created an intolerable schism.

After the collapse, a number of ex-socialist countries' achievements were thrown out together with the proverbial bathwater. Replaced by the structural adjustments of our current era, the new policies aimed to achieve alternative (though implicit) utopia, the capitalists' promise of material abundance and endless personal choice. It seems that even explicitly anti-utopian political projects need some level of utopianism in order to mobilise people to help bring about social change. That such a capitalist utopia is also temporary, fleeting and available as a reality to only a minority of the world's population does not make it any less attractive or real. For the 72 days the Paris Commune existed it was probably as real as our own reality, as were all the other socialist–communist achievements. During its existence, the particular utopia was not only aspirational, it produced a new reality – it was generative and positive, creative and transformational. This is equally true for a number of other, already mentioned, socialist and communist utopian aspirations, despite their final – often violent – collapse.

This later interpretation of utopia is in agreement with Hertzler's argument (1965, p.266) that while 'not all of any of the utopias has been realized ... much of them have been, as is the case in any improvement scheme.' Likewise, it agrees with Fred Polak's argument about yesterday's utopia often becoming today's social philosophy:

> Many utopian themes, arising in fantasy, find their way to reality. Scientific management, full employment, and social security were all once figments of a utopia-writer's imagination. So were parliamentary democracy, universal suffrage, planning, and the trade union movement. The tremendous concern for child-rearing and universal education, for eugenics, and for garden cities all emanated from the utopia. The utopia stood for the emancipation of women long before the existence of the feminist movement. All the current concepts concerning labor, from the length of the work week to profit-sharing, are found in the utopia. Thanks to the utopists, the twentieth century did not catch man totally unprepared (Polak 1973, pp.137–38).

Power exists only at the point where it is implemented, argued Michel Foucault; it 'exists only when it is put in action' (1982, p.219). Similarly, the power of utopia fails only once it is no longer used: as 'a vision, a way of life and a tool' (Boulding 1986, p.365). In the end, communist utopia produced some positive shifts, some progressive movement, even though these too were temporary:

> [despite the word 'socialism' recently acquiring] dramatically new connotations ... nonetheless, some socialist ideas deserve respect and retention. In its original form, socialism was an admirable attempt to assist laboring peoples relentlessly exploited by capitalism in its early, oppressive stages. Many people have found the fundamental socialist ideal of universal social equality and justice a source of moral strength. Since capitalism and liberalism might not have survived without the influence of certain socialist ideas, to refer to what happened in the Soviet Union and East Europe as the triumph of capitalism is an oversimplification (Ikeda 1995, p.45).

Attributing mass killings during Stalin's era to utopianism may also be an oversimplification, a straw-man argument or replacement of thesis. The actual numbers of deaths, of course, were staggering. In the Soviet Union alone, between Stalin's ascent to power and the end of communism in 1991, it is estimated that tens of millions died, were shot or perished in prisons or in exile. Unlike similar massive death tolls that often occur in inter-ethnic conflict or inter-state wars, which seem more 'acceptable', these were examples of a totalitarian society running amok against its own citizens. In addition to these tens of millions in the Soviet Union, millions more were killed by this and other communist regimes in other times and other places, making communism 'not merely an abstract idea but ... a global tragedy that brought grief to millions of victims throughout the world' (Bestuzhev-Lada 1996, p.132).

At the same time, Stalin, rather than being somebody inspired by a particular utopian ideology, was by most accounts a pragmatist (Phillips 2000), a person who was more interested in maintaining power and utilising a particular style of government to meet those ends. Like many other pragmatists he believed that higher goals justify sacrificing human lives and that resorting to violence is an acceptable political strategy. This mythology has, among other occurrences, resulted in 'huge colonial genocides and massacres, the millions of deaths in the civil and world wars through which our West forged its might, [all which were sanctioned by] ... the parliamentary regimes of Europe and America' (Badiou 2010, p.3). Stalin's methods of repression were not new, nor were they the tools of communism alone. They were borrowed from previous regimes, have been used in non-communist totalitarian regimes as well, and thus have nothing in common with the utopian impetus of desiring differently.

Stalinism was perhaps more a result of not enough utopianism than too much, or about each utopia's unintended and unavoidable detrimental consequences. Utopia is about improvement, and thus it can be measured only by overall social progress. For societies to move forward utopia and utopian sentiments are paramount. It is only when a system/society proclaims 'the end of history', seeing itself as a pinnacle of social achievement and the best of all worlds, that utopianism is weakened and the decline imminent. If utopia is to provide 'as much freedom and happiness for its inhabitants as is possible to human life' (Breton 2010, p.284), if it is to visualise a world 'free from poverty, strife, [violent] conflict, economic struggle and competition, hunger, disagreement, and disorder ... with every member of the citizenry enjoying a corresponding inner peace' (2010), then surely Stalinist repression had nothing to do with it. Mass killings, on the other hand, are a marker of a social and civilisational regression, and a sign of a society declining. Rather than being about the unintended consequences of utopianism, mass murders are in every way a departure from utopian sentiment, which requests better ways of organising human affairs. Each and every time humans choose to engage in such violent behaviours – despite the ideology that informs them – they are regressing from better ways of being, from which such extreme examples of direct violence are absent. In other words, neither utopianism nor mass killings exist as abstract and timeless states of being; they exist only once the actions and principles are set in motion. They manifest only once certain behaviours, by real human actors in the real time/space dimension, are put into action.

Blaming a positive vision of an improved present/future for social manifestations that are exactly its opposite may not be logical; however, it has certainly been very effective. In a similar manner that utopianism is blamed for manifestations of its exact opposite, dystopia, pacifism has been blamed for violence, feminism for the patriarchal backlash, multiculturalism for the rise in ethno-nationalism and socialism for the return of conservative social policies and the dismantling of the welfare state. At the same time, the long-term negative impact of repressive violence is most commonly conveniently forgotten. It is forgotten that, for example, repressive violence against the Paris Commune worked, in more ways than one, even though Marx's later statement that 'the working class cannot simply lay hold of the ready-made state machinery, and wield it for its own purposes' (Marx 1871) was to have huge repercussions for even more violent historical episodes further down the track. Despite this, the recognition of previous violence causing further violence is commonly brushed away when totalitarian communist regimes are discussed. Rather, the worldview behind the system that those regimes sought to transform points the finger of blame towards the 'last refuge of the dispossessed' and the suppressed: hope. Not only has this discourse discredited utopian sentiment by and large, it has also managed to convince many about the undesirability of all that is in some ways connected to socialist and communist visions. Good and bad lumped together, such discourse engages in the either/or categorisations and black-and-white thinking, which are, (not so) coincidentally, the exact crimes of which communist utopia stands accused.

In: Mira

Mira Weinberger was ten when she left for the Soviet Union with her mother and brother. Born in Ljubljana in 1920, in a house overlooking the River Ljubljanica, she officially became Frida Franklin in 1930 on newly received documents. This name was to help her cross borders. Overnight she became the daughter of Pavlina Maslova Ivanovna, born in Bucharest, a narrative which terrified Zinka because, 'Anybody wanting to check my identity would soon enough find out it was fake, given that I spoke neither Romanian nor Russian!' Mirko had earlier become Mr Franklin, a Canadian with Slavic first and second names (Josip Karlovič) in his documents. These fake identities could have easily been exposed and created additional anxiety for the family. They were never given any rational explanation for the practice of renaming when Soviet bureaucrats issued the documents. With these new identities they started their life in Moscow. But the new, better life did not last long, if it eventuated at all.

When Mira turned 17 she was fatherless. When she turned 19 she was a widow with a newborn baby girl – her husband Boris perished when the plane he piloted went down during the Soviet Union's attack on Finland in 1939. Soon after the outbreak of the Great Patriotic War (as the Second World War was known in Russia), she was expelled from the university where she was studying economics for being a 'foreigner'. A day after she turned 22, Mira gave birth to her second daughter, when she was in a camp for displaced persons in Engels, a port town on the Volga River in the Saratov region of Russia. A number of the women living in her barrack advised her to 'expose' the baby, because she looked unlikely to survive and Mira was malnourished. Mira's attempt to abort the baby during early pregnancy had failed when the doctor was arrested by the Soviet regime before the scheduled appointment – unlike in the early days of Bolshevik governments, wartime demanded the replenishment of nation-state citizens and abortion was made illegal. The baby, Jelena-Lena, survived both potential early endings of her life. In the end, Mira could not put her baby in harm's way.

By this time the father of her second daughter, Vasiliy, was also pronounced dead, killed when his plane was also shot down but this time during the battles of Operation Barbarossa. This was the battle that helped German forces enter deep into Russian territory – by November 1941 they were only 24 kilometres from Moscow. Numbers of pregnant women and children were by then relocated to communal camps further east. Mira and her firstborn daughter, Svetlana, were in different camps. Svetlana went to a *detskii dom* (children's home) run by The People's Commissariat of Enlightenment or Narkompros. These children's homes, mostly for abandoned, homeless or orphaned youngsters, proliferated, especially through the duration of the Great Patriotic War. Without Boris, the state became, as a bureaucrat put it, Svetlana's father. Her mother was no longer Mira, but the 'whole worker–peasant society'. Svetlana spent some years in one of those homes in deep silence, refusing to talk. When the danger passed and she was reunited with Mira, she no longer recognised her mother.

When Mira worked as an announcer on Radio Free Yugoslavia, she met Veljko, a Spanish war veteran and Communist Youth International secretary. In 1944 their son was born. In 1945 Mira, Veljko, her two daughters and their son, went back to the now officially socialist Yugoslavia. She died in 1988 and is buried at the same Belgrade graveyard as Veljko, but they are buried at different locations. Personal and political scandals were to separate them in death, as in life.

Out: Raising children and worldview

Maybe the circumstances of their burials were not so incongruous, given how much family functioning was influenced and disrupted by politics during time of wars as well as during Bolshevism and Stalinism. Stalinism has been explained and theorised in countless books and articles over the last 80 years or so. Why and how it took place are crystallised into various standpoints, such as:

- Stalinism was an inevitable continuation of Leninism and Bolshevism and their promotion of communism (and due to communism being, perhaps, intrinsically evil), including the promotion of the centralisation of the state and totalitarianism in general

- Stalinism was a consequence of his own personal characteristics, including manic-depressive illness with paranoid tendencies (Hershman & Lieb 1994), which in part may have been due to the way he was raised as a child (violent, alcoholic father) (Ihanus 2007; Shakhireva 2007; Dervin 2008) and/or his family background (Georgian minority, 'humble peasant stock') (Phillips 2000, p.4)
- Stalinism was a consequence of broader historical forces (world wars, the socio-economic culture in Russia, industrialisation, urbanisation, structural changes in the communist party, Russian traditions and the legacy of the Tsarist regime, etc.).

Given that one of the main themes this book deals with is the issue of intergenerational trauma in the context of political upheavals and violence in its various forms, of particular interest here are explanations that focus on family relations.

Looking at the factors that may have contributed to the violence that took place during communist times is important in better understanding the dynamics between personal and political – and not only in terms of how the latter influenced the former. As the political sphere influences the personal so do personal and family spheres infringe on the realm of the political. If it was not communist utopia per se that killed my great-grandfather Mirko and set up a chain of events impacting on at least three later generations, as concluded earlier, where else could we look for some underlying causes of that violence?

New approaches to peace and conflict studies over the last several decades may be a starting point. One example is research conducted in the second half of the twentieth century, which moved beyond looking solely at the realm of the political when investigating causes of large-scale violent events (for example, the Purges). Women peace scholars in particular started looking at ways in which violence, or the expectation of violence, is reproduced within family life. While various peace and conflict theories have initially emerged from the robust 'masculine' field of international politics, eventually, argues Chadwick Alger, it would be 'women peace researchers who would sharpen our capacity to perceive the roots of militarism, violence, and other forms of peacelessness, within our own families, neighborhoods, schools, churches and professions' (1996). Keeping in line with that tradition, potential links that helped create the events that in some way shaped my family's as well as my own story need to be investigated.

The separation of my grandmother Mira and my Aunt Svetlana during the Second World War, for example, was influenced not only by the general events of the war but also by some long-standing historical narratives in regards to the betterment of family relations. Historical narratives, including ideas and visions, are never ideologically innocent or politically neutral. All (historical and current) futures and utopian visions likewise have the power to influence politics, policies and people's everyday lives. They are never without consequences. And sometimes the utopian visions of some people become the nightmarish experiences of others. Going back to family relations it is perhaps pertinent to remember that one of the common themes in old utopias/dystopias of the Plato, More and Campanella variety, was the abolition of the family: 'The Platonic idea is that the family should be completely obliterated. No child will know its parents, no parents their child. Children will be reared exclusively by state officials, the unfit and weaklings being destroyed' (Carey 1999, p. xvi).

Twentieth-century totalitarian regimes of the Stalinist and fascist variety seem to have embraced this 23-centuries-old idea, which has throughout Western history consistently reappeared in both theory and practice as a method of producing 'ideal citizens'. From the practice of separating infants in their most vulnerable years and sending them to wet nurses and other carers among European upper classes (1999), through sending children to boarding schools or youth camps, to the mid-twentieth-century practice of removing Aboriginal children from their parents in Australia, the (modified) Platonic pattern has persisted. Furthermore, the Platonic recommendation that unfit weaklings should be destroyed is now accepted widely in both European/Western and non-Western nations via the use of medical screening techniques followed by selective abortions. During communist times, families were further weakened by the regime's encouraging of youth to spy on their parents and report them to authorities if transgressions were noticed.

But growing up in a family was, for most of European history, also violent, which may partly help explain a history with a high prevalence of violence. In fact, collectivist raising of children, as the literature on peaceful societies shows (Lawlor 1991; Bonta 1996; Boulding 2000; Kemp & Fry 2004; Grille 2005a, 2005b; Kelleher 2010) may not be a reason behind early childhood traumas and the subsequent 'playing out' of them in the adult years. Violence in its various forms (physical, emotional, psychological, spiritual), in both collectivist and private family settings, on the other hand, has been consistently linked with both the development of self-destructive behaviours as well as with the development of the 'authoritarian personality' (Adorno et al. 1950; Barash & Webel 2002, p.134). This type of personality is commonly characterised by 'hierarchical and authoritarian parent–child relationships, a dichotomous view of social relationships leading to the formation of stereotypes, conventionality, exploitative dependency, rigidity and repressive denial, all of which may culminate in a social philosophy which worships strength and disdains the weak' (Abercrombie et al. 1984, pp.23–24).

These hierarchical and authoritarian parent–child relationships, enforced by violence in its many forms, most commonly result in the childhood victim in later years transforming into an aggressor, 'either directly or indirectly by supporting aggression on the part of others' (Barash & Webel 2002, p.134). A number of studies (for example, Milburn & Conrad 1996) show that 'individuals who were brought up in punitive, authoritarian families tend to favour harsher aspects of law and order policy – such as the death penalty' (Grille 2005a, p.187) and are more likely to support war in general. Another set of studies (Miller 1998; deMause 1990; Grille 2005a; Ihanus 2007; Shakireva 2007) focused on the connection between traditional Russian childhood and the Stalinist regime, hoping to shed some light on why the regime was so violent, irrational and brutal. This traditional raising of children overwhelmingly included practices such as infant ice-bathing, baby swaddling, corporal punishment (flogging, beating, kicking, whipping, etc.), shaming and belittling. These practices slowly started to transform in Russia only in the 1930s (Grille 2005a).

The history of not only Russian but also more broadly European/Western childhood, argues Lloyd deMause is 'a nightmare from which we have only recently begun to awaken. The further back in history one goes, the lower the level of childcare, and the more likely children are to be killed, abandoned, terrorised, and sexually abused' (2005a, p.17). The abuse is most commonly attributed to the continuation of the cycle of violence that family life enables, as well as to the necessity of lower level attachment to offspring during times when high rates of infant mortality were prevalent (Carey 1999, p. xvi). The statement by deMause, however, has been challenged by the 'ethnographic and archaeological records' (Kelleher 2010, p.382) of early gatherer-hunter[3] or foraging societies. Most of those societies seem to have been more peaceful than violent (2010), challenging the Hobbesian hypothesis of the natural state in which there is *bellum omnium contra omnes* ('war of all against all') and the life of humans thus 'solitary, poor, nasty, brutish, and short' (Hobbes 1651), the hypothesis that perhaps underlines some aspects of deMause's argument. Nonetheless, despite some problematic generalisations, the work of Lloyd deMause and Robin Grille does provide important evidence connecting violent societies and the violent child-rearing practices prevalent in them. In other words, evidence shows that 'comparatively permissive societies seem to be less warlike than those with high levels of physical punishment of children and of sexual repression' (Barash & Webel 2002, p.135). If these conclusions are accurate, the implication is that the peaceable raising of children, peaceful/peace-oriented socialisation and peace education are as crucial to the establishment of peaceful international relations as diplomacy.

Of course, a particular society, group, culture or civilisation's *raison d'être* influences the purpose and function of its childrearing practices and the philosophy behind them. Depending on the priority the concept of peace has within a particular society and the degree to which childrearing reflects that priority will also vary. Therefore, another set of explanations investigating links between social and family violence focuses on the omnipresence of an underlying worldview that exists within a particular family and society. One fundamental fact emerges upon examination of conflict resolution among peaceful societies and their culture of peacefulness, argues Bonta: 'the peacefulness of their conflict resolution is based, primarily, on their world-views of peacefulness – a complete rejection of violence' (1996, p.74). Consequently, their worldviews of peacefulness inspire them to develop 'cultural technologies for dealing with difference peacefully' (Boulding 2004, p. ix). This cultural technology of peace – the development of 'ideas, mores, value systems, and cultural institutions that minimize violence and promote peace' (Kemp 2004, p.10) – is what distinguishes peaceful societies and families from violent ones. Even though the latter claim to be peaceful and even though we can indeed find 'hidden peace building strengths' in every society (Boulding 2000, p.91), violent societies (and families), by and large, develop different cultural technologies for dealing with difference and conflict. In other words, violent societies can be defined by the degree of maintenance of a 'technology and an orientation toward war, as those in power seek to preserve the right of violence as an instrument of power and conflict resolution' (Kemp 2004, p.10). This cultural technology is always supported by a particular underlying worldview.

As argued by Riane Eisler (1987, 1997, 2000), a particular worldview prevalent in a society can be located on the continuum between two Weberian ideal models of partnerships/more peaceful or dominator/more violence-oriented systems. Eisler further argues that even though societies that subscribe to the violence-promoting worldview may seem very different – for example, a tribal society like the Maasai of nineteenth-century Africa, an industrial society like twentieth-century Nazi Germany or Stalin's Soviet Union, and a religious society like Khomeini's Iran or the European Middle Ages – they all actually have the same core configuration. According to Eisler this core configuration is based on a particular worldview that she terms 'dominator/androcracy', in which the following similarities exist:

> They [those societies] are all characterized by authoritarian rule based on fear of pain in both the family and the tribe or state, rigid male dominance, and a high degree of socially condoned violence, ranging from child and wife beating to brutal scapegoating and [chronic] warfare (Eisler 2000, p.33).

In our contemporary Western societies, this worldview is endorsed by many traditionalists and those on the conservative right-wing end of politics. In his analysis of discourses promoted by these groups in the United States and other Western nations, George Lakoff focuses on thought patterns; that is, 'mental structures that shape the way we see the world', or what he terms 'cognitive frames' (2004, p. xv). He also shows the internal logic of the conservative cognitive frame or, in other words, of the violence-promoting worldview. First, the underlying assumption is that 'the world is a dangerous place, and it always will be, because there is evil out there in the world' (2004, p.7). Further, in families and communities informed by such a worldview, it is commonly believed that 'children are born bad, in the sense that they just want to do what feels good, not what is right. Therefore, they have to be made good' (2004, pp.7–8). Consequently, what is required of the child in such families, communities and societies is above all obedience (2004). Furthermore, it is assumed that a family based on the 'idealised strict father model ... [who is] a moral authority knowing right from wrong' is the best way of protecting its members within the 'dangerous, competitive and difficult world'. This right and wrong is reinforced for children through 'punishment, painful punishment, [any time] ... they do wrong. This includes hitting them, and some authors on conservative child rearing recommend sticks, belts, and wooden paddles on the bare bottom' (2004).

To maintain a coherent structure, the dominator/more violence-promoting worldview thus puts into operation a whole range of practices that reinforce hierarchical relationships between humans, always maintained via violence (including threat of violence), as well as the supremacy of humans over other living beings. These practices, supported by the violence-promoting worldview/thought patterns, influence a wide range of occurrences – from family relations and childrearing to the way international relations and even the global economy is structured (Henderson 1990, 1995, 1999, 2006; Eisler 2008). In short, if the worldview sees violence as normal, natural and necessary, it puts into practice a whole range of strategies – including how children are to be raised – that in turn reinforce it.

Due to the issue of scale, it is difficult to accurately and empirically verify some of the previously mentioned generalisations, such as that children raised violently (by and large) perpetuate cycles of violence. Logically and intuitively the link may be obvious, and yet violent families and societies have also raised children who in their adult years choose transcendence over the re-enactment of trauma. Perhaps a distinction between socialisation to aggressiveness determinism and its influence may be useful here. This distinction can help us understand when, in the context of a dominator worldview, wherein violent childrearing practices take place and create conditions for humanity to 'proceed from domination to domination' (Foucault 1984, p.85), members of these societies and families still choose to discard early and/or dominant influences. Postmodernists have highlighted ways in which dominant discourses are created and re-created or alternatively changed by the marginalised one/s. They have stressed that even in the context where 'there are individuals and organisations that rule over other people' (McPhail 1999, p.861) resistance is also always possible. As Foucault has argued, the process of normalisation, including of the perception that violence is both normal and normative, is never fully complete; other views and ways of being in this world are not and can never fully be co-opted. Rather, he concludes that 'there will always be subjugated forms of (power/)knowledge [within a particular, dominant, normative worldview] that can be used to resist prevailing and hegemonic forms of (power/)knowledge' (1999, p.854). These alternative views can (and do) exist both at the smaller group as well as at the even more micro, individual, levels.

Not only are these alternative (utopian?) practices possible, given that they have existed and continue to exist (albeit in marginalised spaces), they may be our best defence against raising future dictators and dictatorial regimes, argues Robin Grille (2005a). The coming of the future 'gentle society' will happen, argues Elise Boulding (1977), through three main leverage points, all of which are connected with more positive childrearing practices. These three main leverage points include family, early-childhood school setting (nursery school and early elementary school) and community (1977). The shift towards a more supportive, or 'helping mode' of parenting and childrearing is already taking place (Grille 2005a). Originating in the 1970s and 1980s and based on 'a number of revolutionary insights in the field of psychology' (2005a, p.83), this parenting mode focuses on children's needs. It is considerate rather than judgmental and aims to enhance compassion and altruism rather than discipline and punishment. Given that it has recently become a dominant discourse in the academic field of educational psychology, we may hope that its positive impact – already being felt in most Western societies, families and schools; for example, the banning of corporal punishment – will continue. Here therefore lies hope that more democratic and peaceful, gentle societies of the future may emerge, replacing the current bellicose world order.

Alternative childrearing practices, which avoid violence and neglect while promoting gentle, caring and empathetic approaches, are critical to counter the influence of dominant hegemonies of violent childrearing. These peace-oriented childrearing practices, present in more peaceful communities and societies, are also supported by a particular worldview. This is based on a shared 'desire to be peaceful' (Kemp 2004, p.6), which consequently orients the culture in that direction and towards development of the cultural means to achieve such aims (2004). Unlike the previous dominator worldview, such efforts and practices are based on a 'nurturant parent' (Lakoff 2004) or 'partnership' (Eisler 1987, 1997, 2000, 2008) worldview instead. This is marked by several features, out of which a minimum of gender-role differentiation and a minimum of dominance patterns taking place stand out (Eisler 1997, 2000; Boulding 2000). Unlike the dominator worldview, which gives high priority to social and cultural technologies that support domination and destruction, the nurturant parent/partnership worldview gives high priority to social and cultural technologies that 'sustain and enhance life' (Eisler 1997, p.141). Peaceful societies 'vary enormously ... in their cultural, religious, social, and institutional practices' (Kelleher 2010, pp.383–84). What they have in common is a particular peace-promoting worldview that manifests in institutional forms and cultural practices of socialisation and 'nurtures a sense of self that avoids and resolves conflicts' nonviolently (2010, p.382). A range of these peaceful societies – whether manifesting in some contemporary Scandinavian nations (Eisler 2000) or in rural settings and as small-scale societies (Boulding 2000) – tend to be organised according to an alternative core configuration that consists of:

> ...a more democratic and equitable family and social organisation, a more equal partnership between women and men, and the absence of a structural requirement for idealizing or building violence into the social system, as it is not required to impose or maintain rigid rankings of domination (Eisler 2000, p.34).

More recently, the emerging 'helping mode' within the broad psychohistorical evolution of childrearing has signified 'more nurturing, and less blame on the child for parental feelings of anxiety or overwhelm' (Grille 2005b, p.40). This mode of parenting is characterised by 'empathic responses to the child's needs, two-way dialogue with the child, and a greater tolerance for children's emotional self-expression' (2005b). Such a helping mode is based on a contemporary 'nurturant parent worldview' that Lakoff describes as:

> Both parents are equally responsible for raising the children. The assumption is that children are born good and can be made better. The world can be made a better place, and our job is to work on that. The parents' job is to nurture their children and to raise their children to be nurturers of others (2004, pp.11–13).

And what does this nurturance concretely mean, asks Lakoff? According to him, it means two things:

> ...empathy and responsibility. If you have a child, you have to know what every cry means. You have to know when the child is hungry, when he needs a diaper change, when he is having nightmares. And you have a responsibility – you have to take care of this child. Since you cannot take care of someone else if you are not taking care of yourself, you have to take care of yourself enough to be able to take care of the child ... Therefore it is your moral responsibility to be a

> happy, fulfilled person ... Further, it is your moral responsibility to teach your child to be a happy, fulfilled person who wants others to be happy and fulfilled. That is part of what nurturing family life is about. It is a common precondition for caring about others (2004).

In summary, the peace-oriented socialisation and education of children focuses on their *needs* and how to satisfy those and the needs of parents and the community via nonviolent methods. Whether such parenting could have prevented Stalinism and the emergence of 'violent leaders and obedient followers ... hard-wired for 'fight' responses (the violent leaders) – and shame-based or fear-based submission (the obedient followers)' (Grille 2005a, p.236) is, of course, a question that can only be raised hypothetically. What we know with more certainty, however, is that a single-cause theory of violence will always fall short, even if some causes may be more influential than others. Consequently, other factors – cognitive frames and behavioural practices – in addition to childrearing and worldviews also need to be investigated.

In: Vasiliy

Vasiliy Skrobov was 12 when he first met Mira. Secretly in love with her for years, ever since this new student arrived at his school, his heart sank when she married Boris straight after graduation. But after Mira's first husband died, Vasiliy reignited the friendship and then married Mira before their 21st birthdays. Six months later, after the war had begun and despite Mira's wishes, Vasiliy sent in an official request to be directed to the front. Like Boris, he too was a pilot. As a general rule pilots were based some distance away from the front. Many wives of pilots accompanied their husbands and so Vasiliy expected Mira to be with him. After he was posted, Vasiliy wrote to Mira, inviting her to join him. She did not arrive. Months later, after her non-arrival created a massive rift between them, Mira received another letter, this one from the officials pronouncing Vasiliy dead. After Mira died in 1988, her daughter with Vasiliy, Jelena-Lena, also received a letter:

> Dear Lenočka,
>
> It was difficult to decide to write this letter to you. Circumstances in our lives developed in such ways that we were always far apart from each other not only because of the physical distance but by something much greater than that. But several months ago I spoke with Sarra Veniaminovna over the phone, one of your mother's friends, she and I studied together at the college. She told me about your mum's death on March 1st, 1988, almost a year after it happened. Since my conversation with Sarra I could not stop thinking about writing something to you. Many times I started to write but then finished after a few lines. I was plagued by

> questions: what should I write? Is my writing necessary at all? Would it be important to you? I don't know about your knowledge of Russian either and whether you'd be able to understand my letter. My handwriting has become harder to read also, years have left their mark. But I understand that opportunities to talk to you are becoming less and less and I would not like to leave with you any vague memory or misunderstanding about myself.
>
> I will try to write as short as possible, certainly not everything about my life, and not as a confession, but only what is connected with you and what you may possibly want to know about me.

The letter was from Vasiliy. Lena found out about the circumstances of her mother and father's separation, of his narrow escape from death, of his many years in prisoner-of-war camps, first in Sevastopol and Simferopol, and then somewhere further inside Poland or Germany. She also learned about how his group was guarded by 24 German soldiers when they attempted to escape, the first time unsuccessfully – for which they were locked up for five days without any food and threatened with assassination if they attempted to escape again. He also wrote to her that, despite these threats, he still attempted to escape again, and he was shot at but fortunately not hit. This escape was successful and so, six months after his plane went down, he became one of a very few dead men to return home. In the letter, Vasiliy also told Lena of his 12 years spent 'working' in Siberia:

> After the war, I have gotten into lots of trouble ... It took me years to fully understand the complete horror of my situation ... I became a second class citizen of the USSR, under the vigilant eye of the 'ideologically pure and committed', without being trusted and without any hope for the future. After demobilisation I have gone through very heavy times. For almost a year I could not get a job and the reason was always the same – my captivity during the Second World War. My condition was awful and I was very lonely. This is how my kind Fatherland[4] has 'repaid' me for all the spilled blood and for all the sunken fighting ships of the opponent and for all the hundreds of enemies destroyed by me. It sounds so awful now, hundreds of destroyed enemies, but at that time the question was who kills who? Either they will kill us or we will kill them. I have loved and will love till the end of my days my Native land, although I spent many years as a sick child wrapped in politicised and ideological nappies. And I had to continue living. After a year of unemployment, I got a job and for about one year worked among swindlers, rascals and thieves. There was another reason why I received such harsh treatment. Your grandfather, the father of your mum, was arrested

> before the war as the enemy of the people. I saw him only once, and we never talked. Still, this was enough for government to be vigilant towards me. In 1942 my navigator admitted to me that he was given a task to watch me and report information about me. After he was killed in 1943 this unpleasant business was assigned to someone else. After Second World War my difficulties continued. After a year without work and a year working with swindlers I wrote a letter to Marshal Zhavoronkov, the chief of the Civil Air Fleet who met with me, remembered me and after talking for a long time decided to allow me to work again as a pilot. He could not restore me to the previous position, I became a civil pilot and went to Eastern Siberia. I do not know what kind of spiritual qualities I possess but people always helped me. Friends from the front would find me after 30–40 years had passed and pilots from the Civil Air Fleet also did not forget me either then or now. In Siberia I worked for more than 12 years and a particle of my heart was left in those stunning terrains.

This, then, was his reward for 'allowing' himself to be captured during the Great Patriotic War, because, as Stalin pronounced and Vasiliy remembered and then transferred onto paper, 'We have no returned captured soldiers, we have only traitors!'

Out: Othering

My biological grandfather, whom I never met, was one of those traitors. The black-and-white thinking underlying many of Stalin's views and which created perpetual divisions with 'in' and 'out' groups, to a large degree, has also underlined much of Western, and perhaps global, history. The prevalence of 'us' and 'them' thinking is so pervasive and of such long duration that, like violence, it too often appears natural.

It is important here, though, to distinguish between the separation between 'the self' and 'the other' that occurs as a psychological developmental process through which each child develops her or his sense of uniqueness and own identity, and the detrimental process most commonly termed 'othering'. This latter process occurs when a separation between the self and the other extends at the group level and an often sharp distinction between the in group and out group takes place. This in/out group distinction could be found perhaps universally in a range of cultural and historical settings. As the term 'identity' is derived from the Latin noun '*identitas* which means "sameness" (from *idem,* "the same") [implying] a "core" similarity between a number of elements, which is said to exist despite apparent differences' (Mikula 2008, p.92), the self imagines other members of her/his in group to be similar to her/him while projecting difference onto the out group. The sharper this distinction, the higher the sense of separateness and alienation from others is. And the bigger the (perceived) gap between us and them – coupled with naturalisation as well as projection of 'the difference' onto the other – the more pronounced is the process of othering. This seems to potentially create a whole range of problems, especially in situations of conflict:

> Phenomena such as prejudice, negative images and stereotypes of the opponent, and distorted perceptions, interpretations, and evaluations of the behavior of members of the other side in the conflict have been identified by researchers as playing crucial roles in maintaining and intensifying intergroup animosity (Maoz & Eidelson 2010, p.102).

All forms of social interaction, argued sociologist Georges Gurvitch, could be deducted onto the existence of 'we/us' and 'the relationships with others'. Depending on the intensity of the union, we could be organised as a Mass, where the connection is the weakest; Community, where the connection is stronger; or as an Alliance of a group of like-minded persons, where connection is the strongest (Gurvič 1965). Sociologists have consistently found that the higher the real or perceived danger from the outside group, the more there is a desire and practice of homogenising the in group. This applies to behaviour within groups organised as a mass, a community and/or an alliance. Once organised, these groups develop a life of their own, behaving in ways that sole individuals would perhaps not. Crucially, 'societal beliefs of unity refer to the importance of ignoring internal conflicts and disagreements during intractable conflict in order to respond forcefully to external threats' (Maoz & Eidelson 2010, p.103). In other words, the more *they* threaten *us,* the conscious/unconscious logic goes, the more we need to homogenise to survive.

Further, psychologist Erik Erikson has postulated that during times of extreme social and economic hardship 'ambiguities and unresolved stresses' at the level of a society may 'combine with the individual's developmental problems to produce totalism, a susceptibility to [and more extreme version of] all-or-nothing simplifications: us versus them, good versus evil, God versus the devil' (Barash & Webel 2002, p.135) and friend versus foe. In this way reality becomes conceptualised in a strictly bipolar way and is dramatically oversimplified (Jahr 2010, p.62). Not surprisingly, stressful parent–child relationships and early emotional trauma create fertile ground for both the inability to feel empathy with others (Grille 2005a) as well as for a deep sense of 'alienation, an acute loneliness and disconnectedness from others [contributing to] the inclination by very alienated people to avenge their pain by acts of extreme destruction' (Barash & Webel 2002, p.135). So while some degree of othering may be unavoidable, certain conditions contribute to the process of othering, becoming if not pathological then certainly extremely detrimental to peace.

The alternative term for othering, developed in the 1930s by anthropologist and sociologist Gregory Bateson (1958) is 'schismogenesis' – a process of differentiation and separation between distinct cultural groups. In summary, the process of schismogenesis can be described as 'the pulling apart from the antagonistic group, the destruction of trust, the vilification, dehumanization, and "pseudospeciation" of the enemy so that it becomes a legitimate and moral act to organize his systematic destruction' (Stevens 2010, p.326). This concept can perhaps help us understand 'how and why groups don't undergo some sort of cultural osmosis when they come into contact with one another, why cultural mixing doesn't result in "melting pot" cultures and why distinction and rivalry are often intensified through contact' (Gregg & Seigworth 2010, p.127). Crucially, such processes play 'a vital role in arousing warlike enthusiasm' (Stevens 2010, p.326) and are prominent in cultures where violent domination and 'antagonistic intergroup contact is an essential element of their general life-world' (Gregg & Seigworth 2010, p.127).

Stalinism was marked by all of the previously mentioned detrimental features of othering. Most significantly it was marked by the mentality of extremely tight we groups of like-minded persons (alliances) that relied on all-or-nothing simplifications as well as on violent methods of suppressing the threatening others. It seems that once a group embarks on destructive in–out grouping during times of extreme stress (some of which may be self-imposed), the perceived threat becomes bigger and bigger and the in group smaller and smaller. As a consequence, many violent conflicts take place in order to establish which exact individuals or groups could claim *true* in-group (national or ideological or even religious) identity. Alternatively, many peaceful initiatives can take place in order to re-establish unity within diversity and the expansion of the in-group identity. The larger the group identity the lower the potential for conflict – as *they* become *us.* A number of humanistic and spiritual movements (and worldviews) expand us to include all (humans, living/sentient being) and in such way serve as one of the best preventions of processes of othering, the latter almost always intrinsically being linked with violence.

The excesses of Stalinism against those that (sometimes literally overnight) became part of the out group are well documented. More surprising is the way Stalin's regime othered not only the official enemies or even its own problematic citizens but also its own soldiers, including people committing violence to maintain the regime itself. Stalinism went above and beyond the more common neglect returning soldiers (especially if in some ways incapacitated and made vulnerable) experience in violent societies; it actively and en masse prosecuted many of them, which may indeed be without precedent in the history of warfare. Consistent with his paranoia are Stalin's 'attitude and [the] actions he took toward most officers and soldiers who fell captive to the Germans' (Maslov 2001, p.45). This attitude was also evident in the military purges of the 1930s: 'Stalin never fully trusted the Red Army officers corps – or anyone else for that matter. Therefore, after war's end his often brutal treatment of Red Army officers and soldiers who had already suffered in German captivity was entirely in character' (2001).

Stalin's treatment of the members of his own army may be a case study in paranoia but, more significantly, it is also a case study of the logical consequences of othering, taken to the extreme. As already mentioned, lessons from the violent end of the Paris Commune included both Marx's conclusion about the dangers of adopting or adapting the 'ready-made state machinery' of a previous regime. As Lenin later concluded, the proletariat *cannot* 'lay hold of' the 'state apparatus' and simply 'set it in motion' for its own purposes. But it can '*smash* everything that is oppressive, routine, incorrigibly bourgeois in the old state apparatus and substitute its *own,* new apparatus. The Soviets of Workers', Soldiers' and Peasants' Deputies are exactly this apparatus' (1917a).

Once again it is apparent here that a particular behavioural practice of violence is more a result of certain interpretations, theorising and understandings of social change, previous violence and how to achieve desired (safe/peaceful) outcomes for the in group than due to anything inherent or natural. The 'smashing' of the old army occurred within a span of two decades, showing both the gradual nature of Stalinism's development, as well as the logic behind the madness. For the outsider in both time and place, such logic is anything but, and yet scores of otherwise possibly rational people participated in it. Neither purges in general nor purges of the military in particular could have happened had not so many people actively participated in them. Like violence, peacebuilding is a process of choosing active participation in different interpretations and practices (worldviews and behaviours), including active restraining from participation in various forms of violence. And like any other violence, the purges took place because the latter set of worldviews and behaviours had, for a majority of the population at the time, less appeal than the former.

Anyhow, the logic and the rationality behind the process of military purges started when, after the Bolshevik revolution took place in 1917, and the means of the old regime, including its army, were acquired. The professional officer corps who had created and run the newly formed Red Army units then needed to be purged, since they represented 'the heritage of czarism', even though their cooperation was initially welcomed. Because skilled soldiers were removed, new staff were needed to replace them. The new staff were, understandably, unskilled, and training was required. This was done with the help of German experts. But then, during the period between 1937 and 1939 when half the entire leadership of the country, the political and military establishment at all levels, was killed, those with foreign connections were especially targeted. Since there was a 'deep suspicion of anyone negotiating with or influenced by outside powers' and since 'the new corps of the Red Army were German-trained' that essentially included all of these people (Weir 2008, p.139). It was perhaps 'this kind of idiocy – creating a corps with German assistance to train the army against the growing German threat, then killing them for consorting with Germans – that passed beyond even the normal barbarism of internal security forces' (2008).Why was the process not stopped at some stage, abandoned or transformed? Perhaps the narrative of othering was so strong that it managed to override even the usual logic of military strategising, let alone empathetic dealings with people, citizens and soldiers alike?

Anyhow, the previously outlined plan resulted in many negative consequences for the Soviets, including huge Soviet losses during the Winter War with Finland. Despite the fact that they outnumbered the Finns four to one in men, 200 to one in tanks and 30 to one in aircraft, Soviet aggression could have not been translated into victory. Besides resulting in the deaths of hundreds of thousands of people, the Russo–Finnish Winter War of 1939–40 killed my grandmother

Mira's first husband and the father of my Aunt Svetlana, partially setting in motion another set of events (re-marriage, the birth of another daughter and then her granddaughter writing these lines), the second and third order impacts that rarely get mentioned in the official war/history accounts. Stalin's decision to wipe out the upper echelons of his own armed forces created other ripple effects:

> The untold millions who died as a direct result of Stalin's tyranny are even to this day highly debated ... Stalin's terror in retrospect was scattered, insane, and in one specific aspect, utterly reckless, with severe consequences not only for those unfortunate victims but for world affairs in general. Leaving aside sheer insanity, it was essentially paranoia and fear that led Stalin not only to dispose of many millions of his own people – many of those who had helped ... win the Revolution – but also on an unprecedented level to wipe out the upper echelons of his own armed forces. The purge of the Red Army left the Russians apparently unprepared to defend their own territory and prompted Hitler to think he could outdo Napoleon and successfully invade Russia. The failure of Hitler's Operation Barbarossa was no thanks to Stalin's idiocy in destroying his own generals (2008).

The processes that took my biological grandfather into the war and pushed my grandmother from Moscow into a camp for displaced persons, where she gave birth to my mother, who by sheer miracle survived the January 1942 cold and malnutrition, could have then been due, in part, to the way Soviet Russia conducted its absurd and ridiculous wars. The regime's paranoia in seeing enemies and traitors even within the ranks of returning captured soldiers also started a chain of events that meant I was to never know my biological grandfather even though, perhaps, those events meant I was to be born in the first place.

Beneficiary of war and violence that I am, I am in very good company. Socio-biological and evolutionary psychology theories postulate that most of us alive today may be descendents of 'proto-human warrior bands [which] ... were a major selective force in our own early evolution, with successful bands killing off those that were less successful' (Barash & Webel 2002, pp.123–24), consequently receiving a reproductive payoff. The downside of this is that the same cognitive and behaviour patterns that influenced our ancestors to use aggression, force and violence in order to achieve and maintain domination over others are passed on to their descendants, who are likely to possess similar 'traits and capacities' (2002). Putting alternative interpretations of human history aside temporarily, if this tendency is extrapolated into the future, and the sheer amount of wars, violence, and human suffering and misery due to them in the twentieth and twenty-first centuries as well as the strength of contemporary weapons added, a very depressing conclusion cannot be avoided. Peaceful utopia is never going to be realised and humanity's self-destruction is imminent.

In: Leon and Danica

Leon Weinberger, son of Mirko and Zinka and brother to Ella and Mira, was born in 1922. When his older sister Ella died, due to a childhood illness and malnutrition, he was not yet a toddler and so did not remember her. Yet he was responsible for all but one photo of Ella disappearing. His mother hid an envelope underneath his clothes, thinking that if she was searched while crossing the border, her eight-year-old son would be spared. Neither was searched, but the package containing precious family memories was lost somewhere between Vienna and Budapest. The only remaining image of Ella was now with Leon's aunt back in Šempeter.

This was not the last time Leon felt guilty for circumstances beyond his control and/or level of maturation. In 1942 he tried to prove that he was ready to fight for the Russian and Soviet cause, and hopefully exonerate the family in the eyes of Soviet bureaucrats. If only he could show how loyal and hardworking the family was, perhaps his father Mirko would come back, would be saved. As soon as he turned 18 he immediately went to the army and volunteered to go to war. He was rejected on the grounds of being a foreigner and was, instead, taken to a weapons factory somewhere in the Ural Mountains. He spent nearly a year and a half there, working impossible and often 20-hour-long shifts, yet struggling in silence as if wishing to redeem himself and his whole family.

Even though Leon was silent, Zinka was listening. She was listening really attentively to all the stories that came her way through official and unofficial channels, especially tales told about factories in the Ural Mountains. There were too many stories of disappearances, only this time from strange illnesses and 'accidents' at work. She had a horrible feeling about the whole thing. She lost sleep and about five kilograms from her already slim frame. She knew she had to do something. She also knew that if anything could save her son it was connections. Fortunately for Leon, Zinka was not only hard working, proper and loyal, she was also a Comrade Connection. Leon came back weighing 48 kilograms, hardly enough for a 175-centimetre-tall boy. Soon after his weight was restored to a level enabling survival and then more strenuous physical activity, Leon volunteered to join the brigades of Yugoslav youth, leaving Russia to fight for communism at home. In doing so he paid off his mother's debt.

The end of the war found Leon fighting at the Sremski Front, in the northeastern part of Yugoslavia. Still not sufficiently redeemed, he soon changed his surname to his mother's maiden name, Martelanc. Even though Weinberger could have also been of Ashkenazi Jewish heritage and the reason why a number of his Weinberger relatives who stayed behind in Slovenia ended up in various European concentration camps, it sounded too Austrian and too Germanic. Martelanc fitted better with his career prospects, which included working for UDBA – the state security administration – or SFRYs secret police. Whether the brutality experienced in his teenage years was carried over to his new post, whether the victim became the perpetrator post–Second World War, is not known. What is known is that Leon's hardships did not end when the Second World War did.

Among his more difficult tasks was finding the name of his first cousin Danica, born in 1923 to Engelbert and Antonija Weinberger in Zagorje ob Savi, on the list of victims who had died in the notorious Croatian concentration camp Jasenovac. Together with her mother and father, who like his brother Mirko was a Slovenian pre-war communist and anti-fascist, Danica was arrested and taken into the largest Second World War extermination camp in Croatia, where hundreds of thousands of other people also perished. Like other teenagers and children that died there, Danica's only crime was a parental sin; in Jasenovac these sins included having parents who were anti-fascist, communist or of Serbian, Roma or Jewish heritage. The last time Leon had seen Danica was before their migration to the Soviet Union when he was eight and she was seven. The image of his playmate back in Slovenia, a blue-eyed lively girl, contrasted starkly with the name written on the paper he held in his hands in the post-war Jasenovac, and would haunt him for years.

Out: The failure and the evolution of utopia

At the beginning of the second decade into European civilisation's third millennium we continue to be haunted by the utopias-turned-dystopias of the past. Without an exit strategy, argued Ashis Nandy (1987), today's utopias often become tomorrow's nightmares, or their exact opposites – dystopias. Paradoxically, an exit strategy from a utopia becoming either stale or nightmarish is in yet another utopia, because whether or not they are explicitly expressed and/or recognised as such, utopias continue to inform *all* politics.

That is, many narratives about the future that aim to represent realistic and pragmatic approaches informing the present also commonly incorporate utopia – what is desired and hoped for. These approaches are disguised as *crypto*[5] utopias, or 'utopia that is hidden, disguised, elided, concealed, covert' (Milojević 2006, p.26). Nonetheless, they also incorporate 'prescriptive and improved imagined states of both collective and/or individual being' (Milojević 2002, p.45). The capitalist utopia, which as a new/old vision replaced the communist one in previously communist/socialist regimes, is, like its predecessor, also firmly rooted in several centuries if not millennia of European philosophy and mythology. Themes of material abundance, individualism, unrestrained freedom and endless choice are extremely common in both traditional and contemporary utopias (Hollis 1998; Carey 1999). Like the communist utopia, the capitalist one has had its philosophers (such as Ayn Rand, Milton Friedman and Friedrich Hayek) and successful/failed utopian experiments (like the 1880s Town of Pullman, Illinois, and perhaps the contemporary globally interlinked capitalist financial sector). While disguised as realistic/pragmatic, the contemporary utopia of capitalist and economic globalisation further focuses on expansion, an unlimited supply of material goods and the successful control of natural and biological processes. At the myth level, this is the idealised future image of *The Land of Cockaygne* – the land of milk and honey, the 'golden age' where nature provides abundant resources and the magic porridge bowl never empties – that was particularly popular in medieval Europe (Hollis 1998). It is a land of unlimited consumption, limitless choice, and ever increasing growth and progress. Another implicitly utopian image of the future, that of a technologically advanced information society, is also located within a particular European/western tradition of 'discovery, exploration, colonization and exploitation' (Bell 2000, p.697). For example, cyberspace has routinely been referred to as a 'new world' or a 'new frontier', even a 'new continent', whose conquest and settlement is often compared to the conquest and settlement of the New World.

These narratives about a globalised cyberworld or globally networked, even post-scarcity society, were especially popular in the 1980s and 1990s – coinciding with the coming of the Christian millennium. As postmodernists remind us, every reality has an author (or authors). The same is true of futures visions, including both utopian and dystopian narratives. Geographically, the globalised cyber utopia originated in Western societies among those who had access to financial, political and technological resources to experience, among other things, the 'shrinking of time and space'. Their utopia promised an 'irreversible shift of power away from the developed countries to the rest of the world ... delivering billions of people from poverty, creating opportunities for choice and personal development, and reinforcing democracy all round the world' (Martin 2000, pp.12–14). As it presented the liberal market economy as 'the summit of human endeavour' (2000), globalised cyber utopia conveniently neutralised anti-capitalist rhetoric by replacing more problematic terms such as 'monopoly capital' or 'world capitalism'. It also helped more concretely name the previously vaguely described New World Order. Crucially, the globalised cyber world envisioned utopia with:

> Material benefits, instant satisfaction of material needs, international democracy globally, more consumer and employment choices, cyber democracy, world harmony, environmental crisis resolved, freedom to create new virtual identities

> and communities, freedom from repetitive boring tasks, more time for leisure, liberation from the limits of time as well as geography, class, disability, race and gender (Milojević 2005, pp.109–10).

True to all utopias, the strategies proposed to achieve this vision have not been desired by all. Furthermore, some have warned about dystopian dangers arising from the pursuit of globalised cyber utopia such as:

> the gap between haves and have-nots, rampant poverty, increase in gender inequality, [a] single culture and society dominating the planet, global sameness, western imperialism, environmental degradation, hierarchical, unequal and insecure social environment, digital divide between info-rich and info-poor, formation of cyber-ghettos, electronic surveillance, total lack of privacy, information feudalism as networked are controlled by few companies, adcult as advertising becomes ubiquitous, infoglut as information overload cultivates stress, confusion and ignorance, temporal and cultural impoverishment (2005).

Others have warned that globalisation may increase the risk of future civil wars that result from higher inequality among people (Collins & Graham 2004) or the risk of terrorism (Lansford et al. 2009) or that economic globalisation is in itself a form of a religious war (McKinley 2007). Most importantly, utopian narratives are reflected in the work of authors who put forward the liberal belief that the main obstacles in the quest for a peaceful global order are only so-called rogue states. This in turn is partly based on a belief in the inevitability of a particular evolutionary pattern and in the direction of liberal democracy (Fukuyama 1992; Burchill & Linklater 1996, p.28). Such a desired (utopian) future, of universally spread liberal capitalism and democratic nation states, incorporates a belief in 'western forms of government, political economy and political community ... [as] ... the ultimate destination which the entire human race will eventually reach' (1996).

Whether labelled and overt or hidden (crypto), utopias continue to inform all narratives that propose political and social change. Even postmodernists, who 'in the tradition of Foucault ... generally refuse to offer a vision of the future ... a solution, ideal or utopian hope' (Fendler 1999, p.185), have indeed developed a desired vision for the future, although implicitly. Unlike modernists, postmodernists in general believe that offering desired futures/utopian visions would not only set limits on possibilities for the future but would also mean assuming 'a position of political authority (intellectual as center)' (1999), a position that is generally declined on ethical grounds. And yet, the crypto utopia of postmodernism can also easily be deducted, argue Siebers (1994) and Doll (1995). For example:

> What postmodernism wants is what has been lacking, which is to say that postmodernism is a utopian philosophy. Utopianism demonstrates both a relentless dissatisfaction with the here and now as well as bewilderment about the possibility of thinking beyond the here and now. Utopianism is not about being 'no where'; it is about desiring to be elsewhere. Postmodernists, then, are utopian not because they do not know what they want. They are utopian because they know that they want something else. They want to desire differently (Siebers 1994, pp.2–3).

Similarly, Bill Doll argues that the postmodern utopian vision takes on a new frame that can be called 'post-liberal' as it refers to its 'move beyond individualism' and focuses on the 'ecological, communal, [and] dialogical' (Doll 1995, p.96). The postmodern vision is born from 'our own collective, creative imaginations' rather than from a 'firmly set, a priori ideology' (1995, p.89). It is a vision built on doubt and irony, a vision that recognises its own limits and the centrality of the dialogic process and dialogic community (1995). In summary, the postmodern utopia is one that focuses on heterogeneity, multiplicity, difference and equality – but not of sameness, rather, on equality of differences.

It is perhaps most surprising that even the promotion and glorification of war is commonly underlined by certain utopian themes. This is plainly obvious in 'rational', 'necessary' and 'pragmatic' interventions by the US military. The codenames used to give a particular war a brand name (Jaramillo 2009, p.186) include examples such as Operation Just Cause, Uphold Democracy, and Enduring Freedom, as well as the even more explicit Restore Hope, Shining Hope and Provide Promise. For some soldiers, especially young men, write Barash and Webel, 'there is something exhilarating about meeting death face to face, perhaps even heroically and for a noble cause, rather than to be overtaken alone in the night' (2002, p.136). Otto Dibelius wrote in 1930s Germany that 'the Joys of War' are not only for soldiers, but for 'all who long for something out of the ordinary' (quoted in Deist et al. 1990, p.44). 'Parades, manoeuvres! Even the most doctrinaire pacifist must feel an electric shock run through his blood when he hears military music!' (1990). When serving the Fatherland, Dibelius concludes, a Christian also serves God – a basic doctrine of Christianity being to obey authorities – and in such way perhaps also gets closer to God and the afterlife heavenly utopia (1990). Attractions of war thus include engagement with both post-life and present-life salvation, together with, paradoxically, the utopia of ever-lasting peace.

It is not only the end result of war, which includes both the desire for pacotopia as well as for the 'spoils of victory that has attracted generation after generation to go to war' (Stevens 2010, p.325). It is also the activity itself:

> War brings out both the best and the worst in us, mobilizing our deepest resources of courage, cooperation, loyalty, and self-sacrifice, and releasing our capacities for xenophobia, hate, brutality, sadism and revenge. 'The comradeship of war, the fact that under conditions of stress, our capacity for identification with our fellow is increased, has been one reason for the continued popularity of war', writes the psychiatrist Anthony Storr. Lacking a sense of purpose in their lives, people 'find an almost religious satisfaction in devoting themselves to one main objective, and in orientating their lives in submission to the single wartime aim of victory' (2010).

The plain truth is, William James argued in 1904, 'that people *want* war':

> They want it anyhow; for itself and apart from each and every possible consequence. It is the final bouquet of life's fireworks. The born soldiers want it hot and actual. The non-combatants want it in the background, and always as an open possibility, to feed imagination on and keep excitement going. Its clerical and historical defenders fool themselves when they talk about it. What moves them is not the blessing it has won for us, but a vague religious exaltation. War is human nature at its uttermost. We are here to do our uttermost. It is a sacrament. Society would

> rot without the mystical blood-payment (quoted in Lawrence & Karim 2007, p.4).

While the plain truth is that *some people* wanted war, by attaching war activity to the inevitability of human nature and social progress, James has not only succeeded in promoting war activity, he has also helped create a discourse by which wars become desirable and thus possible. Furthermore, his 'paean to war heralded a new age of American expansionism [a means by which] ... [f]or most of the twentieth century, the U.S. government attempted to export its values and its products throughout the world' (2007). The alleged realism, pragmatism and radical empiricism, once again, colluded with the 'truth = power to assert one's own biases as the objective reality' or, in other words, to describe one's own desirable vision as the inevitable outcome for all.

The sanitised romanticising of war and violence found in many contemporary 'children's cartoons and toys, movies ... music, art, and literature' (Barash & Webel 2002, p.138) further enhances war's utopian appeal. This is coupled with narratives in which war is seen as something that 'brings the best out of men', enhances their deep comradeship and sense of belonging, enables sacrificial deeds for others, explores the boundaries of their capacities, brings forward novelty and a certain 'underlying stream of clarity, energy, and freedom that ... emerge(s) from within yourself ... [and] that is to be found hardly anywhere else in ordinary life', according to de Chardin (2002, p.136):

> We [soldiers] are liberated from our individual impotence and are drunk with the power that union with our fellows brings. In moments like these many have a vague awareness of how isolated and separate their lives have hitherto been ... With the boundaries of the self expanded, they sense a kinship never known before. Their 'I' passes insensibly into 'we' ... At its height, this sense of comradeship is an ecstasy (2002, p.137).

The exaltation, the exhilaration, the thrill, the rush of adrenaline and the ecstasy, especially for a number of human males (Stevens 2010, p.325), from time to time, becomes 'irresistibly seductive'. Often coupled with a 'compelling sexual component' (Barash & Webel 2002, p.136) 'the delight in banding together to train and arm themselves for battle' (Stevens 2010, p.326), a utopia of war continues to inspire and motivate many. For why else would collective acts of violence and wars still take place if they were not in some ways, by some people, still deemed desirable? Hiding between 'inevitability' and 'being forced' narratives is a thin veil that can be easily removed, for no collective human activity takes place unless it is believed sufficiently attractive. Within a context of violent/dominator societies, such inspiration gets replaced with a desire for peace only after war's 'exhaustion, destruction, and grief have [finally] taken their toll' (2010, p.325).

What can be concluded from the previous discussion is that despite all the efforts to kill it off, utopia has survived into the twenty-first century. It can be found in both realistic and pragmatic as well as some more commonly considered dystopian places, such as war. Historically, and in the context of mainstream politics, both left and right, both radicals and conservatives have tried to destroy it, although for different reasons. For conservatives, utopia challenges the present order – which is what they want to avoid. They thus argue for realistic projects for the future, whose aim is, in general, to bring about business as usual and more-of-the-same futures, or alternatively back-to-the-(idealised)-past scenarios. They thus label all progressivist politics as utopian, to be understood as naive and unrealistic, if not dangerous. Such politicking has long roots and history. 'The representatives of a given order', argued Mannheim in the 1930s: 'label as utopian all conceptions of existence which *from their point of view* can in principle never be realized' (Mannheim 1936, pp.176–77). They also point at the failures of such (progressive) utopias, or, alternatively, argue that they are no longer needed because, due to advances in technology and in general knowledge, almost 'any form of the concrete world, of human life, any transformation of the technical and natural environment is a [real] possibility' (Marcuse 1970, p.62):

> The greatest irony of the concept of Utopia is that people are still searching for it when, at the dawn of the 21st century, most citizens of the world's industrial democracies are already living in one. If we could communicate with even the wealthiest people who lived much before 1900, and told them we live in a time when even ordinary people have clean clothes and houses, nutritious food and portable water, the freedom to quit any job we dislike, the ability to hear symphonic music and watch dramas without leaving home, and vehicles to transport us anywhere in the world in a matter of hours, who can doubt that they would cry out, 'you live in paradise!' (Anonymous 2000).

Perplexingly, on the one hand, utopia is seen to have disappeared because it has failed miserably to bring positive social change (such as, for example, communist utopia). On the other hand, utopia is seen to have failed because it is no longer needed (such as, for example, both feminist and materialist abundance utopias). But even those interested in radical social transformation have attacked utopia. Karl Marx perhaps started this trend when using the concept 'in the fight between Marxism and non-Marxian socialism ... [and] to differentiate between his scientific socialism and what he felt were the dreamy abstractions of others' (Ozmon 1969, p. v). Despite his thought having all the elements of the utopian (including its potential dystopian downfall), Marx became instrumental in creating a cognitive frame that differentiates between scientific and realistic/pragmatic versus utopian approaches while engaging with social and political change. Somewhere in that process, the utopian was simultaneously equated with unrealistic, naive and unfeasible even within the left-wing side of politics. Being labelled utopian would consequently delegitimise a political project by default.

The political implications of such delegitimisation are many, not least the emergence of crypto utopias promoted by conservatives and the simultaneous weakening of social progressivism. By arguing that crypto utopias are about realism and not the desired, their champions manage to convince about their inevitability. While at any given time in history there are numerous, often competing, utopian and dystopian visions that are constantly being negotiated, locally and globally, realistic approaches manage to be privileged mostly because they fit into the worldview that legitimates. Their biggest success may not lie in either the quality or practicality of their own utopia, but rather in the ability to convince about their own inevitability, as well as about the dangers, impossibility and naivety of other (perhaps more marginal) visions. To be perceived as realistic a particular futures-oriented project must present the continuum of the present realities, including the continuation of the androcracy/dominator (Eisler) or violent society. These realistic policies and politics are almost always constructed as if their implementation is also inevitable. Their proponents often push the narrative of being left without a choice, of simply having to – being forced to use violence, for example, as in the dilemma faced by Western democracies and leaders of the free world when dealing with dictators, totalitarian governments or global terrorist networks. It is this group – that continues the most common approach to dealing with conflict (that is, classic diplomacy which incorporates wars as diplomacy via different means) – that benefits most from the discrediting of utopian sentiments. Non-violent peace-promoting actions and worldviews, on the other hand, have more to lose by the disappearance and the discrediting of utopianism. This is because overt, explicit utopias have traditionally always been on the side of marginalised social groups and worldviews wishing to change their own disempowerment and disrupt the status quo.

Extending this principle also means that there will always be a social group in need of an explicit utopia – as an expression of the hope that the future can, indeed, be different. Communist and socialist utopias historically spoke for people struggling with poverty and socio-economic exploitation, and those wishing to create more egalitarian societies. Likewise, pacotopias spoke and still speak to all people who have suffered from the negative effects of violence as well as to those who object to it on either moral or pragmatic grounds. Without the hope for a more peaceful future, the belief that it is possible, what is left to motivate nonviolent change? What is to break the 'realist's' preference for 'peace through strength' approaches (Harris & Morrison 2003, p.16), a preference that is based on a belief that 'humans are violent and the world is competitive' or 'war etched in our genes' (Barash & Webel 2002, p.122)? What is to disrupt the process by which such preferences influence the choosing of particular actions (that is, 'arms, balance of power, force, deterrence' [Harris & Morrison 2003, p.16], support of militarism, mistrust of others, othering and so on) and in such a way help create realities in which the belief is affirmed in the first place?

The rescuing of utopianism is therefore indispensable if more peaceful futures are to materialise. In other words, only critiquing violence-promoting discourses, or only arguing that nonviolence also works and is also realistic, may not be sufficient. This is because the perceived realism of war and violence versus the utopianism of peace and nonviolence also means that the first set of political strategies are often seen as the only ones that are workable. No matter how much pacifists argue about the practicality of their own strategies, within the discourse of realism, and also within the context of a dominator society, war and violence will always be perceived as more realistic. Despite the many utopian themes that underlie collective acts of violence expressed in wars, as discussed earlier, such collective acts of violence are currently commonly justified on the grounds of necessity rather than desire. Yet if certain groups and individuals did not desire it, did not promote it and did not justify it, collective acts of violence would be as absent from our present realities as they are from historical peace societies and communities, or from peace-promoting worldviews. Reframing war debates from discourses on inevitability or practicality towards discourses on desirability ('*who* wants it', '*whom* do these strategies *serve* and whom don't they') are consequently as crucial in weakening those 'realistic' futures narratives as are more pragmatic peacebuilding approaches. In other words, in addition to showing why and how nonviolence also works or is even superior, a 'force more powerful' (Ackerman & DuVall 2000), exposing utopian character of all futures visions is also necessary. This focus on desirability may further weaken the determinism – backed by a belief in the ubiquitous character of historical and social structures that leave little space for human agency – of which the belief in the ubiquitous strategy of violent conflict resolution is but one example. Consequently, the alleged inevitability of war and violence, unlike the utopianism of peaceful society, remains a legitimate discourse. This is extremely problematic because:

> There is a special danger in the belief that war is inevitable, because it is likely to discourage

> people from seeking to end war and to promote peace ... it can also serve to *justify* war by making it appear somehow 'good' because it is natural. [And this] naturalistic fallacy [is based on] the mistaken belief that '*is* implies *ought*' (Barash & Webel 2002, pp.129–30).

By simultaneously delegitimising utopianism and attaching it to pacifism, violent societies further marginalise, even eliminate, this alternative. Hegemonic futures discourses often eliminate alternatives not by making them 'illegal, immoral or unpopular', but by making them 'invisible and therefore irrelevant' (Postman 1993, p.48). As utopianism in general became invisible and irrelevant, so did the political projects connected with it. In such a socio-cultural-political climate, even peace activists have often struggled to picture an (utopian) alternative, and utilise an image of a desired future in its important function of being an 'agent of social change' (Boulding 1995, p.95). Such struggles posed difficulties with creating a 'positive imagery of a possible desired world, rather than [re-creating] negative images of a feared world' (1995, p.97). Coupled with the prevalence of the dystopian genre within the twentieth-century Western world, difficulty with engaging with the utopian dreaming has in some ways legitimised fear at the expense of hope, further argued Elise Boulding.

Perhaps due to the perceived failure of previous utopian experiments, people nowadays want to be realistic; however, they simultaneously take it as 'axiomatic that fears are realistic and hopes unrealistic' (1995, p.100). The prevalence of the dystopian genre, both in fiction and especially in the news, images of 'natural disasters, accidents, crime, war, disease, social injustice ... [which] convey a picture of a world where nothing works – in short, dystopia now' (Jennings 1996, p.212), has had a profound negative impact on both the general population as well as on young people in particular (Hicks & Holden 1995; Hutchinson 1996; Slaughter 1998). This is especially disheartening because it is usually the role of younger generations to revitalise each society, including society's progressivist politics.

The enhancement of progressivist politics is, crucially, necessary for the continuation and enhancement of peace cultures. This is because, historically, 'virtually all political movements of the far right (and even some moderate right-wing or conservative parties) have rarely if ever professed peace as an important national political goal' (Barash & Webel 2002, p.21). On the other hand:

> ...most left-wing (progressive and/or radical) thinkers and parties have traditionally claimed a strong association with world peace [even though] ... many of the less radical, more liberal members of progressive political movements and parties have frequently approved of war under certain conditions (2002).

In that process of creating and practising progressivist politics, a degree of utopianism has historically within Western civilisation always played a prominent role. The utopian sense of 'human empowerment sets in motion a powerful dynamics' argue Elise Boulding (1995, p.96) and Fred Polak (1973):

> Through their daily choices of action, individuals, families, enterprises, communities, and nations move towards what they imagine to be a desirable tomorrow.... [On the other hand] in eras when pessimism combines with a sense of cosmic helplessness, the quality of human intentionality declines and, with it, the quality of imagery of the not-yet. (Boulding 1995, pp.95–96).

'Utopia is the principle of all progress and the essay into a better future', further argued Lester Pearson (1972). As such it is necessary for the promotion of 'the ideal of world peace and security through international action and institutions' (1972). Without overt paxtopias then, all we are left with is realist politics that limit our choices to those that are repeating the violent presents/pasts. To break this cycle, investigation and articulation of alternative peace histories, present peace/nonviolent practical strategies *as well as* the articulation of overt utopian (desired futures) peace-oriented visions are all simultaneously necessary.

The critical re-evaluation of utopia that took place in the twentieth century was not, however, without positive, perhaps unintended, consequences. Even though the hope may be 'superior to fear' because it is 'neither passive like the latter, not locked into nothingness' (Bloch 1986, p.3), our societies also need a healthy dose of dystopian thinking, providing that such thinking represents insight arising from healthy scepticism. Dystopian thinking, argues Jennings (1996, p.211), can take two basic forms or functions. It can be expressed as a description of 'a place or condition in which everything is as bad as possible', or take the form of anti-utopias (1996). In the first form, dystopias play the important role of emphasising 'the serious problems that may result from deliberate policies, indecision and indifference, or simply bad luck in humanity's attempts to manage its affairs' (1996). On the other hand, as anti-utopias, dystopias are 'satirical or prophetic warnings against the proposed 'improvement' of society by some political faction, class interest, technology, or other artefact' (1996). In this latter sense, dystopias can 'poison our outlook on the present, or even prompt us to give up trying to do better' (1996). Even though the dystopian in its anti-utopian meaning as well as realistic thinking about the future became the normative futures discourse, they too need to be critically evaluated. That is, concludes Jennings, taking a critical view of both dystopian (based on fear) and utopian (based on hope) visions is necessary to balance the need to perhaps 'prepare for the worst with a desire to achieve the best' (1996, p.212).

Another positive consequence of the critical evaluations of previous utopian discourses that took place in the twentieth century has recently manifested in the emergence of two new concepts – those of *eutopias* (decisively good not perfect places) and *heterotopias* (places of otherness). Eutopia represents a shift from previous understanding of utopias as 'perfect societies' that 'eliminate real people' (Carey 1999) towards utopias understood as marked by self-doubt and questioning. The new term implies that while it is not possible to create perfectly orderly societies – a desire that reflected modernist, industrialist civilisation – it may still be possible to create better ones, improvements on the past and the present. As such, eutopias can adopt the function of being safe(r) spaces for speculation, social dreaming, subversion and critique, an expression of a desire for different (and better) ways of being. The postmodern era further demands 'heterotopias', which Michel Foucault (1986, p.27) initially defined as 'a space of illusion ... a space that is other'. Literally translated as other or different places, this term has more recently come to denote imaginary place of otherness, multiplicity and diversity – insisting on the *plurality* of spaces of otherness. In such a way heterotopias reconceptualise nineteenth-and twentieth-century utopia by including flexibility, questioning and work in progress. Such a conceptualisation is extremely important in every pluralistic society – and every society is always in essence pluralistic – because it can further open up the possibility of developing alternative, including peace-promoting, discourses.

Such new utopias are understood as 'self-limiting, partial and plural' (Alexander 2001, p.579). In this way they also represent an attempt to replace the previous 'rage for order' in utopianism with diversity and even chaos. This is critical if peaceful societies and peace cultures are to be created because the very definition of peace cultures in the simplest possible terms (Boulding 2000, p.1) assumes 'a culture that promotes peaceable diversity'. Peace culture is 'a mosaic of identities, attitudes, values, beliefs, and patterns that leads people to live nurturantly with each and the Earth itself' (Boulding & Forsberg 1998, p.36). As such it includes an:

> appreciation of difference, stewardship, and equitable sharing of the earth's resources among its members and with all living beings ... [it would] offer mutual security for humankind in all its diversity through a profound sense of species identity as well as kinship with the living earth (Boulding 2000, p.1).

In a nutshell, imagining peace cultures and societies, imagining pacotopias, is as important as a critique of the violent alternatives. Merely opposing is not enough since, 'To say something is not true, valuable, or useful without posing alternatives is, paradoxically, to affirm that it is true, and so on. Thus coupled with this negative project, or rather, indistinguishable from it, must be a positive, constructive project: creating alternatives' (Grosz 1990, p.59). This is because in a 'vacant space after one has resisted there is still the necessity to become – to make oneself anew' (Hooks 1991, p.15). Coupled with 'the negative or reactive project of what currently exists' (Grosz 1990, p.59), it is thus always necessary to offer 'a positive alternative, a vision of a better future that can motivate people to sacrifice their time and energy towards its realization' (Alcoff 1988, p.418). The role of utopia, evolved into eutopias and heterotopias of our era, in this way neither provides a blueprint that forecloses the future nor prediction or prophecy but, rather, is in an 'imagined possibility' (Boulding 2000, p.257) for times ahead of us.

If such a project is (consciously/intentionally or unconsciously/unintentionally) abandoned, not only will one travel without knowing where s/he wants to go, but also we may all find ourselves engaging in actions that are bringing us exactly those futures that we least desire. Indeed, we may all continue to be haunted by what only a handful considers attractive and desired but package as realistic and inevitable. We may all remain hostages of their dystopian-utopian dreaming.

CHAPTER 2

War, dystopia: The holy trinity of militarism, imperialism and nationalism

> War is not about victory or defeat. It is about the total failure of human spirit. When you see the things I see, you would never support war ever again (Fisk 2005, p. xix).

Udah: Jama[1]	In: The Pit[2]
Krv je moje svjetlo i moja tama. Blaženu noş su meni iskopali Sa sretnim vidom iz oşinjih jama; Od kaplja dana bije sni oganj pali Krvavu zjenu u mozgu, ko ranu. Moje su oşi zgasle na mome dlanu.	Blood is my daylight, and darkness too. Blessing of night has been gouged from my cheeks Bearing with it my more lucky sight. Within those holes, for tears, fierce fire inflamed The bleeding socket as if for brain a balm – While my bright eyes died on my own palm.
Sigurno još su treperile ptice U njima, nebo blago se okrenu; I şutao sam, krvavo mi lice Utonulo je s modrinom u zjenu; Na dlanu oşi zrakama se smiju I moje suze ne mogu da liju.	While played, I never doubt, God's feathered creatures, Reflected still in them, and clouds' procession; But all I felt were my blood-spattered features, Bruised gulfs in that once brilliant profusion. How radiant lay my eyeballs in my hand, Yet from those eyes no tear could more descend!

Udah: Jama [1]	In: The Pit [2]
Samo kroz prste kapale su kapi Tople i guste, koje krvnik nadje Jos gorşom mukom duplja, koja zjapi Da bodež u vrat zabode mi sladje; A mene dragost ove krvi uze, I şutio sam kaplje kao suze.	Then ever other fingers ran the warm Coagulating blood my slaughterer found By the profounder agony of holes he formed For better grip, more sensuously to wound; But me the softness of my blood enthralled, And I rejoiced as blood were red tears falling.
Posljednje svjetlo prije strašne noşi Bio je bljesak munjevita noža, I vrisak, bijel još i sad u sljepoşi, I bijela, bijela krvnikova koža; Jer do pojasa svi su bili goli I tako nagi oşi su nam boli.	The final light before the frightful night The lightning swooping of the polished knife, The cry too white still in my blinded sight, The bleach-white bodies of the murderers, Who stripped their torsos for their sweaty task – Was dazzling even to my blinded mask.
O bolno svjetlo, nikad tako jako I oštro nikad nisi sinulo u zori, U strijeli, ognju; i ko da sam plako Vatrene suze, s kojih duplje gori: A kroz taj pako bljeskovi su pekli, Vriskovi drugih muşenika sjekli.	O painful daylight, never so hard yet Or penetrating did you break the East With fiery arrow; I might have thought I shed Teardrops with leaping flames that seared my cheeks Through all that hell so many lightnings burnt, So many cries of other victims cut.
Ne znam, koliko zar je bijesni trajo, Kad grozne kvrge s duplja rasti stanu Ko kugle tvrde, i jedva sam stajo. Tad spoznah skliske oşi na svom dlanu I rekoh: "Slijep sam, mila moja mati, Kako şu tebe sada oplakati..."	What time that furious conflagration fanned, All that I knew of time were callouses for eyes, Hard-grown and aching; and could hardly stand. And only then my slippery eyeballs fingered And knew – and cried: My sight, O Mother mine, is gone. How shall I weep when your life too is done?

Udah: Jama[1]	In: The Pit[2]
A silno svjetlo, ko stotine zvona Sa zvonika bijelih, u pameti Ludoj si-jevne: svjetlost sa Siona, Divna sv-jetlost, svjetlost koja svijetli! Svijetla ptico! Svijetlo drvo! Rijeko! Mjesece! Svijetlo ko majşino mlijeko!	Then dazzling daylight like a myriad carillons From endless gleaming bell-towers in my crazy Brain illumined like the lights of Zion, A lovely light – a light which sanctified – Bright birds, bright river, trees and, brilliant Boon pure as mother's milk, still brighter moon.
Al' ovu strašnu bol veş nisam şeko: Krvnik mi reşe: "Zgnjeşi svoje oşi!" Obezumljen sam skoro preda nj kleko, Kad grş mi šaku gustom sluzi smoşi; I više nisam ništa şuo, znao: U bezdan kao u raku sam pao.	Now came a torture I had never guessed – My murderer commanded 'Break your own eyes!' I nearly prayed for mercy to the beast, But slimy-fingered spasmic hands obeyed – And then no more I heard, no more could tell, To empty nothing faltered, and [into the Pit] I fell.

Out: Knives, guns and beyond

I think I was about eight when I found out during one of my classes at school that in the Second World War some people slit other people's throats and gouged their eyes. Not knowing what to do, I decided to stare at my shoes. 'Look, brand new and shiny. The colour is lovely: kind of chestnut brown, similar to the colour of the trees in our street. In particular, I like the shoelaces. The soles are not too bad either. I like that they are made of rubber and that they have all those ridges. My mother said those ridges will keep me safe from slipping.' It felt good to know I was so well protected.

When my father heard that people slit each other's throats in the Second World War he was also eight. Unlike me, he did not hear it during class. He was there, living that history. The fact was conveyed to him by a man who had moved forcefully into his parent's house during the war along with his fellow fighting mates. The family was relocated into one room, and soldiers occupied the rest of the house. 'Look at my knife,' the man told Zoran, the eldest son of his 'hosts' Zorka and Stanoje-Staša Milojević and who later became my father. 'Can you see all the indentations?' Zoran nodded. And he counted seven. 'Each one of these gashes', the man proudly stated, 'matches the line on the throat of an enemy I personally made.'

Trophy taking, in the form of carved lines on knives, or in the form of 'heads ... scalps ... foreskins ... notches on guns ... or "kills" painted on the fuselage of a fighter plane' was widespread in 'premodern war' and the 'vestiges of this custom can [also] be seen in modern times' (Barash & Webel 2002, p.151). The main difference between the customs during 'premodern' and 'modern' times, argue Barash and Webel is that 'indiscriminate killing of old people, women, and children is rare in premodern cultures, even in the most heated of wars'. Further:

> self-renown, rather than death to one's enemies, was widely considered the highest goal. The 'war hero' is valued among technological peoples as well. The difference between pre-modern and

> modern peoples in this regard is that personal aggrandizement – for wealth and/or glory – is not supposed to be the most important reason for engaging in contemporary warfare; rather, the individual combatant is ostensibly acting as a defender of public security, national honour, and/or human rights (2002).

It seems that the more 'civilised' we get, the better we are at justifying our own violence. One way by which this is done is by arguing that one fights for higher goals, or that one is willing to sacrifice their own life for the survival/wellbeing of the larger community (in wars). Yet another way of justifying and minimising their violence by the civilised is to present their killing techniques and motivations as somehow superior to or more advanced than those of others, which are perceived and defined as barbaric. This subtle difference, though, may be irrelevant to potential victims. In other words, whatever the articulated reasons behind trophy taking, for a powerful life taker (in the form of a trophytaking warrior) this custom may signify glorious, or even civilised behaviour, but for a defenceless child (that is, an eight-year-old) any method of killing signifies an external demonic threat and reminds of one's own vulnerability. Rarely, however, does the perspective of a child enter political texts and history books, which have for centuries, in their own way, facilitated glorification of (discriminate) trophy taking as well as the perception by the mighty warriors.

The (real or potential) victimisation of the weaker and more vulnerable was to be suffered in silence. This rule extended to wounded and disabled soldiers who, no longer powerful, often suffered the similar fate of post-trauma neglect and invisibility. The only exemption to this general rule of silencing the cries of the less powerful seems to be through the use of their vulnerability and trauma to promote a particular political agenda. Only then is the narrative of victimisation at the hands of the 'evil' other aired openly. This too has negative consequences. Most importantly, selective victimhood narratives are often (ab)used to encourage revenge and/or pre-emptive violent interventions against potential or real enemies – evil others.

Like most societies, the former socialist Yugoslavia (1945–91) in which I was born and raised dealt with trauma from the Second World War and other wars by selective remembering and selective representation of trauma/victimhood. In post-Second World War society, Yugoslav peoples were surrounded by traumas, only some of which – that is, those fitting the overall political agenda – were allowed to be recognised. Politics therefore did not only influence what was going on in society as a whole, but also what went on in people's everyday lives as well. Even the suppression–expression trauma continuum was politically mediated. To this day, all over the world, this remains a rule with very few exceptions.

One case in point regarding selective remembering and the political mediation of how trauma is expressed is the poem '*Jama*' by Ivan Goran Kovačić, which was studied in primary schools all over the former Yugoslavia. I include it here because not only did it have a traumatic effect on me when I was forced to memorise it as a child but the pit metaphor for me is crucially linked to some of the things my two grandfathers experienced during the Second World War. Further, the (actual) pits were dug up again during the 1990s wars in the former Yugoslavia – wars that destroyed the society I used to belong to. To me the metaphor symbolises end states rather than new beginnings, which wars and other collective acts of violence inevitably bring. When even a single person dies in a war – which is understood here as an organised and premeditated activity of collective violence – their personal phoenix never arises later. Dystopian personal endings, where some people are wounded, killed and tortured, always accompany wars no matter how 'civilised'. Furthermore, physical and mental injuries continue many years later, negatively impacting on those unfortunate individuals and their families and communities, even the society as a whole. Despite all the utopian narratives that make wars not only possible but also openly or secretly desirable, for the vast majority of people the reality is that wars are the pits of humanity's lost/taken hopes and dreams, where bodies as well as human spirits are often buried.

If one can bear to read it, the poem *'Jama'* can, through words, help visualise images of horrors that commonly result from the injuries inflicted during collective acts of violence. Like many similar poetic expressions it also reveals some common delusions that help deliver such horrors in the first place. Many horrors of the twentieth century were in part carried through delusions supported by, most significantly, metadiscourses of militarism, imperialism (including eurocentrism and discourses of social Darwinism) and nationalism. In addition to the overall dystopia of war, it is these discourses that are of central concern here. Another critically important metadiscourse, patriarchy, is so intimately linked with violence that its analysis warrants a separate section (Chapter 3).

Within my broader analysis of various historical and contemporary metanarratives that support war and collective acts of violence, as well as narratives that support peace, a discussion of the poem *'Jama'* is relevant for several reasons:

- it expresses the dystopia of war
- it is an example of dealing with trauma from violence through writing and poetry (the strategy I have also chosen)
- it is an example of political mediation and selective remembering of trauma and victimhood
- it raises issues around appropriate pedagogical practices in post-conflict societies

- it raises issues relating to the perception of the distinction between more and less barbaric methods of torture/killing during violent conflict.

To start with, '*Jama*' is possibly one of the most horrific poems written in the Croato-Serbian/Serbo-Croatian/Croatian/Bosniak/Serbian/Montenegrin language. The poem, from which only the first section (out of seven, or nearly 70 verses or about 2500 words) is reproduced here, could be seen predominantly as an example of anti-war and anti-fascist poetry. Given that the nationality or religion of executioners and victims is never mentioned, its message against torture, mass murders and war crimes could be seen as universal:

> As long as a last man speaks Croatian and the language of humanity in general, *The Pit,* with its reach of artistic strength, is going to be an everlasting condemnation of crime and a hymn of human freedom, truth and beauty, a hymn to human dignity (Kaštelan 2012).

In that sense the poem is among 'the most poignant and terrifying poetical responses to the war' (Cornis-Pope 2004, p.148). But the life, work, death and interpretations of the legacy of Kovačić, the poem's author, are somewhat more complicated.

Kovačić was born in Lukovdol, Gorski Kotar, Croatia, in 1913. He was a former student of the Zagreb Faculty of Philosophy for Slavic Studies, where he studied history and Croatian language but dropped out mostly due to poverty and illness, and later devoted himself to writing and journalism. At the end of 1942, in the socio-historical context of a strong Croatian nationalistic movement and German occupation, Kovačić joined the anti-fascist and communist-led (Yugoslav) national liberation army or Partisans. A mere six months later, on 12 July 1943, at the age of 30, he was killed by (Serbian) Chetniks, the same ideological and political group the man who showed off his knife to my father belonged to. Kovačić wrote several well-known poems, including the prophetic *'My Grave'* – foretelling in it that his grave would remain unknown – but his most famous poem remains *'Jama'.* In the former SFRY the poem was studied at school not only as an example of anti-war poetry but also because Kovačić's life, work and death made him 'a symbol of Yugoslav unity' (Naumović & Jovanović 2004, p.245). During those six months that he was with the Partisans, Kovačić witnessed many atrocities or aftermaths of atrocities, including those against local Serbs in Croatia and Bosnia by Croat Ustashe and Bosnian Muslim forces. His poem was partially a protest against crimes 'his own people' have committed against others, whose alleged 'representatives' (that is Serbian Chetniks) then ended Kovačić's life. Unlike Kovačić who, by most accounts, channelled his trauma away from recreating it or repeating it and attempted to, albeit briefly, deal with it with poetry, the latter group chose the strategy of revenge and of recreating cycles of violence and trauma. More specifically, at the beginning of the Second World War the region of Foča witnessed the murders of prominent Serbs at the hands of Ustashe (Stenton 2000, p.327). Foča was one area in eastern Bosnia where 'in the summer of 1941 the genocide against the Serbs ... acquired broader proportions ... particular targets were Orthodox priests, wealthier citizens and intellectuals, with the goal of morally and psychologically disarming the Serbian population and alarming them' (Redžić 2005, p.78). This goal was fulfilled, the alarm was obviously raised and the Serbian uprising followed (2005, p.79). The cycle of violence continued during the Second World War: 'The massacre of Muslims in Foča, in eastern Bosnia, was the most dreadful. The Ustaše had killed the leading Serbs in the town; when the Chetniks took Foča the ensuing massacre of Muslims was far worse' (Stenton 2000, p.327). To avenge the violence, Chetnik Serbs also systematically raped Muslim women and slit the throats of over 2000 men in the region of Foča alone (Hart 2011), the very same place where Ivan Goran Kovačić was also later killed.

After the Second World War and after communism won in the former Yugoslavia, partisan literature (poems and novels), to which *'Jama'* belongs, 'had been one of the central genres for the propagation of post-World War II supranational Yugoslav identity' (Wachtel 1998, p.198). During those socialist times the underlying message was clear: the poem describes atrocities committed by those the Partisans fought against, both foreign fascist and local Ustashe and Chetnik groups. In such a political climate, Kovačić's trauma was on 'the right side of history' – thus its inclusion in the elementary school curricula. But Kovačić's overall message also reflected the universal desire to create and maintain peace (especially pertinent after major violent conflicts), and to avoid future dystopias. Further, his life and work reflected transcendence of ethno-nationalism, refusal of fascism and the promotion of values of humanism, all of which were relevant to both the former Yugoslavia as well as Europe immediately post Second World War. These values were crucial to support both collective healing as well as a vision for a new multicultural Yugoslav society.

After the 1990s Yugoslav wars, however, Kovačić's trauma suddenly found itself on the wrong side of history in Croatia and Bosnia but simultaneously on the right side of history, though reinterpreted, in Serbia. Despite Kovačić's own anti-violence, anti-fascism and humanistic stance, common interpretation of the poem in Serbia is now (mis)used to promote nationalism, including the idea of a victim, and to negatively mark the (ethnic, no longer ideological) other (Veličković quoted in Gočanin 2011). This shows that motivations for the study and interpretations of texts are fundamentally more important than, perhaps, the actual texts that are studied. Motivations and interpretations are, in turn, always influenced by the dominant ideology and worldview. Once nationalism had overridden discourses of humanism and multiculturalism, the previous (socialist Yugoslav) interpretation of this particular text also had to change. No longer could the poem describe atrocities committed by those the Partisans fought against – both the foreign fascists and the local Ustashe and Chetnik groups – which had been the underlying message and interpretation during socialist times. No longer was the distinction between different methods of killing – that is, barbaric killings of fascists, Ustashe and Chetniks, versus the cleaner and less sadistic methods of execution (by guns) preferred by the Partisans – necessary, for those who controlled the discourse to justify their violence. And no longer were the atrocities committed by communist-led Partisans kept invisible; for example, those towards the end of and after the Second World War against local ethnic Germans and Hungarians, as well as other 'domestic traitors and enemy collaborators'. But the change in the dominant discourse within the Yugoslav successor states did not bring about a more objective picture of the past, nor a more pacifistic interpretation. Equally skewed, albeit in a different (pro-nationalistic, but still bellicose) direction, the biases and (mis)interpretations continue.

Given the violence that occurred on a massive scale during the twentieth century, it comes as no surprise that the underlying interpretations and worldviews of literary texts were rarely pacifistic. Rather, militaristic, nationalistic as well as imperialist narratives most commonly prevailed. Taken to the extreme, these narratives led to fascism (including Nazism), an ideology that explicitly and openly glorified war 'not only as a means to alleged national political goals but also as a desirable end in itself' (Barash & Webel, 2002, p.15). The consequences of such developments were many, not least the poem *'Jama'* and the events it described/condemned.

Even explicitly taught anti-violence lessons could, however, potentially be a catalyst for further violence. Most disturbingly, another poet, Bosnianborn Duško Trifunović (1933–2006), has argued that *'Jama',* instead of being a deterrence from violence as was initially intended, served as a 'textbook to those who, after certain passage of time, gouged eyes in a manner similar to that which Goran described' (Trifunović 1998). Which begs the question, how could future generations be warned about the horrors of war without, simultaneously, naturalising and normalising violence as part and parcel of human history and social change? Should or shouldn't texts like *'Jama'* even be studied?

Research by Hava Shechter and Gavriel Salomon (2005) in the context of Israeli–Palestinian conflict shows that exposure to graphic descriptions of violence does not automatically create empathy towards the distress of an adversary. If accompanied by nationalistic lessons, the 'vicarious experience of one's own group's suffering' does not necessarily mean 'one's empathy towards the suffering of others' (2005 p.125).

Likewise, the contact hypothesis, which proposes 'negative attitudes toward other groups are rooted in limited knowledge of them, which generates anxiety' (Niens 2010, p.592) and suggests a solution of becoming acquainted with experiences and perspectives of adversaries, has not been confirmed by the empirical studies:

> Despite its obvious intuitive appeal, research has not unequivocally supported the contact hypothesis in the context of political conflict ... One of its main weaknesses was that even if positive attitudes were formed toward individual out-group members, these attitudes often failed to generalize to the out-group as a whole. (2010, p.593)

In other words, perceptions of inter-group membership seem to override more human-centric and compassionate responses.

My own observations of different groups from the former Yugoslavia watching and commenting upon graphic descriptions of violence are that a particular cognitive template always mediates emotional responses. Empathetic responses were present when those victims of violence were perceived to be part of the in group. On the other hand, empathetic responses towards victims of violence who were perceived to be part of the out group were usually arrested, unless the cognitive frame of pacifism and humanism was used. However, most commonly it was a just-war theory or attributional biases that took precedence, and the empathic response did not occur. More specifically, the just-war theory, that proposes 'our war is just', and attributional biases that cause someone to see one's own group in a more positive light than the out group, prevented development of empathy by either psychological processes of justification (*we* were forced to do it) or of disbelief (*we* couldn't possibly have done it).

To empathise with the suffering of others you need to perceive them as human beings, first, and only after that in terms of their ethnicity (or in terms of other characteristics that differentiate them from the us group). When the discourse of nationalism is present this order is reversed, and so a person is perceived as a member of an ethnic (religious, etc.) group, first, and then as a human. What follows in the narrative are lines such as, 'What about *our* own suffering?' and '*They* did worse'. This may explain why lessons about the dangers of inter-ethnic violence during socialist times in former Yugoslavia failed to prevent future animosities. Once the dominant multicultural discourses (*we* are united in brotherhood) was weakened and replaced with nationalistic ones (*they* are no longer *us),* history was reinterpreted and selective remembering as well as selective victimhood was elected to represent 'the only truth'. This also means that graphic descriptions of violence are useful and can help deter further inter-ethnic violence only if alternative interpretations to the nationalistic and bellicose ones are offered. Discourses of humanism, pacifism and multiculturalism, for example, influence selection of poetic texts that highlight altruistic and empathic behaviour among former and/or potential enemies, focusing less on the graphic descriptions of violence and more on the prevention of attitudes that may lead to violence in the first place.

Poems, like other literary texts, tell a story and generally help to create meaning, and this is particularly so with regards to violent conflict. It may be important here to distinguish between constructive and destructive storytelling, because each plays a role in both dealing with trauma from violence as well as preventing engagement in violent activities. By and large, destructive storytelling is damaging because it is 'associated with coercive power, exclusionary practices, a lack of mutual recognition, dishonesty, and a lack of awareness' (Senehi 2010, p.111). Examples of this type of storytelling exists in most national European mythologies – as expressed in poems, folklore, stories, songs, national epics, proverbs and fairy tales – any time humans are portrayed as generally 'bad, cruel, violent and selfish' (Eisler 2000, p.27). Fairy tales and traditional myths in the European context are 'full of cruelty, trickery and violence', including violence against women, children and those who are deemed 'different' (2000). This is in contradiction to the messages parents and teachers try to communicate to children, specifically, to be 'good and kind, nonviolent and giving' (2000). Such destructive storytelling, whether in the form of poems or longer literary texts, can be helpful when addressing issues of discrimination, prejudice and violence, if it is critically evaluated from a peace-oriented worldview.

Simultaneously, storytelling is a powerful, flexible, accessible and inexpensive method that, if done constructively, can be utilised directly for peacebuilding (Senehi 2002, Tanaka 2005, McKee 2008, Neile 2010). Unlike destructive storytelling, constructive storytelling is 'inclusive, and fosters shared power and mutual recognition, creates opportunities for openness, dialogue, and insight, brings issues to consciousness ... can be a means of resistance ... and an important means for establishing a culture of peace and justice' (Senehi 2010, pp.111–12). It is an especially powerful method when working with young people because of universal human receptiveness to stories and because storytelling is typically 'a more indirect and respectful rather than prescriptive and didactic method of teaching' (2010, p.112). In other words, alternative, peace-promoting literary texts should form the backbone of the curriculum if schools and societies are serious about preventing *all* violence. If not, even an anti-war poem such as '*Jama*' can still be used to promote the underlying templates of 'we' are good/'they' are bad' and 'violence is necessary in order to defend ourselves against evil others', or the very templates that facilitate collective acts of violence in the first place.

Whether the alternative pedagogical approach – focused on constructive storytelling – could have created somewhat better results than the one that occurred during the former Yugoslavia's collapse is far from certain. What is known with more certainty is that the back-to-the-past, nationalistic ideologies of the late 1980s and early 1990s glorified traditional weapons, such as knives, as part of their overall warrior iconography. This return of 'almost all irrational delusions of the past ... in our Yugoslav space [and] the "vampirisation" of national-chauvinism' (Čolović 2002, p.261) also encouraged the return of the knife as a symbol of previous suffering as well as of the traditional (male) warrior power. Inspired by ethno-nationalisms and their past proponents (Ustashe, Chetniks) some nation-ethnicity defenders picked up knives, rather than guns, as their weapon of choice. Knives regained their previous significance because:

> the wars in Former Yugoslavia were often fought not between soldiers but between soldiers and civilians who were branded as enemies. It was literally a war of slaughter; knives were important weapons. This retreat to such unsophisticated arms seemed to many in the West evidence that the state was not involved, but it surely was (Duyvesteyn & Angstrom 2005, p.171).

The involvement of state in promoting nationalism and militarism has been critical during the twentieth century, but was not limited to former Yugoslavia. Likewise, the distinction between knives, guns and more advanced weapons did not end with socialist

Yugoslavia. A similar underlying template was (and continues to be) used when justifying various interventions by 'clean', 'precise', 'surgical' and 'smart' new technologies of destruction. Those on the 'right' side of history (and power) – for example, NATO's involvement on the territory of the former Yugoslavia – claimed to fight a 'clean/cleaner' war. Precision weapons – in this case, depleted uranium ammunition – seemed to have verified superiority, development and civilisational involvement almost by default. Despite dozens of blunders, injuries and killings of innocents, the 1999 NATO intervention was 'nevertheless':

> a very clean war ... There were two essential features of this conflict ... the first was technological. A significant number of the munitions were precision guided or 'smart bombs' (35 per cent compared to 8 per cent in the US-led war against Iraq in 1991) and the unprecedented accuracy of these weapons significantly reduced collateral damage (Reus-Smit 2004, p.197).

But even if the prospects of 'war without casualties (i.e. deaths)' are to move from fantasy into reality '...some of these weapons (blinding lasers for example) may not kill, but have an exceedingly nasty consequence for their victims. And in the end a disabling weapon works only if it leaves an opponent vulnerable to full-scale deadly force (Cohen quoted in Brown 2003, pp.100–101).

A perception that being blinded by lasers rather than knives is somehow preferable may or may not make sense, depending on the underlying cognitive template used. If progress is measured solely by technological development, the following conclusion is inevitable: being killed by smart bombs is definitely preferable to being killed by guns or knives. If, on the other hand, progress is measured by the development of 'alternative, nonweapon "instruments of peace", any alleged "advance" from stone axe to hydrogen bomb' (Barash & Webel 2002, p.67) is seriously undermined. Given the extraordinary inventiveness of people in 'developing fast, efficient, and devastating means of destroying other people (as well as animals, plants, buildings, and land), with ever increasing ease and at everincreasing distances' (2002), it seems logical to me that the only way to minimise casualties in the future is to refrain from using *all* and *any* weapons. In fact, more sinister and infinitely more dangerous consequences of modern weapon technologies make it imperative that the overall 'progress via technology' narrative be undermined. In this process, supplementing measurements such as GDP (gross domestic product) and HDI (human development index) with HPI (happy planet index) and GPI (global peace index) is a start. Alternatively, non-existent 'GMK' (global mutilation and killing index) and 'NCW' (short and long-term negative consequences of the use of all weapons) should be the true measures of all and every 'barbarism'. By changing how progress and regress is measured, locally and globally, perhaps new, more peaceful realities could be better supported. These new peace-promoting narratives need new measurements and new stories, including the (age appropriate[3]) stories that portray collective violence as it really is: a very concrete and real dystopia of horrors.

Sadly, whether it is via the 'cult of the knife', 'the cult of the gun and the bombs' or the cult of 'invisible state violence' hidden from the public eye (Duyvesteyn & Angstrom 2005, p.170) dystopias of horror have continued well into the twenty-first century. Bellicose states and societies continue to play a pivotal role in creating the conditions for violence to occur as well as post-violence justifications. They do so by exposing the violence of others as unjust and barbaric and also by providing reasons why *our* retaliation is necessary. This means that the underlying templates of militarism and nationalism are still the most powerful narratives influencing war/peace debates. In doing so, these templates obscure the real message of literary texts such as *'Jama':* the necessity of preventing the potential future agony of the mutilated, wounded and dying, agony that transcends all artificially imposed human divisions.

In: Veljko

I am about six or seven and am sitting on my grandfather's lap. We don't see my mother's adoptive father Veljko much. He is busy with his career as a high-ranking politician in the Yugoslav government and travels internationally a lot. But this is not the only reason I am sitting apprehensively on his lap. My grandfather is a tall and imposing man, a charismatic and warm presence. And yet his walking stick gives away the fact that one of his legs is made of wood, I was told, replacing the real one he lost in the war. So I am worried: if I am sitting on his wooden leg will any sudden movement do further harm? Consequently I sit stiff and quiet and wonder which of the two legs – the real or the artificial one – I am sitting on. I would like to touch the leg with my fingers, poke it a bit or even ask about it, but I don't dare. Wooden legs frighten me and so do their carriers, despite their softly spoken voices and their general demeanour of kindness. Fortunately, I don't stay on that lap for long. Once down and away from the wooden leg I can finally breathe with ease again.

Many years later I read my late grandfather's reflections upon being wounded and mutilated:

> They are taking me from the first front line with three wounds, each as heavy as the lead in them. Three sources of hot blood tell that a few minutes ago three red-hot pieces of iron pierced through my body. The size of the blood sources indicates whether the bandits used ordinary or dumdum bullets. They were mixing both ... Hospital ... muffled groans and gritting of teeth. Next to me is a sixteen-year-old boy. My bed is numerated with the number 6, his with the number 7 ... The

hospital is overcrowded, and there is enough space in the building for less than a third of the arrived wounded. The rest are arranged in the courtyard, under the clear sky. I am taken into the operating theatre, to have a couple of bullets taken out of my right hip and around ten pieces of shrapnel ... Just before midnight, when I was on the table in the operating theatre, fascist planes arrived and spilled their deadly cargo above the hospital. Two bombs fell in the hospital's courtyard and finished off around a hundred injured. The light disappeared. Staff working in the operating theatre temporarily left. I was lying alone in the darkness of the operating theatre for more than half an hour. Through the broken glass of the hospital windows I could hear the screams from the courtyard of the re-wounded injured. Staff, who came back to the theatre, finished their job on me in haste as they needed to prepare the room for the other difficult cases. They relocated me into the basement, into the room in which, like in a can of sardines, more than 40 other wounded also lay. Here too there were screams, groans, swearing, delirious and incoherent talk, and shouting for nurses' attention. It was pitch black all around us. But the hardest thing to bear was a foul smell of alcohol mixed with the smell of unattended wounds that festered ... Once upon a time I imagined dying at the front line differently, in a majestic and splendid, glorious and epic way. Is this how Byron died? Is this how Paris

Communards and heroes of the October Revolution died? Is this how my uncle and his uncle died? But this situation here is much more prosaic, mundane, and simple. Instead of grand music and speeches, battle symphonies, yelping of machine guns and explosions of dumdum bullets, there is only an occasional scream or an irksome cry, and then a shortlived silence. In those moments of sudden silence what prevails is the smell of the freshly dug up earth from the trench my friend and I were digging all night, up until dawn. This is how earth also smells after pits and graves are freshly dug up. Did we dig our own grave last night, without knowing what we were doing? Will our friends know how we died? I observe the blood, my own and of my own friend, how it is absorbed and sinks into the loose soil. Only the dark stain remains. I wonder if from this blood the next year's olive trees will be more bountiful? And then, suddenly I remember the verses we sung in jail: 'Lots of blood will be spilled, but still the day when every man will be happy and free will come' (Vlahović, 1981, pp.22–27).

Out: Bellicose fantasies of glory

A coward dies several times in his life, a hero only once.

> He who dies honorably is remembered for one hundred years, and he who dies without honor is forgotten [even] by his own children.
> A proper hero does not die at home.
> An honorable death celebrates your life.
> These tombs are not graves, but the cradles of new forces.
> (Pešić 1994, p.69)

Given the socio-historical context he grew up in, it comes as no surprise that my grandfather Veljko, like many others, glorified dying on the battlefield. At least, until that moment when he almost experienced it firsthand, in which the actuality of inconsequential irksome cries replaced previous fantasies of splendour. Despite such realities, which repeat themselves in each and every violent conflict, fantasies and delusions of glorious fighting and dying for the cause persist. There are currently few indications that these fantasies and delusions supported by androcratic (bellicose and militaristic) worldviews are being radically transformed within the mainstream western–global society. There are also few indications that glorifications of violent conflict resolution in general and the relentless promotion of 'our cause' will diminish in the near future. Notwithstanding the successes of peace movements, the globalisation of militarism continues unabated. Despite militarism at the beginning of the twenty-first century becoming less 'extreme', or perhaps even because of it, the 'ideology of militarism or "warism"' (Zimmerman 1994, p.150) continues to threaten our common futures.

This is a consequence of our recent social and political history. To 'unprecedented degree', the twentieth century proved to be 'The Age of Militarism' (Nisbet 1982, p.221). Of particular interest here is *social militarism* or the presence of 'military values and mentalities percolating into a civilian society' (Berghahn 2010, p.27). This definition includes the 'prevalence of military sentiments and ideals among a people' (*Oxford English Dictionary* quoted in Berghahn 2010, p.27). Understood in this sense, social militarism can be further described as:

- the belief or desire of a government or people that a country should maintain a strong military capability and be prepared to use it aggressively to defend or promote national interests (*Oxford Dictionary* online 2012)
- a policy of glorifying military power and of 'maintaining a strong military organization in aggressive preparedness for war' (*Collins English Dictionary* 2003)
- 'the aggressiveness that involves the threat of using military force' (Dictionary.die.net 2012).

Overall, militarism is understood here as 'the use of force at the expense of alternative solutions' (Mirra 2008, p.94).

The use of force and violence requires preparation both in terms of developing certain social or cultural technologies (that is, promoting bellicose narratives and worldviews) and in terms of investing in and developing certain physical technologies (weapons). Militarism has historically been an important building block of both imperialist and expansionist states as well as within those old/new states liberated from the rule of such expansionist states. Despite various impetuses for demilitarisation over the last century, militarisation and militarism continue to be significant forces in 'The Age of Terror'. And despite the recent global depression (2009–), the amount the world invests in tools for killing increased by 1.3 per cent in 2010 to a record high of over US$1.6 trillion (SIPRI 2011). It seems that an earlier prediction by Robert Nisbet (1982, p.228) made in the 1980s that 'the future almost certainly belongs to the military' has come true, as well as the much earlier statement by Friedrich Engels that 'militarism dominates and is swallowing Europe' (Engels 1877).

The post-Cold War demilitarisation trends in Europe of the early 1990s have been since reversed and the European military organisation, NATO, is increasingly flexing its muscles. Since Operation Deliberate Force (in Bosnia and Herzegovina 1995 – an earlier involvement started in 1992), NATO has militarily intervened in other non-NATO countries such as the Federal Republic of Yugoslavia (the so-called rump Yugoslavia, which at the time included Kosovo, in

1999, Operation Allied Force), Macedonia (operations Essential Harvest, Amber Fox and Allied Harmony, 2001– 2003), Afghanistan (operations Eagle Assist and Active Endeavour, 2011), Iraq (NATO training mission, 2004), Somalia, Gulf of Aden (Operation Allied Protector, 2009) and Libya (Operation Unified Protector, 2011). Not all of these interventions have resulted in collateral damage (the killing of civilians), but certainly interventions in the former Yugoslavia as well as recently in Libya show clearly that European leaders no longer consider civilian deaths resulting directly from their military involvement to be an obstacle to militarily disciplining violent regimes. Military interventions, of course, are always done at the expense of other, usually less-expensive and long-term-oriented alternatives.

Whether policing wars, 'deterrence and even confrontation are the only way' (Mueller 2010, pp.328–29) to deal with some countries/regimes is disputable, but what is more certain is that 'once systems for waging war are created, it is difficult to dismantle them: they become apparently permanent social institutions' (Vissing & Moore-Vissing 2010, p.344). Even before these interventions NATO 'as a military alliance relying heavily on nuclear weapons [was] ... the major obstacle to the creation of nuclearweapon-free zones in the western parts of Europe ... jeopardiz[ing] the peace-building initiatives of the Council of Europe' (Boulding 2000, p.245). Its military 'successes' since 1995 make it less likely that such strategies will be abandoned in the near future. NATO is currently leading an expansionist policy and future enlargement swallowing most of Europe is planned. These military operations and policies are supported, in turn, by militaristic narratives that are both a result and one of the causes of NATO's survival and expansion. In our globalised era Engel's statement could also be extended to argue that militarism is now dominating and swallowing the world – not only in terms of the ever-increasing funds poured into the military–industrial complex but also in terms of the continuation of violence-promoting sentiments heard within current nation-states and dominator-based cultural worldviews.

Full immersion within a militaristic worldview, as well as the omnipresence of this worldview in warrior–androcratic societies, make it really difficult to recognise and practise pacifistic alternatives. Although 53 years separated my grandfather's birth and mine, we were both born and raised within a bellicose culture. My own direct encounters with militarism started in primary school and continued throughout my higher education studies. The quotes mentioned at the beginning of this section (reproduced in Pešić 1994) were from Yugoslav textbooks that were used in all schools across former Yugoslavia. Other popular quotes/well-known sayings included *'bolje grob nego rob'* (better grave than slave) and *'bolje rat nego pakt'* (better war than pact). Used during protests in times of violent conflict, or just prior to one, these sayings were taught in times of (relative) peace, as the militaristic worldview demanded that the curriculum rationalise and prepare the people for violence. Narratives explicitly stated in textbooks are significant because they continue to play an important role in many parts of the world where they are still the only books available to children. Further to this, textbooks:

- in concise form express mainstream knowledge and the mainstream value system, they show which knowledge is selected and attains the status of 'socially legitimate' narrative
- represent a standard, a norm which school systems aspire to achieve
- are conscious means for socialisation
- are a part of a powerful system which attempts to model future generations in accordance with desired images, whether that means a continuation of a current society or the creation of 'new nation-state citizens'/a new society (Pešić 1994).

Militarism was omnipresent in European nation-state curricula during the last century:

> Militarism in the upbringing particularly of male children is a phenomenon characteristic of the nineteenth and twentieth centuries. After conscription was introduced in many European countries in the course of the nineteenth century, not only the composition but also the perception

> of armies in European societies changed considerably. The soldier became a role model for a growing number of young boys, primarily from the middle and upper-middle classes, and military values came to play an increasing role in the education of male children (Levsen 2010, p.215).

As socialist Yugoslavia promoted gender equality, militarism was extended and played a role in the education of female children also. As a consequence – that is, because the militarisation of the former Yugoslav society extended beyond the limits of gender – I was trained to use weapons as part of obligatory 'defence classes', including the use of real ammunition. For 40 years, in between the end of the Second World War and the end of SFRY, all school children, irrespective of gender, were taught a rudimentary military and defence training in primary and high schools and this included first aid, in case of an injury during an enemy's attack; protective jackets and masks usage, in case of a nuclear/chemical weapons attack; as well as how to fire weapons (pistols and rifles). Drills on how to escape from the classroom and into a nuclear bunker were also a common practice, as were the lessons on how to recognise 'a foreign enemy' in the first place – all with an underlying message of not trusting foreigners and needing to remain always vigilant against 'the other'. Parallel to this, national war heroes were worshiped for 'giving us our freedoms and way of life'. Steeped in a history of wars and violence, both multicultural

Yugoslav as well as Yugoslav predecessor and successor nation-states, which are based on more narrow ethnic identities, organised (the only) legitimate narratives around notions of their respective peoples' 'freedom', 'victory', 'national independence' and 'strength' for centuries. These identities have also been constructed in the context of the earlier mentioned politics of victimhood. The Chosenness-Glory-Trauma syndrome (Galtung 2002, p.23) almost universally present in European nation-states and countries (and beyond) was part of Yugoslav 'deep culture' as well.

Narratives that portray Yugoslav peoples as victims of foreign oppressors have been ingrained in literature, education and the predominant worldview (Rosandić & Pešić 1994). The subsequent conclusion stemming from such a view has been, to avoid being a victim you have to always be ready to defend (by means of fighting in wars) life, family, territory and nationhood. This, of course, requires preparation, and that preparation – military training – is to involve every capable young man. All of my male relatives and friends had to do a stint in the army. For most of its existence Yugoslav government drafted only men – girls and women, however, were mostly spared, as somebody had to take care of the 'homefront'. Nationalistic ideologies enhanced gender divisions – the quintessential soldier was of the male gender. Liberal feminist efforts notwithstanding, female soldiers remained an exception to the general rule. Within the context of militarism, coupled with its Siamese twin patriarchy, whether women do or don't participate is probably inconsequential as, once militarised, women soldiers become honorary men. Like their male colleagues they must denounce all 'feminine' traits, particularly those that are in some way connected with pacifistic qualities. Whatever his or her biological sex, a soldier has culturally always been of the 'male' gender. This phenomenon – of all men by definition being soldiers – influenced the blurring of boundaries between civilians and soldiers, most notably in the horrific crimes committed during the 1990s (for example, the Srebrenica massacre).

A heavily militarised culture does not give a (capable) man the option not to be a soldier. In the context of violent cultures in the territory of former Yugoslavia, every man of a certain age has been a soldier by default. Only very recently – post the 1990s war – is this slowly but surely changing with the creation of a professional army. Further examples of militarism, in both the former Yugoslavia as well as all over the European continent are not difficult to find. Glorification of soldiers in nineteenth-and twentieth-century Europe is forever enshrined in the continents' city squares, argues Johan Galtung. The quintessential 'man on a horse' statues – of men holding weapons, a monument and an artefact that contains a deeper message (Galtung 2002, p.14) and which signifies dominance over others as well as over nature – are a lasting reminder of European militarism. Further:

> This makes the male warrior or statesman highly visible, instead of the most significant of all events; a woman giving birth to a new human being, to life. By the same token there seems to be no monument dedicated to a family, mother and father, children, just being sweet, loving to each other. In this there is a deep message, carried just as much by the positively present monuments as by the negatively absent monuments (2002).

Particularly up until the First World War, European society as a whole 'from capital cities to small villages, from Britain to Germany, from France to Russia, had been dominated by European "men of violence" who worshipped militarism' (Weber 2008, p.9). This was only weakened during post-Second World War Europeanisation, 'with the gradual dissolution of nation states' (2008). If this was a general trend in western Europe it certainly wasn't present in the former Yugoslavia. CGT or Chosenness– Glory–Trauma syndrome has been and remains the key archetype within most former Yugoslav deep cultures. In the context of Serbia the strong belief in being 'a Chosen People (C), with a Glorious past and/or future (G), but at the same time a people suffering from countless Trauma (T) ... inflicted by Others' (Galtung 2002, p.23) has been at the core of the very definition of Serbian nationhood. From the socialist CGT syndrome that existed during SFRY, ethnic-based CGT dominated prior to and came to dominate after the dissolution of Yugoslavia. The more bellicose the ethnic culture, the stronger the CGT syndrome has been. Like most other nations, Serbian identity and nationhood has been born 'on the killing fields' and, although a 'masculinist birth' and in this way 'a mission impossible' (Lake 1992), patriarchal appropriation of what has been predominantly women's activity does not pose any problems within the context of militarism. Even though Serbia gained independence from the Ottoman rule through nonviolent means this is rarely registered within collective selective process of remembering. To this day negotiation and nonviolent conflict resolution are commonly equated with weakness and passivity, even sleaziness and danger. This underlying worldview and rationale for violence is exhibited in a [contemporary] Serbian history textbook:

> The *moderate and peace-loving* ruler Stefan Uroš III Dečanski (1321– 1331) was not captivated by conquest and his goal was to maintain the state he inherited from his father. Neighbours understood his *peacefulness as weakness,* and so Bosnia, Byzantium and Bulgaria *attacked* Serbia. (Kočić 2007, p.135, italics added).

Likewise, the ruler who brought Serbia partial independence from Turkish rule is often portrayed within various products of culture as sleazy. This is because:

> Practically without fighting the Turks, Miloš [Obrenović, reigned from 1815–1839 and 1858–1860] used money, skill and diplomacy to obtain considerable concessions for Serbia, such as a constitution and hereditary monarchy. The foundations of a state government were also created – a judiciary and administration. Miloš allowed 'neither the Turks to oppress the people, nor the people to insult the Turks' and he confirmed this compromise, which brought great concessions to Serbia, with gestures such as repairing the Jagodina mosque. It is also said that he gave alms to the 'Turks in the masses' (the poor) and 'showed respect for their religion' (Pešić 1994, p.69).

As this does not sit well within the worldview of militarism the narrative is barely present in textbooks nor is it seen in the collective selective remembering within, for example, mainstream media and popular culture. Likewise, as a historical analysis of Yugoslav/Serbian textbooks in 1994 has shown, there are 'almost no pacifist messages, whereas the militant ones accentuate bravery, reaching as far as brutality, death as the source of life, honor and standing achieved through bravery, remembering defeat and taking an oath, and general harmony (for discord is always the reason for defeat)' (Rosandić 1994, p.7). More recent studies have shown that history textbooks in Serbia, Croatia and Bosnia continue with the narrative in regards to the necessity of defending oneself via military means, as well as with narratives that project blame for wars on others: 'it is "the other" who is guilty for war, he started it, we defended ourselves and had to endure the greatest sacrifices' (Dakić & Palić 2011). It comes as no surprise then that as recently as 2011 Minister of Police and deputy of Serbian Prime Minister Ivica Dačić publicly stated that no one in Serbia is allowed to say that Kosovo (the province that proclaimed the independence in 2008) is lost (to Serbia) and that s/he does not want to wage a war for the province. 'We have lost and regained Kosovo several times during history. The [current] attacks on Serbs in Kosovo are also attacks on Serbia as a whole which Serbia cannot and does not want to observe peacefully' (B92 2011). His statements were supported by several political and military commentators who agreed that 'militarily defending our own territories is legal and recognised under international law' as well as that 'wars remain an important part of overall diplomacy'. Hope remains that the discourse proposed by the only person voicing the opposition to the above bellicose narratives, vice president of the Democratic Party Jelena Trivan, who stated that 'our country should not use war to fight its battles because its victims would be people' (2011), will become the dominant discourse in the future. She also added that Serbia can no longer afford the luxury of losing yet another generation in wars because then there would be no Serbia. This is why 'we need, instead, to use intelligence and diplomacy when fighting all future battles' (2011). Sadly, within the context of a strongly bellicose culture, even peace promotion seems to be relying on militaristic metaphors.

These practices of schooling and 'taught taking' in media are dangerous because they educate and prepare people for future animosity. Another dangerous practice in most bellicose societies is not only the selective interpretation of history – that is, the marginalisation of the history of inter-ethnic peace to the benefit of wars and violence – but also the overwhelming focus on history rather than on the future. For example, the year 1389 continues to play a crucial role in the mythology of Serbian nationhood. Of course, as 'everybody knows', that was the year the Battle of Kosovo took place. Serbian 'Tsar' Lazar's army suffered a defeat and thus the fate of Serbia was sealed. The Serbian identity/nationhood is very much formed around this myth of the birth of the nation at the killing fields of Kosovo (Trauma) – as it is on the myth of a highly advanced and powerful society of the fourteenth century: 'when we ate with forks and spoons while the English still had food dripping down their fingers' (Chosen People). But then 'the Turks' defeated the Serbian forces in two decisive battles: first on the river Marica in 1371, where the Serbian noblemen in Macedonia lost, and the second in Kosovo Polje in 1389, where Prince Lazar's army perished. The Ottomans continued their conquest until they seized the entire territory of the Serbian state in 1459, when the town of Smederevo fell. Serbia was then:

> ruled by the Ottoman Turks for nearly 500 years. During this period the conquerors had particularly persecuted the Serbian aristocracy, and physically exterminated the social elite. Since the Ottoman Empire was an Islamic and theocratic state where Christian Serbs were second rate citizens suffering all sorts of abuses, exploitation and humiliation, the Slavic population slowly abandoned the developed urban centers where mining, trade and crafts had flourished, and retreated to the inaccessible mountains, where they lived mostly on cattle (Savković 1998, p.17–18).

The past-oriented narrative, which proposes both victimhood and 'liberation' must be mediated through violence – as during the early twentieth-century Balkan Wars and the first and second world wars – remains strong. Once liberated from various oppressors, previously colonised nation-states, in accord with the overarching template of social militarism, predominantly recognised the military means by which this liberation took place. As a result, social militarism became further perceived as a necessary discourse to put into practice during even more peaceful times ('lest we forget'). Violence – threat of violence and preparation for violence – continues to dominate the former Yugoslav and now separate nation-states' security discourses, which is in turn supported by social militarism. It seems that within this discourse of militarism no escape from violence, either during conflicts or during more peaceful periods, is possible. In that, Yugoslav and Serbian case studies are not unique examples. Rather, most contemporary nation-states suffer from CGT syndrome, with further militarisation commonly presented as the most 'obvious' solution to threats to nationhood potentially arising in the future. And so, despite all the empirical evidence to the contrary, bellicose fantasies of glory continue to be nationalists' holy grail.

In: Stanoje

Unlike my maternal grandfathers Vasiliy and Veljko, my paternal grandfather Stanoje-Staša did not care to volunteer for war. In the 1930s he was a budding capitalist who established his own business, employed workers and invested in the market. As well as this, his new family was growing. During the first seven years of his marriage to my grandmother Zora, three children, two sons and a daughter arrived. Both his business and his family were expanding and the future looked bright and promising. But in 1941 war came to him.

After the invasion and dismantling of Yugoslavia in April 1941, Stanoje and his family became citizens of *Militärverwaltung in Serbien* or 'Military administration in Serbia', a period also known as 'Serbia under

German occupation'. He was given new documents, logically in German, which stated:

> *Hadwerker-Vereingung für Stadt und Bezirk Kruschewatz, 30.VII.1941. AUSWEIS. Herr Stanoje Milojević, Sneider, geb. 21. II.1911 aus Čitluk ist Mitglied der Innung der Hadnwerker in Kruschewatz. Derselbe ist berechtigt, sicher Stadt frei zu bewegen and seine arbeit auszuüben. Präsident der Hanewerker-Verein Strahinja Budinovič. Für den Feldkommandanten, Oberkriegsverwaltungsrat.*

Even though he did not know German, Staša understood that these papers, arranged by the association of craftsman that he belonged to, would allow him to freely move around his own town. This 'freedom' did not last long. In 1942 he was taken into the work camp to dig up minerals the Nazis needed to maintain and continue their rightful occupation of the 'lesser people', of the *Untermenschen* – the subhuman race that Staša learned he also apparently belonged to. During his absence Zora and their children relocated to her parental home. It was two years before the family were to see their husband and father again. Those two years felt like 200 to Staša.

Labouring in the camp was hard but being called to dig the pits was harder. He never knew whether any of those pits he was digging were, perhaps, meant for him. It wasn't logical that he should be killed at that time. But then again, it wasn't logical that some of his relatives and neighbours were to be killed either, and yet they and many others were. He was also never sure if being called to close the pits brought revulsion or relief to him. He would not look into the pits; he never looked anywhere but into the earth he was shovelling. His captors seem to have liked that. They seem to have liked that he always hung his head, looked down, that he was not proud and feisty like some others. They called it 'cooperation', a workable compromise for all. You don't complain and perhaps we'll spare you, spare your life so that you can return home to your wife and children.

Staša covered the bodies of those who did not return, those randomly taken so the deaths of occupying German soldiers could be avenged. Similar to the other parts of occupied Europe, the going rate was 50 to 100 communists, Jews, Gypsies or local other people for one German soldier. Staša knew there was very little he could do, except to look down, into the earth, the dirt he came from and into which he would return. Looking into the earth had always brought comfort to him, since his childhood. But even that seemed to be failing him now. He knew earth was very good at covering death, of people, plants and animals, he'd seen it many times before. But now, earth allowed the evidence of what had just happened show. Nowhere in the land that he was aware of, nowhere in this land that he was familiar with, was there layer upon layer of dead bodies directly beneath a thin coating of soil. Nowhere else, but here, were there so many bodies whose blood would be soaked up by the earth and brought to the surface. Years later, even decades later, gazing at the earth was never again to bring comfort and reassurance to Staša.

After the war ended, Zora said, Staša was never the same. He took to occasional drinking, and lost the gentleness and kindness he exhibited during the first seven years of their marriage. Before the war he was a pleasant and optimistic young man. After the war he suffered in silence but his whole demeanour changed. It did not help that his store was nationalised by the socialist regime or that all his pre-war market investments went up in flames. It did not help that he became one of the state employees in what had been his very own store. The affection he had showed his children early on disappeared only to return with the arrival of his grandchildren, myself being one of nine. The new generation helped heal him but by that time his health was already damaged. He suffered a stroke in his early fifties, a consequence of a fall from a bicycle and the fall a consequence of a loss of balance due to alcohol intoxication. Staša hated the taste of alcohol but it was the only strategy available to him that promised much-needed relief when the stress of post-war living simply became too much to bear. Staša died in 1984, on Djurdjevdan,the Eastern Orthodox holiday that celebrates a Christian saint and the beginning of spring. Still holding lilies of the valley that he had just picked from his garden – the flower that symbolises new beginnings – his last vision was possibly of the loose earth of a small ditch into which he finally collapsed.

Out: 'We' of the 'lesser' people

The idea of 'lesser' and 'higher/more advanced' people was central to the doctrines of imperialism, Eurocentrism and social Darwinism. It reached its peak in fascism and Nazism. By extension, any time this idea creeps in, even in a less overt and more-subtle way, to the political decision-making processes, what we have is mini fascism, or fascism and social Darwinism thinly veiled. Sadly, racism, ethno-nationalism and imperialism-based politics have not influenced only fascism. Rather, these ideologies have significantly impacted the whole contemporary world. The arena of international politics, in particular, is built on hierarchical relations between lesser/higher people, of which the latter have not only more wealth/power in general, but also more influence in political decisionmaking processes locally and globally.

Within the boundaries of Europe, it has been the area of the Balkans that has, by and large, been inhabited by the lesser people. 'A specter is haunting Western culture – the specter of the Balkans,' begins Maria Todorova's seminal text *Imagining the Balkans* (1997, p.3). What she means by this is that:

> All the powers have entered into a holy alliance to exorcise this specter: politicians and journalists, conservative academics and radical intellectuals, moralists of all kind, gender, and fashion. Where is the adversarial group that has not been decried as 'Balkan' and 'balkanizing' by its opponents? Where the accused that have not hurled back the branding reproach of 'balkanism'? (1997).

The discourse of balkanism makes politics within the region, within Europe and globally, further argues Todorova (1999), 'significantly and organically intertwined' with a construction/invention/imagination of the Balkans as lesser. From an innocuous geographical term – denoting the area surrounding the Balkan Mountains, or the Balkan Peninsula in Southeast Europe – the construction of the Balkans at the beginning of the twentieth century meant that:

> Europe had added to its repertoire of *Schimpfwörter,* or disparagements, a new one that, although recently coined, turned out to be more persistent over time than others with centuries-old tradition ... That the Balkans have been described as the 'other' of Europe does not need special proof. What has been emphasized about the Balkans is that its inhabitants do not care to conform to the standards of behavior devised as normative by and for the civilized world. As with any generalization, this one is based on reductionism, but the reductionism and

> stereotyping of the Balkans has been of such degree and intensity that the discourse merits and requires special analysis (Todorova 1997, p.3).

This special analysis is pertinent to the area of peace and conflict studies because the conceptualisation that Todorova critiques is widely present within the field. One example is *The Oxford International Encyclopedia of Peace* (Young 2010b), where there are no less than 23 entries in some way directly related to the 'Balkans'. To start with, the term 'Balkan Conflicts' is defined in the following way:

> In the 1990s Yugoslavia witnessed the worst violence Europe had seen since 1945 in a series of wars that devastated large parts of the broken federation. Several hundred thousand people – mostly civilians – died. Millions fled abroad or were displaced internally. Chauvinism, fuelled by the conflict between Serbia and Croatia, the two longstanding South Slav rivals, engulfed Bosnia. Eventually, after years of equivocation, the West intervened to prevent the wholesale deportation of the Albanians of Kosovo. The scale and intensity of the crisis *forced* the Atlantic democracies to base much of their security strategy after 2000 on the integration of the Balkans into common Euro-Atlantic structures with the European Union (EU) increasingly taking the lead in shaping policy (Gallagher 2010, p.168, italics added).

Not only is this entry written by a non-Yugoslav, non-Balkans-based author, but also none of the bibliographical entries accompanying it (with titles such 'The Balkans' [twice], 'The Balkans after the Cold War: From Tyranny to Tragedy', 'The Balkans in the New Millennium', 'The Balkans: From Constantinople to Communism' and 'The Balkans in World History') is by a Yugoslav or Balkan-based author. And while Balkanbased authors may also be guilty of balkanism, it is still less likely that they will theorise themselves as 'inferior'/'uniquely problematic'. Barash and Webel's *Peace and Conflict Studies,* an influential text, is likewise full of references to balkanisation and 'the Balkans'. For example, 'Following the establishment of nation-states in Western Europe' low levels of various kinds of violence existed, 'at least until the resurgence of genocidal ethnic cleansing and xenophobia during the 1990s in the Balkans' (2002, p.177). They also state, 'Furthermore, it is not clear that further *Balkanization* – of Africa, India, or anywhere else – will necessarily further the cause of peace. Certainly, the Balkans peninsula, known as the "tinderbox of Europe"...' (2002, p.169). The implication, even most likely not intended, is clear: without its 'tinderbox', (western) Europe would have been fine, peaceful and tolerant, so it is obvious here who the problem is! The claims of 'primordialism' and 'perennialism', long abandoned when explaining the behaviours of western European and other 'developed' states, continue to be used for the Balkan ones. Incidentally, Todorova's argumentation and writing, as well as that of many other authors, have been published within the context of *Slavic,* rather than political or peace/conflict, studies. But to better understand a whole range of issues within this region, cross-pollination is necessary.

Foucault's observation about power-knowledge systems that determine how reality is perceived and defined is apparent in the discursive construction of the Balkans. For example, the 1976 *Popularna Enciklopedija* (*Popular Encyclopaedia)* by BIGZ in Beograd (Belgrade) defines Balkan as:

> BALKAN (Turkish 'mountain'), mountain system in eastern Serbia and Bulgaria, composed from various mountain ranges, 530 kilometres long, 21–45 kilometres wide; it can be divided between Western one (see *Stara Planina),* Middle one (see *Shipka)* and Eastern one (up to the Black sea); highest mountain tops: Botev (2376 m), Vezen (2198), Midzor (2169). Sheep raising is developed and there are coal, copper and gold deposits.

The Hutchinson, Softback Encyclopedia's (published in Oxfordshire, United Kingdom, in 1994) definition is:

> BALKANS (Turkish 'mountains') peninsula of SE Europe, stretching into the Mediterranean Sea between the Adriatic and Aegean seas, comprising Albania, Bulgaria, Greece, Romania, Turkey-in-Europe, Macedonia and Yugoslavia. It is joined to the rest of Europe by an isthmus 1,200

> km/750 mi wide between Rijeka on the west and the mouth of the Danube on the Black Sea to the east. The great ethnic diversity resulting from successive waves of invasion has made the Balkans a byword for political dissension. The Balkans' economy developed comparatively slowly until after World War II, largely because of the predominantly mountainous terrain, apart from the plain of the Sava-Danube basin in the north. Political differences have remained strong – for example, the confrontation of Greece and Turkey over Cyprus, and the differing types of communism prevailing in the rest – but in the later years of the 20th century a tendency to regional union emerged. To 'Balkanize' is to divide into small warring states.

Despite some tendencies towards regional union then, the term Balkans remains a signifier of disunity. Further, the question could be raised as to how confrontation between Greece and Turkey over Cyprus differs from confrontations over other parts of greater Europe (that is, the dispute over Alsace-Lorraine between France and Germany, 1871–1945 or Northern Ireland between Ireland and the United Kingdom, 1920–99). Nor is there mention of the fact that the colonisation of the region by various European (Austro-Hungarian, Nazi German) and non-European (Ottoman) empires contributed to the 'Balkans economy developing comparatively slowly' until after the Second World War (when the area was largely decolonised). Instead, geographical ('eternal' as in 'mountainous terrain') conditions are presented as the main reason for the region's economic 'backwardness'.

The Hutchinson is significant both for what it says and also for what it does not. Given that it defines the Balkans in political as well as geographical terms it could be expected that it would provide some additional information and interpretations such as: that the poverty of the Balkan region occurred largely because of colonisation by the Ottoman and Austro-Hungarian empires; that people living at the Balkans experienced invasion and brutality by Nazis during the Second World War; and that the eighteenth-century Balkan question actually refers to the competition and struggle between western European nations to get territories and spheres of influence on the peninsula during the decline of Ottoman empire, etc. However, the cognitive template of balkanism overrides such alternative discourses. Interestingly enough, the cognitive template of the colonised (nation-states within the region) focuses predominantly on the blaming of imperialist policies for its own political or economic difficulties. Both cognitive templates – of balkanism as well as anti-imperialism – are a result of imperialist and nationalist practices that have contributed to the various forms in which violence took place in the region. And both templates continue to underlie policies and politics still impacting upon millions of people living there.

One example of this can be seen in the way *the construction of the Balkans* – that is, being defined not only in geographical but also in cultural and political terms – impacted on both the practices as well as perceptions of violence that took place in twentieth-century Europe. The geographical definition or understanding of the Balkans is not very precise and correct; for example, in the case of Yugoslavia, none of the three Yugoslavias that have existed thus far was completely within 'the Balkans'. The mountains in Slovenia are part of the Alps mountain chain; Slavonija and Vojvodina are north of the Danube and Sava, in Panonska nizija (the middle European Pannonia depression). Thus neither area, strictly and geographically speaking, belongs to the Balkans. Most importantly, the common understanding of balkanism forgets about not only the peaceful coexistence of many ethnicities in the region but also about various political projects of the twentieth century that aimed at regional unification. Within the discourse of balkanism there is, for example, no mention of *pan-slavism,* or of an historical movement that attempted to *unify* all Slavs within one nation-state (within the Balkans in particular and Europe in general). Nor is there mention of the Balkan Leagues (I in the 1860s, II in 1912–13) that temporarily unified Greece, Bulgaria, Serbia and Montenegro in their efforts to overthrow the Ottoman occupation. Other alliances and treaties that deserve but rarely receive a mention include the Balkan Pact (1934), a treaty signed by Greece, Turkey, Romania and

Yugoslavia, wherein signatories agreed to suspend all territorial claims, and the Balkan Bled Agreement (1954), an agreement between Yugoslavia and Bulgaria recognising distinct Macedonian ethnicity and language. The idea of a Balkan Federation manifested on and off from the late nineteenth century up until 1948. Other shorter-or longer-lived organisations and projects such as the League for the Balkan Confederation (1894), the Balkan Socialist Federation (or Socialist-Democratic Conference) (1910), the Revolutionary Balkan Social Democratic Labour Federation (1915), and the Balkan Communist Federation (1920–33) all involved Balkan people working together and cooperating on a range of issues.

The area, like the rest of the Europe or indeed the rest of the world, has therefore seen both diversifying and unifying political movements. It has been moulded in particular political units and formations in accordance with the political climate and the mainstream discourse of the time. And, these units, formations, movements, ideologies and politics were changing through time and space. They are thus neither 'eternal' nor 'primordial' but socially, politically, culturally and historically constructed. However, the mainstream discourse has captured the notion of the Balkans within particular interpretations, according to the needs of those that help promote it. Balkanism and its subjects are:

> imprisoned in a field of discourse in which 'Balkans' is paired in opposition to 'West' and

> 'Europe', while 'Balkanism' is the dark other of 'western civilization'. When the Balkans were part of the scatter pattern of invective aimed at the east and 'Orientalism' was the other necessary for the self-essentializing 'West' and 'Europe', there existed the prospect of their rediscovery in a positive fashion. With the rediscovery of the east and orientalism as independent semantic values, the Balkans are left in Europe's thrall, anti-civilization, *alter ego,* the dark side within (Todorova 1994, p.482).

The term has thus become useful in conveniently exempting 'the West' from:

> charges of racism, colonialism, Eurocentrism and Christian intolerance: the Balkans, after all, are in Europe, they are white and they are predominately Christian (1994, p.455) ... Balkanization not only had come to denote the parcelization of large and viable political units but also had become a synonym for a reversion to the tribal, the backward, the primitive, the barbarian. In its latest hypostasis, particularly in American academe, it has been completely decontextualized and paradigmatically related to a variety of problems (1994, p.453).

The violent conflicts of the 1990s in *one* (now former) country *partially* geographically based in the Balkans have brought this discourse to the front of mind, transforming it into 'one of the most powerful and widespread pejorative designations in modern history' (Todorova 1997, cover page). This is because, as Todorova once again astutely remarks: 'The Balkans are usually reported to the outside world only in time of terror and trouble; the rest of the time they are scornfully ignored' (1997, p.184). This allows for this region – 'geographically inextricable from Europe, yet culturally constructed as "the other"' – to continue to serve as 'a repository of negative characteristics upon which a positive and self-congratulatory image of the "European" has been built' (1997, cover page). Even though ethnic homogenisation within nation-state has been one of the basic themes of European history overall, and conflict in the former Yugoslavia, as Todorova has argued, the 'ultimate Europeanization of the peninsula' (Stokes 1997), the discourse on balkanisation won. In other words, considering the 'extent of the devastation that Europeans have wrought on each other, to say nothing of the rest of the world, in ... "the century of expulsions" ... the rhetorical ... attempts to distinguish "the Balkans" from "Europe" ... are suspect' (Hayden 1996, p.797) and should thus be rejected.

Nonetheless, the balkanism discourse influenced not only Europe's relationship with the region, but also debates within former Yugoslavia. That is, Balkans/Europe dualism has been 'central to much of the political discourse over the legitimacy or necessity of political acts concerning Yugoslavia's collapse and subsequent wars, both by Yugoslav politicians and by those on the world stage who have had to deal with them' (1996). Within the former Yugoslavia and its successor states, 'the designation of the "other" has been appropriated and manipulated by those who have themselves been designated as such in orientalist discourse' (Bakić-Hayden 1995, p.922). Accompanying socialist and multicultural Yugoslavia's collapse was not only the questioning of the 'common-identity-through-common-communist-state but, lead by their political and intellectual elites', the restoration of '"original" identities that predated the common state' (1995). These original or 'real' identities were not only to be found in the pre-Yugoslav past, their (re)construction also followed 'the familiar orientalist pattern of 'unchanging truths' ... exhibit[ing] a curious mixture of culture and politics' (1995, p.926).

The portrayal of Yugoslav peoples as a whole or some particular groups of subject-victims within Western media as 'powerless victim of circumstances, deprived of all political identity, reduced to bare suffering', argues Slavoj Žižek, represented 'a certain naturalization, a purely racist perception of what went on in Yugoslavia, treating things there as a kind of almost natural catastrophe, as if a kind of primal ethnic hatred exploded there, tribal war, everywhere against everyone else' (Žižek 1999). Instead, a more accurate perception is that even a 'subject-victim to whose aid NATO intervene[d] [was] a political subject with a clear agenda' (1999). Indeed, many citizens of Yugoslavia were actively participating in the dismantling of the country. In doing so they too utilised the discourses of superior/inferior peoples. Concretely, early in the 1990s the battle to locate oneself high(er) on the 'hegemonic western scale' and geographically and/or culturally closer to 'the centre' or western Europe started:

> From the standpoint of the 'northern republics', Slovenia and Croatia, centuries under Habsburg rule have qualified them to 'join Europe' at the present [post Yugoslavia] time. Historical circumstances which led to industrial development in western Europe have been appropriated by Slovenes and Croats as the product of their superior qualities, and western-like participation in the cultural circles of mittel Europa is stressed, without consideration of *how* they participated – as equal actors or otherwise (Bakić-Hayden 1995, p.924).

These republics proclaimed that they 'belong' to Europe; simultaneously, however, there was a strengthening of the 'popular perception in the north and west of Yugoslavia that there is a southern, "Balkan burden", which has slowed if not prevented entirely the non-Balkan parts of the country from [being] what they "really are" – European' (1995). Further to the east/south, Serbs and Montenegrins tried to position themselves as historical defenders of Europe, European civilisation and culture from the invasion of oriental barbarians: 'the last barrier to the ongoing onslaught and aggression of Islam' (Šarić 1990, p.68). Therefore 'Serbs, Montenegrins and, to a lesser extent, Macedonians ... felt compelled to defend their "other" Europeanness by stressing their complementary contribution to the European cultural heritage and the cultural discontinuity created by the Ottoman conquest of their part of Europe' (Bakić-Hayden 1995, pp.924–25). Yugoslav Muslims also needed to position themselves within the overarching narrative of balkanism. While Serbia reinvented the Kosovo myth as the historical proof of its ties to Europe, Kosovo Albanians (the majority of whom follow the Islamic faith) reiterated the myth of Balkan indigeneity, or the national myth about Illyrian descent.

Further to this they positioned themselves as victims of Slavic occupiers – the non-Slavic people imprisoned in South Slavic States (that is, Yugoslavia, Serbia). This enabled them to create effective political strategies that eventually also led to secession and the formation of the independent state. Especially efficacious in this process were the nonviolent methods of civil disobedience Kosovo Albanians implemented under the leadership of Ibrahim Rugova (1944–2006). Their ten-year, nonviolent campaign, which took place during most of Slobodan Milošević's reign, gained them respect and sympathy internationally, paving diplomatic paths for achieving secessionist political goals. Muslims in Bosnia found themselves in the ambivalent situation of having to simultaneously confirm and denounce their own balkanism. Geographically closer to the European 'centre' (than Serbs, Montenegrins and Macedonians) and yet culturally (via religion) connected with the Islamic 'orient', their main hope lay in contrasting their unique culture against the barbaric Serbs (and occasionally even Croats) – for which Serbs provided plenty of empirical evidence. Their somewhat closer (but also highly ambivalent) ties to Croatians were partially connected with what Muhamed Filipović terms 'tutorial, patronage relationship towards Muslims and Islam ... into the national corpus of Croatian people' (quoted in Bakić-Hayden 1995, p.927).

Due to the strength of the Kosovo myth and the 'defenders of European civilisation' narrative, Serbian attitudes towards Bosniaks (Bosnian Muslims) were more negative. Often pejoratively called 'the Turks', they have most commonly been perceived by Serbs as 'traitors ... converts ... whose weakness and opportunism deprived them of the religious and cultural identity bequeathed to them by their forefathers in Kosovo' (1995). Lastly, all these groups could position themselves as higher than the true 'untouchables' of Yugoslavia, 'Gypsies' or Roma people. If all else failed, victimised and voiceless, Roma people could always be used as a reference point denoting the superiority of other, more 'European' ethnicities. Another shared characteristic within the region of the former Yugoslavia has been the internalisation of balkanism in discourses that demanded 'no generation in the

Balkans could live their whole lives without experiencing war at least once', that war is somehow entrenched in 'our hotter blood and temperament', or that '*all* previous transitions between different systems of government were violent'. Even though none of those statements is empirically true (has anybody actually measured the difference in blood temperature between various European people?), nonetheless, this internalised balkanism has proved popular and resilient. Most importantly it created cycles of self-fulfilling prophecies wherein these discourses finally found validation in reality.

After these narratives of 'nesting orientalisms' (Bakić-Hayden 1995) collided in the wars in Slovenia, Croatia and Bosnia and later Serbia and Montenegro, Europe's lack of enthusiasm to provide unequivocal support for the 'defenders of its civilisation' confused Serbian nationalists. To explain what was perceived as unequivocal support by western European nations towards Slovenia and Croatia, narratives stressing divisions between Catholic-Protestant and Eastern Orthodox European Christians were evoked in Serbia. Due to the promotion of these narratives, after a while large sections of the Serbian population started to believe that salvation from the (real and perceived) injustices committed by their immediate neighbours was no longer coming from western Europe but from their Eastern-Orthodox ally, Russia. True to the CGT syndrome, the rumour went around that conflicts over the former Yugoslav territory *have always* caused world wars, and large sections of the population expected Russian involvement against NATO, which was, apparently, to trigger yet another larger European war. Milošević's regime waited for nearly three months while NATO bombed Serbia and Montenegro, but the Slavic brothers did not come to the rescue. The political leadership around Milošević was most likely truly surprised that neither the narrative of 'Europe's defenders' nor of 'eternal brotherhood with Russians' yielded the expected results. In the end, Milošević's regime proclaimed 'victory', a proclamation that most likely the regime itself – like the majority of the population – failed to believe in. To this day, Serbia is confused, even split down to the middle, in terms of which narrative to tap into when envisioning its desired future.

Slovenia, on the other hand, quickly benefited from positioning itself as part of Europe, the furthest northwest, the most economically developed and the least 'polluted' by the heritage of the Balkan and balkanism. Given that Slovenia was ethnically the most homogeneous Yugoslav republic (population around 90 per cent Slovene at the time), and unburdened by 'other inferior people', it was relatively free to go. The Yugoslav army threw a tantrum, possibly more out of a habit of repressing dissent rather than out of attachment to Slovenia itself. The Yugoslav army command's closest ties were with Belgrade, which had no claims to parts of Slovenian territory. One of the rare quick wars took place, of low duration (ten days) and intensity. Still, around 60 people were killed and more than 300 wounded.

Another legacy of this war was the further disintegration of the Yugoslav army, Yugoslav communist party and the Yugoslav state. Slovenes and Croats left all these institutions, even though at the time the president of the rotating Yugoslav presidency (Stjepan Mesić) as well as the prime minister (Ante Marković) were of Croatian descent. Mesić's alleged statement that he would be 'the last president of Yugoslavia' was widely circulated in Serbia. The motion by then Yugoslav president Borisav Jović (from Serbia) to block Mesić's becoming a new president based on constitutional automatic rotation rule was not circulated at all. Neither was Jović's discussion with the Yugoslav defence minister-commander of the Yugoslav army (1988–92) Veljko Kadijević and President of Serbia Slobodan Milošević (1989–97) about the redrawing of boundaries after Slovenia's and Croatia's secession. The public was never to hear that the military option was proposed to both quench opposition to Milošević's rule within Serbia as well as to 'push out' Slovenes and Croats while retaining sections of Croatian territory wherein Serbian people were in a majority. The careful choosing of narratives also did not include reports on Milošević's meeting with Croatian president Franjo Tuđman in which they agreed to divide Bosnian territory between Serbia and Croatia (the Karađorđevo agreement, 1991).

Instead of transparency about political processes and the competing visions for the future by multitude of players and actors, the Yugoslav public was pulled between the trinity of CGT syndrome for the multiplicity of particular needs or issues. Packaging and repackaging of narratives became a full-time occupation for government officials, and for the intellectuals and journalists who were close to regimes. Underlying narratives of 'belonging', 'victimhood', 'rightful place', and so on, were always present, albeit in different guises. It was not uncommon that a new narrative was formed almost overnight, even if it was contradictory to the previous one (that is, retention of Yugoslavia versus creation of ethnic nation-state, or alliance with Europe versus alliance with Russia). Relentlessly promoted, the old–new narrative would almost completely obliterate the previous one. This testifies that despite the eurocentric cliché, 'according to which people in the Balkans have this very long memory, [that] they never learn anything new, they never forget anything old', the reality of the ground confirmed that, on the contrary, 'the Balkans, if anything, is the area where people forget extremely quickly, extremely fast' (Žižek 1999).

This last sentence may represent reverse essentialising (even though I actually agree with Žižek's point here) because, like in any other geographical place, in the Balkans some people have longer, and others shorter, memories. Most often people identify with narratives that they receive in families, schools, from governments, or through media and other cultural means (for example, literature) and then filter (remember or forget) new information through those narratives. Underlying cognitive frames, paradigms or worldviews play a critical role in this process. Europe–Balkan dualism, long present as a method of ascertaining superior/inferior or lesser people, was an archetypal narrative that experienced its logical consequence during the Yugoslav wars of the 1990s. The choice of narratives is important because 'even if something is a purely manipulative ideological invention, nonetheless it produces certain material effects' (1999). In other words, the imaginations of superior/lesser people, coupled with a nationalistic imagination of homogenous communities, facilitated a process that produced 'real victims' (Hayden 1996, p.783). Killings, tortures, wounding and abuse of real people followed, with the well-publicised 'summit' of genocidal ethnic cleansing.

Within this process of ethnic cleansing one group disappeared with the most ferocity and velocity – the 'Yugoslavs'. Imaginations of allegedly primordial, homogenous and 'pure' communities made the existing heterogeneous, intertwined, intermingled and diverse multicultural Yugoslav community unimaginable (Hayden 1996, p.783). Especially in the areas where the mixing of people (with the exception of Vojvodina) was high, 'where the intermingling of the populations was most complete ... forced unmixing of peoples' (1996, p.790) took place. In the end it was the multicultural Yugoslav community that had existed in real life in many parts of the country that became first part of the lesser and then 'nonexistent' people. Where the mixing was greatest, where boundaries between people were the most blurred, as they represented a 'living disproof of the nationalist ideologies' (1996), the violence had to be at its most ferocious:

> To reverse Benedict Anderson's evocative phrase (1983), the disintegration of Yugoslavia into its warring components in 1991–2 marked the failure of the imagination of a Yugoslav community. This failure of the imagination, however, had real and tragic consequences: the Yugoslav community that could not be maintained, and thus has become unimaginable, had actually existed in many parts of the country ... In a political situation premised on the incompatibility of its components, these mixed territories were both anomalous and threatening ... For this reasons, the mixed regions could not be permitted to survive as such, and their populations, which were mixing voluntarily, had to be separated militarily (1996, p.788).

'We', the lesser people of thriving inter-ethnic collaborations, have been successfully obliterated and ethnically cleansed but not even one monument marking this tragedy has been erected. It is as if the shame of unnatural coupling should best be forgotten as soon as possible. Even a memory of those interminglings of people is to disappear for fear of being accused of futile, perhaps damaging, nostalgia at best. And, at worst, of being seen as a potential threat to a newly established order or even evidence of possession of a psychiatric condition. For Yugoslavs, myself and others, there is no return home, a return that is perhaps possible to the other communities ethnically cleansed during wars of the 1990s. As argued by, among others, Olivera Simić, this return of Yugoslav refugees is not possible because home has been completely swallowed by the flames of war:

> I was born in a country that exists no more. I speak a language that exists no more. I did not lose a close family member, but like many Yugoslav people, I lost so much. The beginning of the war in my country meant the end of my physical belonging to the country I was born and grew up in, the country I loved, the country I left and abandoned. I tried to move on, to forget destruction and war, to run away from it all. But, the further I was from home, home was closer to me, to my heart, to my mind. The smell, the sound, the sky and the sun of my home haunt me. They are always with me. I carry them in my smile and in my sorrow. And I know I am not the only one (Simić 2011, p.248).

The disappearance of the Yugoslavs as a national minority, as a consequence of the wars of the 1990s, is only partially due to balkanism. In fact, the continuation of these multiethnic, multicultural Yugoslav identities was made impossible by the long-standing historical processes of 'Europeanisation' – denoting homogenising into nation-states prior to potentially entering larger unions. As these processes are not limited to Europe or its lesser cousin the Balkans, a better term for them is 'state ethnicisation'. Ethnicisation here is understood as 'a dialectical process by which meaning is attributed to socio-cultural signifiers of human beings, as a result of which individuals may be assigned to a general category of persons which reproduces itself biologically, culturally and economically' (Miles & Brown 2003, p.99). Ethnicisation occurs within states, across states and even globally, so it is important to stress that state ethnicisation denotes efforts to homogenise within the territory of a (new or old) state, impacting on all its instruments as well as on the overall mindset within it. State ethnicisation therefore stands in direct opposition to efforts to envision particular states as multiethnic, multicultural, intercultural or diverse.

While state ethnicisation has also been a reaction to the imperialism and colonialism of previous eras and is in itself perhaps 'positive' in reinforcing local identities, it is simultaneously an antithesis of more global and universal notions of human identity, as, for example, proposed during the European Enlightenment period. Such antithesis is, by and large, detrimental to the maintenance and continuation of peace for two reasons. First, state ethnicisation goes against the voluntary mixing of people, as its primary goal is to maintain 'pure' boundaries. In that sense, state ethnicisation goes against empirical reality and human history marked by the constant movement of people. Arresting these movements is then only possible through more or less violent measures. And second, the narrow frameworks of ethnically pure states will always make sections of its population somehow 'inferior'. This is a particular form of violence, wherein inferior peoples are constructed as having lesser quality and thus being ontologically of a lesser value. Such demarcations and rankings of people make perfect sense within nationalistic, imperialist and militaristic discourses. However, these practices are in direct opposition to building positive and more lasting peace. Consequently, if positive and lasting peace is a goal, practices of homogenising ethnicities within nation-states go directly against it. Instead, more inclusive identity markers within states – perceived not as bearers of nationhood but as bearers of citizenship; that is, in their purely administrative function – are needed.

Understanding processes in the former Yugoslavia through these (state ethnicisation) notions rather than through lenses of balkanism is important. Minor differences in interpretation count. For example, in the 1990s both Croatia and Serbia wished to retain their territories where other ethnic minorities (Serbs in the former, Kosovo Albanians in the latter case) lived, minus these ethnic minorities. Serbia also wished to broaden its administrative territory to include 'their' people living within administrative territories of Croatia and Bosnia. Unlike the previous two republics that interpreted the Yugoslav constitution's allowance for 'selfdetermination' of people to mean the self-determination of republics, the Serbian regime interpreted this clause to mean the self-determination of the 'constitutive people' who created Yugoslavia. This minor difference in interpretation influenced the processes that resulted in several hundred thousand deaths, millions of individual displacements and migrations, economic collapse, environmental destruction, massive mental health costs, an increase in ethno-nationalism and chauvinism, and even the increase in local fascism.

Likewise, whether the former Yugoslav peoples were seen as rational, political actors or irrational 'Balkans people' influenced the type of strategies used to address past violence in the region. The consequences of this minor difference in political imagination were also many. It was crucially important when in the eternal battle between the civilised and the barbaric (some time post Cold War) that the category of Eastern Europe and communism was replaced by the notion of inferior, dangerous Balkans. True to other European traditions, that is, of militarism, the barbaric other was seen to be in a need of strategic discipline. In the new post-Cold War climate, 'post-communist societies have been roundly represented as "younger" siblings of the West' and nowhere was this more pronounced than 'during the secessionist and political conflicts in the post-multicultural society of the former Yugoslavia during the 1990s' (Murawska-Muthesius 2006, p.305). As 'the notion of political immaturity and moral baseness had been fixed and historicized as an essential feature of the Balkans, and the legacy of both Ottoman and Byzantine absolutisms' (2006), disciplinary interventions by the civilised were apparently required.

Once again, deep cultural stories of superior and lesser people manifested behind the mask of rational and political decision-making processes. But behind this alleged rationality an unconscious fear existed: that unless the Balkan is 'disowned', the discourse of 'democratic' and 'developed' states of Europe no longer fighting each other post Second World War would have been weakened. Perhaps if a narrative similar to the one of democratic and developed states not fighting each other could have equally been invented for the territory of both the former Yugoslavia as well as the Balkans, this too would have become a self-fulfilling prophecy. Such an invention does not have to gather inspiration from the realm of fantasy because it can easily gather information from the realm of empirical reality. For example, a narrative highlighting the duration of *actual peaceful cohabitation* of the multitude of ethnic players in the Balkans, as well as within the former Yugoslavia, could have been offered. Not only would this narrative have been more accurate, more in line with the historical and empirical realities of the region, it could have provided strong support for maintaining peace. Stressing the long periods of history within which Balkan people have collaborated, unified, created treaties, cooperated and above all lived peacefully together would have significantly undermined narratives of primordialism and perennialism of the 'Balkan conflict'. Sadly, within the context of a highly militarised continent these alternative narratives would have redirected attention away from bellicose and militarised politics; another reason why, to slightly paraphrase Hermann Keyserling, if 'the Balkans did not exist it would have to be invented' (quoted in Todorova 1997, p.133).

Alternative, peace-promoting narratives would have also dramatically disturbed the, often unconscious, beliefs about the superiority/inferiority of European (and the world's) peoples. This would have prevented the 'civilised' from justifying their own violence while simultaneously denouncing the violence of others. And, perhaps, it would have prevented Western democracies from justifying their alleged superiority of culture, civilisation and even violence. As pointed out by Jan Oberg in response to 'human-rights' based interventions at the turn of the century:

> When democracies fight wars and make interventions they legitimate it with reference to highly civilized norms such as peace, human rights, minority protection, democracy or freedom – and they do it as a sacrifice, not out of fear. In contrast, 'the others' start wars for lower

> motives such as money, territory, power, drugs, personal gain, because they have less education, less civil society, less democracy and are intolerant, lack humanity or are downright evil (Oberg 2001).

Whatever the reasons behind the de-politicised 'militaristic humanism' of the 1990s (Beck 2006, p.127), in which violence was again justified on the grounds of higher civilised goals (in this instance, of 'universal human rights'), in the case of former Yugoslavia it was ultimately the deep story of balkanism that made such humanism possible. As well, it was the internalised balkanism that influenced the detrimental behaviours of a number of Balkan and non-Balkan (former) Yugoslav peoples and their governments. Avoiding the discourse of balkanism, in all its forms and guises, in the future thus remains crucial for avoiding further violence in the region. Coupled with alternative narratives that put forward the 'radical' proposition of all people being of equal value and narratives that highlight the Balkan's peaceful histories and presents such discursive practices remain the best guarantors of the region's peaceful futures.

In: Zora

By the time 'Clinton's war' came, or when in 1999 NATO conducted a three-month-long bombing campaign on much of the territory of Serbia and Montenegro, my paternal grandmother Zora was in her mid eighties. She did not care much about Clinton nor 'his war' – 'I heard the bombs and the explosions, of course'. She would sit on her sofa bed, the same one she'd been sitting on for over 60 years, and listen. 'Sometimes the explosion was to the right, sometimes to the left ... If they were to drop the bomb on my house, why would I care? ... I've been ripe for many years now, it's about time.'

My grandmother's fondness for nature-based and agricultural metaphors – even when on the subject of her own death – was inspired by her early life experiences. Born the year the First World War broke out in most of Europe, she felt safe and secure while growing up on a rural property attached to the town of Trstenik. Her father, Lesa Pavlović, was a wealthy farmer who managed that rural property as well as acres of land located on the rich soil of the West Morava River. The early years spent in Trstenik were my grandmother's utopia; all that came later was a fall from this paradise. Until her death in 2010 Zora was never to erase Trstenik as her image of a perfect place; and the life she lived there as the only sensible way to live.

A true image of Arcadia, Trstenik is the epitome of Arcadian mythic space – described/promoted by the ancient Greeks, Renaissance humanists and today's various (that is, ecological, New-Age and antiglobalisation) movements, wherein 'nature is bountiful but humans do not indulge themselves beyond their needs' (Hollis 1998, p.14). Gently sloping hills, rich vegetation, beautiful trees, luscious grape vines and succulent raspberry patches during the season, coloured with the richness of roses, petunias and geraniums planted by the houses with their white walls and terracotta roof tiles was, for Zora or her selective remembering, never to be replaced or surpassed by any other beauty, of any other human settlement. The industrial and economic development the town of Trstenik experienced throughout the twentieth century brought ruin to my grandmother's utopia. 'Once they put the factory in,' she said, 'they destroyed the whole lot.' Her father, Lesa, sensing the end of agriculture and the rise of industry, arranged her marriage to Staša and move 'into the town' in 1933.

Upon marriage Zora moved to Kruševac, where numerous reminders of Serbian CGT remain concreted in the geography of the town. The monument in the centre of Kruševac – where my grandfather owned a store before the communist system took it away from him – would always remind them of the losses their people suffered during 'centuries lasting fights for freedom' (Politika 2008). Furthermore, their house in Balšićeva Street is but 200 metres from the ruined walls of the Serbian medieval fortification of 'Tsar' Lazar's compound. The church within that compound, and in which they baptised my father, is claimed to be the one that offered a spiritual ceremony to Lazar and his soldiers prior to their departure for Kosovo Polje in 1389.

The personal stories my grandmother Zora listened to throughout her life were of her own people's suffering. She and Staša had numerous relatives killed in the first and second Balkan wars that took place just before Zora was born (1912 and 1913 respectively), during the First World War (1914–18) when they were babies and children, and during the Second World War when they were in their prime (1941–45). The trauma from the Second World War was such that Zora spoke about it only in her nineties and only after being repeatedly asked about it by her nosy granddaughter. Her overall estimation was that there was no fairness nor logic nor meaning in that war, only horror upon horror that further damaged her perfect place: 'Somebody would like somebody's property and the next day that second person was gone,' allegedly on 'political' grounds. Her and Staša's nephews were murdered in revenge attacks by German soldiers: 'What were they, those young boys, guilty of?' One day they were their family and people's future, the next day they were no more. 'Let's not talk about it any longer.' Fifty years later the pain was still there.

The Second World War represented the single major threat to her life, to the lives of her children, husband, family, as well as being a major threat to her property, her land and her house, all of which she cared about deeply. She was not in the least bit interested in the political processes during the Second World War, which made her move, seek refuge, and find it, once again, in her ancestral land. Despite this obvious lack of political interest, my grandmother managed to change her citizenship during her 96 years of living no less than nine times. Even though her only permanent migration involved a journey of about 30 kilometres from Trstenik to Kruševac upon her marriage, she managed to live in ten officially different states: the Kingdom of Serbia (1882–1918); the Kingdom of Serbs, Croats and Slovenes (1918–29); the Kingdom of Yugoslavia (1929–41); *Militärverwaltung in Serbien* or Military Administration in Serbia, better known as Nedić's Serbia (1941–45); Democratic Federal Yugoslavia (established in 1943, officiated in 1945–46); the Federal People's Republic of Yugoslavia (1946–63); the Socialist Federal Republic of Yugoslavia (1963–92); the Federal Republic of Yugoslavia (1992–2003); Serbia and Montenegro (2003–06), and the Republic of Serbia (2006–). Fortunately, some of those transformations were nominal and administrative and thus not all of these nation-state creations were through wars and other acts of collective violence. Too many, however, were.

Out: Nation-states and nationalisms

The year my grandmother Zora was born, 19-year-old Gavrilo Princip, a proclaimed Yugoslav nationalist, became committed to the idea of killing and dying for one's own nation, one's own people. Had he known the chain of events the successful assassination he carried out on Franz Ferdinand, an heir to the Austro-Hungarian empire, in Sarajevo on 28 June 1914, was to trigger, perhaps he would have thought twice. But then again, when a 'narcissistic injury' gets projected onto the 'fictive kinship' (Barash & Webel 2002, p.125) of a larger group (such as a nation-state) and once a large group of us is perceived to be under threat from them, the narcissistic injury most commonly turns into a 'narcissistic rage', which then often 'involves an unrelenting compulsion to undo the hurt; in the pursuit of this vengeful "justice", great violence may be self-righteously employed' (2002). As further elaborated by Barash and Webel:

> ...when the individual associates himself or herself with a larger group, especially with the nation-state, slights or injuries to the group are easy to perceive as injuries to one's self ... Many of the most destructive wars in the 20th century were perpetrated by people seeking to retake territory that had been wrested from them by others (e.g., the French yearning to recapture the provinces of Alsace and Lorraine from Germany, which was a major reason for World War I, or the Vietcong and North Vietnamese, who sought during the Vietnam War to reunite their country). Other wars have been instigated by ethnic groups seeking to secede from a central governmental authority, only to precipitate intervention by armed forces from the nation-state from which they

> hoped to disconnect (as in Nigeria, Ethiopia, Indonesia, the former Yugoslavia, and Russia) (2002, p.125).

But Gavrilo Princip had not heard of the psychoanalytic interpretation of his motives – nor was that even possible given that the explanations of narcissistic injury and rage were developed later in the twentieth century (by Sigmund Freud, Heinz Kohut and others) – and had thus persisted with the *obvious solution* to all the problems that plagued his people. Once the man who opposed the liberation of Bosnia and the unification of Yugoslav peoples was gone (even though this particular man was by most accounts a progressive reformist as far as the rights of minorities go) salvation of his own people would certainly be achieved. Salvation was, however, not to come the way he thought it would occur. In fact, the chain of events that his act triggered took millions of his own people into the various pits of dead-end nothingness.

The assassination of Prince Franz Ferdinand resulted in 'the ultimatum' presented by Austria-Hungary to Serbia and then the subsequent attack by the Austro-Hungarian Empire. While the 'Serbian army bravely defended the independence of its country and won a series of great victories' in the face of 'the overwhelming enemy forces of Germany, Austria-Hungary and Bulgaria, it [still] had to leave its national territory and withdraw across Albania' (Savković 1998, p.23). Then, 'having recuperated and regrouped, these same forces continued the war on the Salonika Front together with the other forces of the Entente which included France, England, Russia, Italy and the United States' (1998, pp.23–24). The result was that, in this war alone, Serbia lost 28 per cent of its total population (1,264,000 out of 4,529,000) and 58 per cent of the male population (1998, p.24). A further 1,700,000 Yugoslavs (10.8 per cent of the population) died during the Second World War (1998, p.30).

Were all these deaths necessary? Did projects of creating various nation-states demand it? In the eternal dilemma of peace versus freedom is violence really often necessary to achieve the latter? Is it true, as the mainstream discourse claims, that without it, *we* would not even exist as a political, cultural, perhaps even physical entity? Were worse tragedies, deaths and humiliations in this way prevented? And, most importantly, could the creation of various nation-states on the territory of the former Yugoslavia (and beyond) have occurred minus the violence?

'Nonkilling nations are not unthinkable' argues Glenn Paige (2009, p.54). As further support for this claim he provides a list of 27 countries without an army, 53 countries[4] that recognise conscientious objection to military service (including all six former Yugoslav republics – now independent states; that is, Bosnia-Herzegovina, Croatia, Serbia, Slovenia, Macedonia and Montenegro) and 93 countries without a death penalty (in addition to all former Yugoslav republics/new states, the list includes other Balkan countries such as Albania, Bulgaria, Greece and Romania – it may be worth mentioning that the newly independent but not universally recognised Republic of Kosovo also prohibits the death penalty in its 2008 constitution). Further, throughout history a number of nation-states have come into existence via negotiation and a nonviolent transition from previous political entities – most commonly cited examples include the dissolution of Czechoslovakia into the Czech Republic and Slovakia in 1989, and the dissolution of the Norway Sweden Union in 1905. Less commonly cited is the *peaceful* separation between two *Balkan* states in 2006 (Serbia and Montenegro) – this is perhaps due to the event being fairly recent. In any case, these examples convincingly show that violence is not *inherently* linked with either the coming into being nor subsequent maintenance of nation-states. Further, most international or interstate interactions are 'cooperative rather than competitive in nature' (Kelly 2010, p.100). Yet, at the same time, the development of nation-states has so far most often gone hand in hand with both violence and ethnic nationalism – 'a doctrine that sustains and legitimizes the modern notion of nationhood' (Mikula 2008, p.134).

There are currently around 2000 'nations' in the world today, estimates Johan Galtung (Galtung et al., 2002, p.126). Within these nations people share values, norms, culture, language, religion and territory. Within the current global system these nations are organised into 200 states, of which only about 10 per cent, or 20, of them are nation-states, 'inhabited by (almost only) one nation'. The other 180 are multinational countries but only one (Switzerland) of those 180 states has managed a symmetric cohabitation of nations residing within it. In all other 179 states there is one dominant nation, 'more equal than the others' (2002). In other words, even though '90 percent of states in the early twenty-first century are "constructed" and multinational, such as the United States or Brazil, and often multicultural as well ... most [also] have a dominant nationality group' (Kelly 2010, p.100). Rather than being purely administrative units, these nation-states and multinational countries usually engage in discursive practices by which some groups of people (that is, dominant national group) are served better than others (national minorities). In practice this manifests as discrimination against minority groups as far as the satisfaction of their basic needs is concerned. Sometimes that means that even their basic need for survival is jeopardised. Most often, however, discrimination against minorities impacts on the needs crucial for their good quality of life; that is, their overall wellbeing, identity and freedom needs may be endangered.

Nationalism generally goes hand in hand with the hierarchical 'ranking of people'. This ranking takes the form of ethnocentrism, 'the belief that one's own ethnic group is in some way superior to other groups' (Mikula 2008, p.64). In other words, and to paraphrase George Bernard Shaw, ethnocentrism (as well as nationalism and patriotism) signifies a belief that this group (nation, country) is superior to all others because one was born into it. Ethnocentrism therefore not only goes 'against the grain of the liberal worldview based on Enlightenment ideals, which attempts to downplay differences by appealing to a universal humanity', it is also dangerous because its concrete expressions often involve 'proselytizing, discrimination, hostility and violence' (2008).

Perhaps distinctions could be made between:

- 'ethnic' (common descent) and 'civic' (agreed principles and values) nationalisms
- nationalism and patriotism (a milder form simply denoting 'love of one's own country')
- 'benevolent' and 'extreme' nationalisms.

Nationalisms could be 'democratic, forward-looking, and generous' – Eugene Kamenka summarises the positive sides of nationalism, as well as the negatives, 'authoritarian, backward-looking, and chauvinist' (1993, p.85). Nationalism could also be 'secular or religious' and 'socialist or conservative' (1993). There are positive sides of 'benevolent nationalism' and ethnic solidarity, conclude Barash and Webel (2002, p.183) in their 'final note on nationalism and ethnocentrism'. The positive sides of nationalism may include transcending the parochialism of other divisions, such as religion, class, gender, and so on. By appealing to a sense of national identity, unity and community, and by including all within borders of this unity/community people could also be motivated to be less selfish and work for the common good. Nationalism can then 'sometimes':

> evoke compassion, love, and community pride and can even serve as a positive force for human cooperation and ecological awareness. Love of the land, the people, the culture, and the ecosystem can contribute to dignity, caring, altruism, and some of the finer emotions of which human beings are capable (2002, p.183).

However, Barash and Webel also contend that while nationalism can, 'in theory, be limited to one's nation in practice, however, it is often combined with antagonism toward other nations' (2002, p.160). Especially when nationalism is activated to support war efforts, attempts to calm bellicose attitudes, engage in rational debates and mobilise for peace commonly become extremely difficult, if not impossible. Therefore, 'one of the great challenges to students and practitioners of peace and conflict resolution is accordingly to channel the benevolent aspects of nationalism and ethnic solidarity while guarding against their horrors' (2002, p.183).

Whether this is where energies are best directed is far from certain. A number of theorists ask the question related to the *practice* of nationhood and the nation 'as a practical category, as classificatory scheme, as cognitive frame' (Brubaker 1996, p.16) rather than questions about its ontological 'isness'. 'We should not ask "what is a nation",' writes Brubaker but 'how is nationhood as a political and cultural form institutionalized within and among states?' (1996). This type of question moves away from understanding nations through the lenses of primordialism (nations as primeval and natural aspects of the human condition), perennialism (nations eternal existence throughout the history), and even ethnosymbolism (focuses on the expression of symbols, myths, traditions and values within pre-modern ethnic communities) (Mikula 2008, p.135) and towards a socio-constructionist perspective. Homi Bhabha, for example, argues that 'nations are imaginary constructs that depend for their existence on an apparatus of cultural fictions' (1994, p.49). Nation is therefore 'constituted through narration, which entails the conversion of a particular territorial space into a place of historical experience' (Mikula 2008, pp.135–36). The best-known proponent of the socioconstructionist perspective, Benedict Anderson, famously proposed 'the following definition of the nation':

> it is an imagined political community – and imagined as both inherently limited and sovereign. It is *imagined* because the members of even the smallest nation will never know most of their fellow-members, meet them, or even hear of them, yet in the minds of each lives the image of their communion.... [As Gellner writes]

> "Nationalism is not the awakening of nations to self-consciousness: it *invents* nations where they do not exist" (Anderson 1991, pp.5–7).

Further, the nation is always imagined as *limited* because:

> even the largest of them, encompassing perhaps a billion living human beings, has finite, if elastic, boundaries, beyond which lie other nations. No nation imagines itself coterminous with mankind. The most messianic nationalists do not dream of a day when all the members of the human race will join their nation in the way that it was possible, in certain epochs, for, say, Christians to dream of a wholly Christian planet (1991).

It is also imagined as *sovereign* because:

> the concept was born in an age in which Enlightenment and Revolution [of the 18th and 19th centuries] were destroying the legitimacy of the divinely-ordained, hierarchical dynastic realm. Coming to maturity at a stage of human history when even the most devout adherents of any universal religion were inescapably confronted with the living *pluralism* of such religions, and the allomorphism between each faith's ontological claims and territorial stretch, nations dream of being free, and, if under God, directly so. The gage and emblem of this freedom is the sovereign state (1991).

And, finally, nation is imagined as a *community,* because:

> regardless of the actual inequality and exploitation that may prevail in each, the nation is always conceived as a deep, horizontal comradeship. Ultimately it is this fraternity that makes it possible, over the past two centuries, for so many millions of people, not so much to kill, as willingly to die for such limited imaginings (1991).

Anderson's brilliant analysis suggests that violence is not an unexpected or accidental result that comes from the way nations are commonly imagined and conceptualised. Bhabha reminds us that 'national culture is not unitary, but rather, ambivalent and disruptive' (Mikula 2008, p.135). In practice, this ambivalence and disruption is most often seen – by nationalists – as a threat to the common, national identity. Within the nationalistic discourse, differences (ideological, political) within their ethnic states are rarely perceived as something positive or even neutral. The likelihood for them to use accusatory labels such as traitors, fifth columnists and foreign conspirators – against other nation-state citizens 'not sufficiently loyal' that they perceive as such – is therefore always on the horizon. Especially during times of violence and conflict (with others), dissent within nation-state is discouraged, often ferociously and violently. As the governments of both nation and multinational states attach and indeed are expected to 'attach priority to the interests of [their] own state, even if its policies are damaging to other nation-states' (Kelly 2010, p.101) this prepares fertile ground for interstate conflict. As these governments, even democratically elected ones, attach and are expected to attach higher value to the interest of the dominant social group (most often dominant by ethnicity, but also by gender, race, class, and so on), minority viewpoints and groups are more commonly excluded or pseudo included (that is, tokenism, marginalisation via invisibility, etc.). In practice nations are conceptualised even more by whom they exclude than whom they include, which means that the very category assumes exclusionary practices.

This imbalance/exclusion most often goes hand in hand with the existence of structural, cultural and epistemic violence that is, in turn, common precondition for the explicit, unmediated use of direct violence. 'Born in iniquity and conceived in sin, the spirit of nationalism has never ceased to bend human institutions to the service of dissension and distress,' Thorstein Veblen (2009, p.38) wrote powerfully nearly a hundred years ago. The material effects of nationalism are, he continued, both 'sinister and imbecile' wherein the 'national mob-mind' mentality of vanity, fear, contempt, and servility' continues to design the 'loyal citizen' (2009). Nationalism, which is above all, 'a state of mind, in which the supreme loyalty of the individual is felt to be due the nation-state' (Kohn quoted in Farnen, 2004, p.45) has thus been linked 'conceptually and empirically to militarism ... ethnocentrism, dogmatism, stereotyping, and lack of cosmopolitan views' (2004, p.57). There is no shortage of theorists who have expressed negative views towards nationalism. Nationalism is a 'great menace' and an 'epidemic of evil' wrote Tagore (1916, p.9). For George Orwell nationalism has been 'inseparable from the desire for power', or, in other words it is about 'power-hunger tempered by self-deception' (Orwell & Angus 1968, pp.362–63). For Eric Fromm nationalism 'is our form of incest, is our idolatry, is our insanity' with 'patriotism' as its cult (1955, p.58). Even in milder forms, patriotism sets up a moral hierarchy' and threatens the peaceful alternatives of egalitarianism, universalism and cosmopolitanism. Any person aiming to lead a moral life must thus abandon it, was Tolstoy's conclusion (Nathanson 1993, p.8). Albert Einstein called nationalism 'an infantile disease' or 'the measles of mankind' (1993, p.187). William Ralph Inge defined a nation as a 'society united by a delusion about its ancestry and by a common hatred of its neighbours' (1949, p.127). Yet another link between nationalism and violence has been proposed by Norman Angell:

> The root of the problem is very simply stated: if there were no sovereign independent states, if the states of the civilized world were organized in some sort of federalism, as the states of the American Union, for instance, are organized, there would be no international war as we know it ...

> The main obstacle is nationalism (quoted in Chitkara 1998, p.79).

Despite this intense critique nationalism remains the 'omnipresent thought in politics, in the minds of ordinary people, politicians and observers in politics, and in international relations' (Harris 2009, p. vi). The current practices of nationalism and ethnocentrism also remain a major reason for violent interstate and interethnic conflict. Imagined ethnic communities too often break up 'actually existing communities' (Hayden 1996, p.793) and create 'real victims'. The mechanism of *how* this is done is brilliantly summarised by Goering's often-quoted explanation at the Nuremberg trials. Whether nation-states such as Russia, England or Germany, whether:

> a democracy, or fascist dictatorship, or a parliament or a communist dictatorship, the people could always be brought to the bidding of the leaders [and into the war] ... All you have to do is tell them they are being attacked and denounce the pacifists for lack of patriotism and exposing the country to danger. It works the same in any country (quoted in Pilgrim 1992, pp.114–15).

This statement was widely circulated via digital social media at the beginning of 'the war on terror', however, the majority of United States and other Western nation-state citizens bought into the bellicose post-September 11 propaganda, at least in the initial stages (see Gallup 2003, p.69; Gareau 2004, p.205; Kashmeri 2007, p.35; Kinder & Kam 2009, p.77).

The role of manipulative elites, who 'act to construct extreme and polarizing identities that are used to consolidate their power and, in the course, to justify the dehumanization and destruction of specific target groups' (Jenkins 2010, p.96) notwithstanding, the process described by Goering is usually enthusiastically embraced, even actively constructed, by the majority (within a dominant national-ethnic group). As this construction is about a particular practice – not essence – it is possible to identify common routes along which the process takes place. In other words, engendering violence via collective participation in practices of denial, marginalisation and justification – within the narratives of nationalism and ethnocentrism – most often follows eight basic steps. This *collective violence pedagogy* seems to be a commonly and easily applied recipe by which nationalisms bring about violence. My own observations in a number of nation-states within which I have resided are that these eight basic steps could be described and summarised as follows:

- Step one: creation-solidification of the category of 'the other' (even if that other was until recently part of 'us').
- Step two: differences (that is, along ethnic, religious or ideological lines) between 'one' and the

'other' are potentiated and similarities are minimised or obliterated.

- Step three: the attribute of 'the lesser' is attached to the other, who has also been construed commonly as 'weird', 'wrong', 'evil' and even 'subhuman'; that is, everything not liked about the self is projected onto the other.
- Step four: a sense of threat of 'them' coming after us is created; the other is constructed as nothing but 'dangerous' – the derogatory images of potential (or long-standing) 'enemy/enemies' are also almost exclusively used.
- Step five: social militarism dominates; heroic fighting and sacrifice for ones' own people/land, is *glorified* – historical discourses are devised with the emphasis placed on data that shows why liberation is necessary and why only the use of weapons will 'work'.
- Step six: active prosecution of opinions/ideologies that are trying to *resist* the above processes (one to five) among 'our own' (ethnic, religious, ideological) group – some useful phrases (depending on the society) include 'traitors', 'enemy collaborators', 'servants of foreign intelligence agencies', 'pacifists empower terrorism', 'pacifism is objectively pro-Fascist', 'the venal pacifism of the politically correct has been shown for the profitable cowardice it has always been', 'bleeding hearts/flowerpicking peace mongers', and the like.

- Step seven: when confronted with our own violent deeds, these are *denied* or *justified;* for example, the harsh facts are met with insistence on us (always) being right and them (always and totally) being wrong – there are many justifications for the violence that can be used and the most potent and powerful ones have so far included 'others are also doing it' and 'it's a war'; numerous other useful phrases are 'they (she/he) deserved it', 'God/morality/justice is on our side', 'in the name of the freedom, democracy', 'sometimes you have to sacrifice the lives of few for the benefit of many', 'they are even worse', 'they are the ones that are evil/demons/devil's advocates/satans', 'they would do (did) the same to us' and (my favourite) 'boys will be boys'.
- Step eight: the whole process is repeated.

The steps have also been used independently, although the whole process is the most potent (and poisonous) when utilised as a package. It is also helpful, and very important, *not* to focus on the future, as this is where more creative nonviolent solutions could be invented. Better to focus on the past, and engage in selective remembering and biased interpreting of all the instances of previous violence between the groups involved.

While more 'universal', this process has been followed to the letter on the territory of the former Yugoslavia and has been liberally used within a number of

Western nations that have been waging war 'against terror' (outside and within their own territories, as per Huntington's *Clash of Civilisations* proposal). Going back to the former case study, the package was extensively utilised, both within the former Yugoslav more multicultural nation-state, as well as within the ethnic nation-state that preceded and succeeded this political-cultural entity. Further, another specific internal nationalistic logic was developed during the collapse of the former Yugoslavia in order to justify territorial claims. This too is perhaps a more universal process that, like the above-described collective violence pedagogy, needs to be resisted if more lasting peace between different people is to result. David C. Pugh summarised this process eloquently in terms of the 'seven rules of nationalism':

- If an area was ours for 500 years and yours for 50 years, it should belong to us – you are merely occupiers.
- If an area was yours for 500 years and ours for 50 years, it should belong to us – borders must not be changed.
- If an area belonged to us 500 years ago but never since then, it should belong to us – it is the Cradle of our Nation.
- If a majority of our people live there, it must belong to us – they must enjoy the right of self-determination.

- If a minority of our people live there, it must belong to us – they must be protected against your oppression.
- All the above rules apply to us but not to you.
- Our dream of greatness is Historical Necessity, yours is Fascism (quoted in Biro 2011, pp.294–95).

The two 'recipes' or processes have been prescriptions for the wholescale disasters that have repeatedly plagued Yugoslav peoples, the Balkans, Europe and the world. The imagined nation-state communities have too often unleashed unimaginable and unspeakable horrors that were avoidable, unnecessary and most often counter-productive. Collective group delusions, fears, narcissistic injury and rage, exclusionary practices, ethnocentrism, competitive sentiments and arrangements, discourses of superiority/inferiority, and so on, while perhaps not inherently linked to nation-states are still most often *practised* within them. Nationalisms, of all kinds, have been notorious for fuelling interstate and intrastate grievances and conflicts, including 'mildly' or 'extremely' violent ones. The imposition of nationalistic worldviews and aspects of culture is so often used to justify direct and structural violence that it is hard to support the view by which nationalism could be viewed as potentially 'benevolent'. Further, the practice of nationalism actively works against and prevents practising of the other, more promising alternative.

One day, perhaps, the alternative of 'the highest form of patriotism' being defined not by the 'boundaries of one's country', but by a 'duty to humankind' (Strauss 1918, p.390) will become the dominant social discourse globally. One day, states may become purely administrative units, without being attached to harmful imaginings of nationalism and ethno-centrism. One day, the recognition of a nation-state as a purely imagined, socially constructed rather than 'real', perennial and 'ahistorical' community, may motivate citizens of civic nation-states to carefully craft those imaginings to promote peace rather than violence. Whether this will materialise largely depends on the strength with which the *real global community* perceives nationalism as neither inevitable nor desirable. It also depends on the strength with which this real global community puts into operation a whole range of alternative discourses that imagine various unification processes, focus on similarities among differences, and devise strategies for satisfying the basic human needs of all Earth's inhabitants.

All of us have indeed inherited certain histories. Most of those, as well as our presents, are the results of human-made political and cultural processes. Given that they are human-made they could be human-remade now and in the future, irrespective of how long these historical practices have lasted. Even those longest-lasting structures–processes are neither eternal nor natural but only as strong as the belief in their eternal–natural quality. In other words, the previous practices of militarism, othering, ethnocentrism, imperialism, and nationalism, frequently utilised within inter-group and intra-group interactions, eventually became embedded in the social structures of nation-states. These structures appear more solid than the practices–behaviours that created them in the first place, but in effect, these structures still rely on the same practices to survive. They are maintained by constant efforts to keep them as they 'are' or by efforts to enforce their 'essence'. So to undo these violent social structures – of militarism, imperialism and nationalism – different discursive practices, such as, for example, of globalism, interculturalism, humanism, neohumanism or social inclusion, are needed. In other words, militarism, imperialism and nationalism are only as real as the frequency and intensity of actions and discourses manifested by their enthusiastic promoters, and rely on the inaction of detached bystanders. Alternatively, the power of militarism, imperialism and nationalism is weakened by the number and the enthusiasm of those who ignore it, choose not to participate in it, critique it, and engage in different ways of being and thinking. Despite its promoters' desire to convince about the inevitability of 'the holy trinity of militarism, imperialism and nationalism', alternatives to these systems and worldviews already exist and have always existed parallel to them. Enhancing those alternative peace-promoting discourses, instead of enhancing nationalism, is not only realistically possible but also infinitely preferable. All that prevents us from doing so, to paraphrase Benedict Anderson, are our own limited imaginings.

CHAPTER 3

Feminism, eutopia: Challenging patriarchy and androcratic masculinities

> Only a different vision, different values, a change in power relationships, and a change in the social construction of [gender] identities – to be grounded no longer in dominance and submission but in harmonized acceptance of differences – can bring about harmony and a future of life and hope, instead of wars and nuclear holocaust (Accad 2000, p.1,987).

In: Persa and Nega

One autumn day in 1943 soldiers came looking for Nega Pavlović's 50-year-old husband, Lesa, to either arrest him or conscript him to fight for some cause. After two years of various armies passing through their village of Trstenik in Serbia, it was hard for Nega to know which of the two possibilities was the case. The treatment she received at the hands or, more truthfully, at the boots of an enraged soldier who could not complete his task gave her a clue. The attack occurred quickly and sharply, as well as unexpectedly.

The whole event deeply disturbed my then nine-year-old father, who witnessed this treatment of his grandmother. After his father had been arrested and sent by the occupying army of the Third Reich to a work camp, his mother had taken him and two other children to the safety of her family. Back in the village of Trstenik, on his mother's ancestral land, my father felt content and safe. But even Trstenik could not protect them from occasional visitations by various fighters' squads and brigades.

Decades later my father still remembered the man and his boots, his slightly built grandmother being pushed onto the ground, the kicks to her stomach and head and the screams to which both she and the man gave voice. Finally, after one of the soldier's mates exclaimed, 'Stop it, you are about to kill her!' Nega was left lying on the ground, bleeding and unconscious. Only after the men were gone could the family come to her aid.

When men came again several weeks later, Nega was still recovering. This time, though, Lesa was on the property. 'Where are you taking him?' demanded Lesa's elderly mother, Persa. By the look on their faces and the silence she understood. The same day 75-year-old Persa decided to look for her son. The whole family, fearing further reprisals, tried to dissuade her. 'He did nothing so he will be back,' many kept saying over and over, perhaps less to convince than to reassure. But Persa had already seen seven other men close to her taken, not 'having done anything'. She lost one of her brothers and four first cousins in the first and second Balkan wars of 1912 and 1913, and she lost another brother as well as her husband in the First World War. She was not going to lose her only son, her own blood, in this one.

The sight of a 75-year-old woman approaching them must have been surreal to the group of dishevelled, smoking and drinking men. None of them moved or said anything, but Persa was not silent. After exchanging the formal greeting *'Pomoz Bog'* ('God helps/May God be with you'), she stated her business. She was there to collect her 52-year-old son. He had responsibilities, extended family and property to take care of. The men looked at each other in astonishment and then at the ground. 'Go home, mother,' one finally said, 'this place is not for women.' But Persa continued to stand in front of them. Eventually, one man stepped away from the group and pulled her to the side, 'Mother, these are bigger things than you or I.'

Persa recognised him, a man from her village whom she had fed when he was a child, more than once, during family visits. She also took care of a wound on his leg once, when he fell out of a tree. She knew his parents and grandparents, and his relatives that had perished in the Balkan wars and the First World War along with her own. She took a deep breath, as if to take in all the spiritual power the fresh air could bring into her lungs, looked him in the eye and said, 'Tell me, is this what I have deserved? After all that has happened, is this how I am to be rewarded?' Then, she lowered her head, turned her back and started to walk away.

'Wait!' the man called her back. 'When the commander comes back I'll see what I can do.' Persa never saw the man again. Her son Lesa Pavlović, despite all of the odds, came back home the very next day.

Out: Mothers and soldiers

The action my great-great-grandmother Persa took on that day in 1943, the story told to me by her granddaughter and my grandmother Zora, was both an act that confirmed her traditional role within a patriarchal society and an act of transgression. As a mother, her role was to give and nurture life, create peace in her family and community, and support others. As both a mother and a woman, she was also expected to stay away from the 'bigger things' of war, violence and politics – considered to be male domains. Persa, on the other hand, entered the male domain of bigger things precisely because she saw it as an extension of her motherly role. She used a different type of power, that of a verbal, psychological and perhaps even spiritual type, to gain a specific outcome. In this particular instance, the power she used succeeded in being 'a force more powerful' (Ackerman & DuVall 2000) indeed.

Patriarchy – understood here as a social system of power and authority that is unevenly distributed between and among genders – has historically undermined both social and individual power exercised by those groups of people marked as 'women', or 'mothers'. In doing so, patriarchy has relied on all forms of violence – physical, structural, cultural, as well as psychological and epistemological. The difference between a man and a woman, wrote Hegel in 1851:

> is the same as that between animal and plant. The animal corresponds more closely to the character of the man, the plant to that of the woman. In woman there is a *more peaceful* unfolding of nature, a process, whose principle is the less clearly determined unity of feeling. If women were to control the government, the state would be in danger (Hegel 2008, p.87, italics added).

Similar examples of epistemological violence, based on essentialist discourse of biologism, abound in political theory and practice. From Sun Tzu's example of the militarisation of emperors' concubines in his *The Art of War* to Machiavelli's treatise on 'How a State is Ruined Because of Women', one theme remains central: 'the development of power begins by bringing the feminine under control by violence' (Goldstein 2001, pp.54–55). Coupled with narratives about the essential nature of female and male, the theme of power, gender and violence identified by Goldstein further supports the view of women as a universal/ahistorical life and pleasure-giving force versus men as soldiers/history creators:

> The true man wants two things: danger and play. For that reason he wants woman, as the most dangerous plaything. Man should be trained for war and woman for the recreation of the warrior: all else is folly ... Do you go to women? Do not forget the whip! (Nietzsche 1977, pp.275–76).

> All my life I dreamt about being in a war, because, I guess, the crucial test of manhood is when a man goes to war. Screw the man who did not serve the army and was never in a war ... that is a real job for a man. There is nothing for women to do there. We know what their duty is: to heal, to cure, and to lie down in bed so that the warrior can relax ... There is nothing else for them. Even as to the cooking and the washing while at war, the men have to do that. The war is a real manly mission (Yugoslav war volunteer from one of the 1991–1999 wars, quoted in Milićević 2006, p.278).

> A real man has to know how to use weapons, and if needed, to protect his family and country, and not to wait for somebody else to do so ... Women carry a child for nine months inside their stomach, why wouldn't men also serve their

> military obligation? (Participants in study, quoted in Milojević & Markov 2008, p.183).

The age-old practice of separating humans into gender-specific roles of mothers or warriors/soldiers meant that, when entering the realm of bigger things, the use of their mother status was one of the more obvious choices available to women. Like Persa Pavlović, a significant number of women peace activists and theorists entered the field of politics via the motherhood discourse. This was especially the case for early feminist theorising during the first wave of feminism (early twentieth century), as well as for essentialist strands of radical-feminism (second half of the twentieth century, second-wave feminism) and pacifist-feminism (both waves). For example, while providing an overview of the history of the US-based movements for world peace and women's rights, over the course of nineteenth and twentieth centuries, Harriet Hyman Alonso in *Peace as a Women's Issue* concludes:

> The motherhood theme, a very real and emotional issue for millions of women has also added a fundamental uniqueness to almost every one of the organizations here – and it is also often used to illustrate just how different the world of men (especially the powerful ones) is from that of women. Although most of the organizations have been careful to define the power problem as 'patriarchal dominance in society,' it is also clear

> that almost every group involved has itself portrayed women as more sensitive, more caring, more thoughtful, and more committed to producing a humanistic and compassionate world than men as a whole (Alonso 1993, p.11).

Groups such as Raging Grannies, *Asociación Madres de Plaza de Mayo,* Another Mother for Peace, *Barış Anneleri* (Peace Mothers), and Mothers for Peace used/use motherhood as a central metaphor for their peace activism. For example, Another Mother for Peace created a *Pax Materna* 'amnesty and understanding among mothers of the world' in 1969, re-realising the original mini-poster from 1985 on Mother's Day in 2005, with the following text:

> I join with my sisters in every land, in the Pax Materna – a permanent declaration of peace that transcends our ideological differences. In the nuclear shadow, war is obsolete. I will no longer suffer it in silence nor sustain it by complicity. They shall not send my son to fight another mother's son. For now, forever, there is no mother who is enemy to another mother (Another Mother for Peace, 2012).

Similar themes featured in Serbian and Yugoslav women's movements of the twentieth century. Like in other parts of Europe, the early women's movement there was organised within two political platforms: those directing their efforts towards Marxist and socialist goals, and those following classic liberalism (Milić 2011, p.52). Peace themes feature within both these platforms, but there was a difference in approach. Marxist/socialist feminists challenged traditional gender roles by promoting the idea of women revolutionaries who would create long-lasting peace by overthrowing violent social structures such as capitalism and patriarchy (by using both violent and nonviolent strategies). Liberal feminists, on the other hand, focused on citizenship issues (such as the right to vote and participation in political decision-making), hoping that once women enter these fields peace will be automatically enhanced. A number of citizenshipbased women's organisations engaged in charity work (Stojaković 2011) that focused on building peace at a micro level by ameliorating problems arising from poverty. Although these two platforms differed in a number of crucial points in relation to the achievement of long-lasting peace, both saw gender equality as a pre-requisite for creation of a more peaceful society. To give women, and mothers, a public-political voice various women's political organisations were formed. One such organisation was the Yugoslav League of Women for Peace formed in 1928. Its president, Danica Zečević, described the goals of the organisation in the following manner:

> By giving lectures and by organising various manifestations during [significant dates for the creation of peace in Yugoslavia] ... our women create public opinion which will always choose

> peace in case the need for such decision arises. We are trying to expel all articles from school's textbooks that promote hatred towards other nationalities ... the Yugoslav League of Women for Peace collected this year 600 000 signatures petitioning for disarmament and peace (Stojaković 2011, p.71).

Peace and anti-war movements often gain prominence immediately before the interruption of war and Yugoslavia was no exception in this regard. For example, a major Second World War women's organisation was the Antifascist Women's Front (AFŽ), which also linked women's empowerment with that of other political goals, such as freedom. AFŽ's primary goals were the liberation of Yugoslavia from Axis occupation, improvement of social and educational status of women, as well as equality between women and men (Sklevicky 1996). After the Second World War, AFŽ's membership surpassed that of the Yugoslav Communist Party, and the latter then decided that, 'since socialism already advocates for gender equality', specialist women's or feminists' organisations were no longer needed.

Throughout the twentieth century this was an exceptionally smart patriarchal strategy – various women's political organisations that were part of some larger political project were abolished either because they were not successful in achieving their specified goals, or because they were no longer needed; in other words, because they were too successful! Following a similar path to that of numerous women's organisations used for certain political purposes and then dismantled once these bigger purposes were achieved, AFŽ was discontinued in 1953. Women's peace activism was then 'not needed' until the dissolution of the SFRY in the early 1990s. Among key peace activists, women once again played a prominent role during this period. In Serbia, Vesna Pešić was one of the founders of the Centre for Anti-War Action, and Staša Zajović among the women who founded the Serbian Women in Black organisation and movement. Zajović expressed her motivation for creating a specifically women's peace organisation:

> Activity within the *Centre for Anti-War Action* was a logical continuation of my antimilitaristic orientation. It was mostly women who worked within the Centre, so I had an impression that efforts to create peace were somehow related to one sex only, as if that is part of our traditional women's role – care about others, consoling, hiding, giving support. This is invisible, hidden and unacknowledged women's work. As a feminist I know that this is an extension of our homework, and that it has a therapeutic effect, but that it does not have a transformational character. Thus it was important for me to start a women's peace group so that women's work is no longer hidden and unacknowledged, as that is unjust (Zajović et al. 2007, pp.16–17).

Zajović further argued that women's peace engagement is not 'our natural role; it is not our motherly duty'. Rather, the women's peace group formed due to a:

> political decision and cultural choice – to be against war, militarists, nationalists, and not to allow them to speak in our name. It was important to me that in the peace movement we do not continue and reproduce patriarchal roles of submission and invisibility, of unequal distribution of power (2007).

Nonetheless, feminist peace activists continued to evoke the motherhood theme, especially during the so-called mothers' movement or mothers' protests in Belgrade in the early 1990s:

> It is not by accident that peace movements' leaders and main activists are women and that mothers of soldiers joined them without any reservations. Women never had the opportunity to make important political decisions, especially not those that are connected with the use of weapons. But at the same time they were always asked to give birth to sons – soldiers whom now impassioned oligarchs irreverently sacrifice for their nebulous, meaningless and unrealizable goals (Ćetković 2003, p.62).

Theoretical links between mothering and peacemaking were also made by a number of other women peace theorists. Sarah Ruddick writes, 'there is a peacefulness latent in maternal practice ... a transformed maternal thinking could make a distinctive contribution to peace politics' (2004, p.166). 'Many women in their own homes and communities,' writes Betty Reardon, 'are making every effort to overcome the violence that pervades society ... In their personal relations and families, they practice constructive conflict resolution. They bring up their children in the knowledge that conflict can be conducted constructively, humanely, nonviolently' (1993, p.146).

Birgit Brock-Utne proposes that one of the three main characteristics of the way women work for peace is that they 'take as their point of departure the concern for, and ultimate value of life, especially the life of children, but also the life of all human beings and of nature' (Brock-Utne 2000, p.1498). Women's knowledge and experience worlds, writes Elise Boulding, 'have equipped them to function creatively as problem solvers and peacemakers in ways that men have not been equipped by their knowledge and experience worlds' (Boulding 2000, p.109). These knowledge and experience worlds have been based on mothering and nurturing, or on 'the historical reality [of] women's work of feeding, rearing, and healing humans' (2000). Like Zajović, Boulding also points out that such work arises not as a result of women's biological predisposition to nurturance and peacemaking (2000), but is based on roles women are assigned to in patriarchal societies, roles that inform who does what type of work. And, like Zajović and Boulding, most other 'modern feminists [also] dismiss the 'essentialised' idea that women are inherently more nonviolent and peaceful then men' (Cortright 2008, p.256). This is because the 'association of femininity with peace is a form of biological determinism that has been used historically to reinforce the subordination of women, to deny women political responsibility' (2008).

At the same time, many feminists and women peace activists do contend that, due to their specific gender roles, women as a social group tend to have a stronger orientation towards peace and nonviolence compared with men, who, as a group, have a stronger orientation towards violent conflict resolution. This assertion is based on research findings that found a gender gap in war/peace orientation – that is, more women favoured peaceful policing and opposed war – in a number of specific settings and historical moments (Pettman 1996, p.83; Amoako & Mwaura 2000, p.141; Goldstein 2001, p.329; Stephenson 2009, p.127). Even though such a gender gap is not universal and is not confirmed everywhere (Tickner 2002, p.286), the discourse that has again linked women with peace has helped shape a particular feminist anti-militaristic tradition in a variety of geographical and historical settings. Which also means that, throughout the twentieth century, women's and feminist's peace research and practice, which focused on the themes of 'caring, nurturing, feeling, intuiting, empathizing, relating' have been and remain 'an important catalyst to challenge militarism' (Forcey 1999, p.19). Their involvement in 'the field of international relations and the peace endeavour is refreshing, comforting, energizing and affirming for women' (1999). The contribution of numerous women's organisations for peacebuilding has been vast, global, and continues well into the twenty-first century.

A number of authors have, however, argued that the association between women and peace must be abandoned. Elshtain, for example, has warned of the dangers of linking women and pacifism, despite the fact that historically pacifism has indeed 'drawn women to its ranks, including pre-First World War feminist internationalists and current feminist anti-militarists' (1995, p.139). For Elshtain, the rationale for the severing of the women and peace link is because, 'given representations of women as pacific Other ... [p]acifist constructions reinforce and reaffirm dominant cultural images of women' or, their role of 'Just Warrior's better half, the Beautiful Soul' (1995, p.140). Such absolute distinctions between women and men when it comes to violence are dangerous, argues Elshtain, because beautiful souls serve as a backdrop against which both a just warrior as well as a brutal, destructive and beastly male is constructed (1995). There is therefore a danger of 'making peace feminine' because that both further 'masculinizes war and draws gender divisions that help soldiers to kill (knowing that they are outside a "normal" world)' (Goldstein

2001, p.331). Lastly, the argument goes, the position that links women and peace ultimately weakens women's peace activism because their views can then be discounted as 'expected', 'unlikely to "get through to" male soldiers or change the gendered nature of the war system' (2001). If disarmament and demilitarisation would indeed be perceived as 'emasculation, how could any "real man" ever consider it?' (2001, p.359).

That peace studies must abandon 'a strict dualism between feminine and masculine development' is also the conclusion reached by Linda Rennie Forcey. According to Forcey, this is partly because 'much of feminists' early observations about women ... their exaggeration of sexual differences ... now seem naive at best, dangerous at worst' and partly because peace studies may continue to be seen as the 'feminine' – read marginalised, voiceless, and hidden – opposite 'of one of the most male dominated of the social sciences fields, international relations' (1999, p.19).

In addition to specific reasons given by Elshtain, Goldstein and Forcey, positions that link women and mothers with pacifism have generally been critiqued on the grounds of being essentialist, meaning that these positions neglect particular socio-historical circumstances in which men and women find themselves and thus universalise experiences of some men and women to humanity as a whole. It is striking, writes Elshtain, how often 'the assertion that men are "by nature" violent, disorderly, destroyers and violators of women, children, and all of nature is simply stated as a matter of fact.' By contrast, 'women are identified with principles of care, peace-lovingness, and attunement with nature. In the more polemical version of a sex polarist argument, the universe itself is imperilled unless peaceful women somehow triumph over violent men' (1996, p.146).

It is Forcey's observation that such a view is common in 'both peace studies and women's studies', fields that 'share basic assumptions about the more peaceful nature of women and the more violent nature of men' (1999, p.14). This contradicts some other observations about the state of both these fields (that is, socio-constructionist perspective in general, awareness of the roles social structure and cultures play) as well as a general disdain towards 'human nature' theories in general. The latter is refuted by both fields as a dangerous discourse that is used for, respectively, promotion of violence and/or gender inequity. At the same time, the peaceful-women/violent-men hypothesis was proposed as a cultural and social phenomenon once gender became more explicit in peace-studies theorising.

This hypothesis was critiqued on numerous grounds. Postcolonial thinkers, for example, challenged the dichotomy of peaceful-women/violent-men by pointing out the role of women from dominant racial and cultural backgrounds in structural violence. Arguments that developed within critical men's studies further focused on this myopia due to the real world existence of peaceful men and violent women. This critique is now a standard and has been directed at 'many analyses of gender and conflict [that] ignore or underestimate the gender-based violence directed against males, and pay little attention to the active roles women play in warfare' (Human Security Center 2005, p.110). Some male activists within various men's movements towards the last few decades of the twentieth century also highlighted women's role in psychological violence within family. Crucially, a number of feminists challenged women's alleged peacefulness by pointing out that women have participated not only at the 'home front' but in combat as well, especially during liberation wars from postcolonial rule. Even early peace theorists, such as Jane Addams, Virginia Woolf, Helena Swanwick and Vera Brittain, pointed out that many women consider war inevitable, even righteous, that women have historically served as vital supporters for war, idealised the hero in battle, been afflicted by militarism and sometimes even looked admiringly upon men in uniforms (Cortright 2008, p.256).

Throughout the twentieth century, feminists also critiqued various 'uses of the motherhood discourse' to promote a patriarchal and warrior agenda. Some of these discourses were of 'suffering mothers' (*our* women and mothers as victims of war) and 'patriotic mothers' (mothers encouraging men to fight for *our* cause/people). The overall awareness arose that the motherhood discourse is a slippery slope, and that it could thus be used or misused to suit a variety of political agendas.

As a result of these and other debates, various theoretical positions within feminism developed in regards to women's active participation in combat – arguably, one of politics' biggest things. On the one hand, a division of feminist peace and conflict theory (FPCT) argues that, 'on the basis of inherent [or learned] peacefulness of women enacted by motherhood and caring, war is not only affecting women disproportionately, it is the ultimate attack on "feminine" non-violent ideals' (Weber 2006). On the other, some other strands of FPCT argue that not participating in 'war is exclusion from decision-making; which particularly affects women. If women are not allowed in the military they are implicitly barred from a primary institution which helps codify and constitute citizenship' (Francine D'Amico, quoted in 2006).

Coupled with the general 'banishment [of] feminism to the margins [of] the discipline(s) of international relations' (Zalewski 2007, p.303), such diversity of viewpoints within feminism – not to mention a diversity of viewpoints within broader/mainstream political debates – creates a situation where gender issues are now often put into the too-hard basket. As such, gender issues are potentially in danger of becoming an area of inquiry not to be touched, even by a majority of peace theorists. But there is a danger here of non-engagement as outdated views remain unquestioned and taken for granted, perpetuating certain gender ideologies and mythologies.

The invisibility of gender and the marginalisation of input by women's and feminists' peace theorising is already the case within most strands of politics, as argued, among others, by Joshua Goldstein (2001) and David Roberts:

> IR [international relations] is unwilling, or unable, to consider that much of the violence that men and women face globally is a product of men's formulations, men's institutions and male-dominated ideational structures and the gender blindness associated with this mono-sex ideational dominance (Roberts 2008, p.163).

One quick look at works within the international relations field (in English) confirms their view. Some examples in which gender is not mentioned or explored as a worthwhile topic include *How Nations Make Peace* (Kegley & Raymond 1999), *After Defensive War* (Rivett 2004), *Sustainable Peace* (Roeder & Rothchild 2005), *Conflict and Peace Building in Divided Societies* (Oberschall 2007), *Metaphors in International Relations Theory* (Marks 2011) and *At War's End* (Paris 2004). In addition to international relations and mainstream political politics, another field of inquiry that also focuses on the analysis of violence, criminology, has had a similar history of 'rather ironically, largely ... gender blindness, where being male has simultaneously been the largest predictor of criminal activity and yet wholly unproblematised in gendered terms' (Edwards 2006, p.59).

Despite the connections of feminism with peace studies, Goldstein argues, 'feminist theory has had a limited impact to date on peace studies overall, and again most of the relevant work is by women' (2001, p.57). Gender continues to be 'invisible in political science and history as well as within peace theorising':

> Feminist political scientists and historians – nearly all women – pay attention to gender in war, but others relegate gender to the dark margins beyond their (various) theoretical frameworks for studying war. Feminist literatures about war and peace of the last 15 years have made little impact as yet on the discussions and empirical research taking place in the predominantly male mainstream of political science or military history. This omission is measurable by counting the number of headings and subheadings in a book's index on topics relating to gender. The typical political science and history books about war – the 'big' books about war's origins and history – score zero (2001, p.34).

Further to this general gender blindness, three other common themes appear in international relations' texts on war and peace, according to Goldstein. First, 'all the gender references concern women; men still do not have gender' (2001, p.35); second, 'when gender occasionally shows up in other mainstream war studies, it does so gratuitously, as a passing note – something that could be interesting, but plays no substantive role in *any* of the main competing theories about war' (2001); and third, the 'author's gender is a highly significant predictor of whether the chapter includes or omits gender ... even in postmodern international relations, gender is ghettoized' (2001, p.36).

Being of female gender *and* being inspired by a pacifist feminist political orientation it is therefore my 'political decision and cultural choice' to bring gender issues to the forefront of the violence–war–peace analysis. As well, I believe I owe it to those earlier peacemaking women in my family whose voices, like the voice of Persa Pavlović, remained marginalised within the private sphere of their family. Not only that but, given 'the universal gendering of war' (2001, p.10) as well as of violence and peace, I believe that peace theorists must theorise gender if they are to better understand these phenomena. Further, in their roles as peace activists and theorists, generations of women helped us understand that constructions of gender and gender relationships permeate not only the so-called 'laundry list of women's issues' (Bunch 1983, p.249), but also the majority of contemporary social practices, including those of the waging of peace/war. The insight that the social practices of waging peace or war are always influenced by society's gender politics is their *legacy*, and it is important that this legacy is remembered and upheld. Not theorising gender, on the other hand, could be seen to constitute yet another 'smart' patriarchal practice of further marginalising generations of women's (and mothers') voices.

The analysis here is informed by feminist theory (and social activism) and the more recent gender theorising within critical men's and masculinity studies (as well as, but marginally, on theorising within gay–lesbian and queer studies). It is predominantly influenced by feminists' – or more precisely pacifist-feminists' – gestalt/holistic view of the world, which provides 'a basis for understanding every area of our lives ... politically, culturally, economically and spiritually' (1983, p.250). More specifically, it is based on insights from twentieth-century and contemporary gender theorising, which connects specific ways of 'doing gender' (Butler 1990 and 2004) with the doing of war and peace. These insights are then useful in seeking answers for two key questions that this section has raised: Should a link between women's and mother's traditional/contemporary social roles of life givers and peacemakers be severed? How can we theorise war and violence as gendered (given that they clearly are) without falling into the trap of inadvertently reinforcing what peace theorists and activists wish to transcend?

In: Zoran's déjà vu

Learning about the violent events of the twentieth and previous centuries was not comfortable for me or my father Zoran. For him, hearing about those events magnified the trauma he experienced during the Second World War, including the beating of his grandmother Nega and his encounters with knife-wielding warriors, and it added some new material. The Yugoslav school curriculum was full of such new materials. Here is a woman running away from the enemy with two twin boys in her arms trying to make a decision which one to leave behind, to give the other one half a chance of surviving. Here is another woman about to witness the gang rape and murder of her 12-year-old daughter. Here is a teacher whose last words just before being shot with his whole class of 16-year-old boys on 21 October 1941 in Kragujevac were, 'Shoot, but even now I am conducting a lesson.' The whole generation of high school (male) children was assassinated in revenge attacks by German defence forces or *Wehrmacht,* together with thousands of civilians. But the Yugoslav curriculum and mainstream political discourse also gave an implicit reassurance that the great victory of the socialist revolution and the Second World War liberation movement had relegated to history violent events like those of the more recent as well as distant pasts. As long as the 'foreign enemy' does not attack once again, peaceful coexistence based on Yugoslav people's 'brotherhood and unity' will continue. Further, the Non-Aligned Movement was to keep us out of Cold War dynamics, enhancing Yugoslav peaceful coexistence with others.

From 1945 until 1989, Zoran was comfortable with these reassurances. Then, in June 1989 (the broadcast of Serbian President Slobodan Milošević's Gazimestan speech) and in January 1991 (the release and airing of Croatian Interior Minister Martin Špegelj's audiotapes) Radio Television Belgrade took away that safety for Zoran, as well as for millions of his fellow citizens:

> *Milošević:* By the force of social circumstances this great 600th anniversary of the Battle of Kosovo is taking place in a year in which Serbia, after many years, after many decades, has regained its state, national, and spiritual integrity[1] ... Through the play of history and life, it seems as if Serbia has, precisely in this year, in 1989, regained its state and its dignity and thus has celebrated an event of the distant past which has a great historical and symbolic significance for its future.
>
> Today, it is difficult to say what is the historical truth about the Battle of Kosovo and what is legend. Today this is no longer important ... What has been certain through all the centuries until our time today is that disharmony struck Kosovo 600 years ago. If we lost the battle, then this was not only the result of social superiority and the armed advantage of the Ottoman Empire but also of the tragic disunity in the leadership of the Serbian state at that time ... The lack of unity

and betrayal in Kosovo will continue to follow the Serbian people like an evil fate through the whole of its history. Even in the last war, this lack of unity[2] and betrayal led the Serbian people and Serbia into agony, the consequences of which in the historical and moral sense exceeded fascist aggression ... Even later, when a socialist Yugoslavia was set up, in this new state the Serbian leadership remained divided, prone to compromise to the detriment of its own people. The concessions that many Serbian leaders made at the expense of their people could not be accepted historically and ethically by any nation in the world, especially because the Serbs have never in the whole of their history conquered and exploited others. Their national and historical being has been liberational throughout the whole of history and through two world wars, as it is today. They liberated themselves and when they could they also helped others to liberate themselves. The fact that in this region they are a major nation is not a Serbian sin or shame; this is an advantage which they have not used against others, but I must say that here, in this big, legendary field of Kosovo, the Serbs have not used the advantage of being great for their own benefit either...

Six centuries later, now, we are being again engaged in battles and are facing battles. They are not armed battles, although such things cannot be excluded yet. However, regardless of what kind of battles they are, they cannot be won without resolve, bravery, and sacrifice, without the noble qualities that were present here in the field of Kosovo in the days past...

Let the memory of Kosovo heroism live forever! Long live Serbia! Long live Yugoslavia! Long live peace and brotherhood among peoples!

Špegelj: ... If necessary, at a decisive moment, organise two or three men for the liquidation of the most dangerous ones. All right. Physical liquidation. You come to somebody's apartment, a messenger – all right, I know. You appear at the door, dum, dum, dum, go downstairs. Afterwards, let them look for the police and let them establish. You walk downstairs, you go to another one and yet another one, or rather at the same time. Those who are the most dangerous ones can be killed on their doorstep. It doesn't matter. Women, children, nothing. Doesn't matter, no questions asked.

As for border posts, when border posts are disarmed, then they will be disarmed, all of them, as many as there are, but leave Albanians five bullets in their automatic rifles, and the rest lock up in cellars and give food and water if this goes on for a few days. As for this, if something happens, then just give instructions to all your people who you know. Kill extremists on the spot, in the street, in the compound, in barracks, anywhere. Just pistol and into the stomach. That will not be a war, it will be a civil war in which there is no mercy towards anyone, women or children. Into homes, family homes, quite simply grenades.

We are going to resort to all resources. We're even going to use weapons. Knin[3] we're going to resolve in the same way. We are going to slaughter everyone. We have international recognition for that – we're going to slaughter them now that this whore won in Serbia. Milošević? Yes. Now the Americans, on the second day when he won, offered us all assistance, and until then everyone was speculating, they would, they wouldn't, this way, that way, 1,000 combat vehicles.

We are going to use all resources. We're going to use weapons as well. Serbs in Croatia will never be there again for as long as we are there and we hope until now too their supremacy is a thing of the past. Their Knin will never be Knin again. We are going to enter Knin too. Knin has to disappear as Knin. All Croats should bear this in mind and we are going to create a state at all costs, if necessary, at the cost of shedding blood (UNICTY).

Out: Masculinity wars

Whether their campaigners were using more-subtle (Milošević's speech) or not-so-subtle cues (Špegelj's tapes) while advocating violence, one thing remains certain: all nationalist ideologies in the former Yugoslavia became intrinsically linked and 'grounded on a purposefully constructed aggressive and violent masculinity' (Papić 1994, p.117). Men, of course, still had a choice to make. My father, Zoran, for example, did not buy into either nationalistic hysteria or the hyper masculinisation of society. Despite being of Serbian origin he was not convinced that the saviour of his people arrived in 1989. He would often engage in arguments with the TV set, exclaiming, 'It is this Milošević again!' or, 'You have no idea what is coming, this is a prelude to a disaster!' His views were shared by my mother as well as by most people in our social circle. The events that unfolded later, though, seemed to show that we were in the minority.

Socialism and humanism-based ideas on gender equity as well increasingly became minority views. Nationalist ideologies, by contrast, relying on the masculinisation and re-patriarchalisation of gender regimes were another déjà vu. These joined discourses helped enhance the desire for a leader who could play the 'father of the nation' role – Franjo Tuđman in Croatia, Slobodan Milošević in Serbia, Alija Izetbegović in Bosnia and Herzegovina. Further, these new–old ideas were necessary for the promotion of just-war/just-warrior motifs, and for bringing back women-at-home and women-as-patriotic-mothers ideology. For example, after the former SFRY disintegrated, and its republics established new 'democracies', the proportion of women members in the just-formed parliaments ranged from 13 per cent in Slovenia, 4.5 per cent in Croatia, 4 per cent in Montenegro, 3.3 per cent in Macedonia, 2.9 per cent in Bosnia and Herzegovina to only 1.6 per cent in Serbia (Papic 1994, pp.115–17). In the same period, the Serbian Orthodox Church introduced the Order of Mother Jugovići – named after a Serbian mythological character whose nine sons and husband all died during the 1389 Battle of Kosovo (to which she responds with no tears or action but dies of a broken heart) – awarding it to Serbian women who gave birth to four or more children. Given that they managed to only give away 16 golden and 14 silver medals in 1993, representatives of the Serbian Orthodox Church publicly expressed their displeasure at the situation: 'Mothers used to be able to equip even nine sons for the Tsar's army, to fight for freedom of their country and their orthodox faith. Today there are mothers like that also, although they are very rare' (Zaharijević 2008, p.88). Since there were even fewer women eligible to receive medals in 1994, the church stopped the ritual, angry that 'fewer and fewer Serbian women are giving birth and fewer and fewer Serbian men are going to the Army' (2008).

During those years of re-patriarchalisation and masculinisation, the asexual socialist *drugarica* (female comrade) was replaced by a saintly warrior mother or a highly sexualised woman. Pornographic material became more and more widely available but the church's spokesmen, finally given a public voice after 40 years of semi-hiding during communism, chose to obsess over abortions performed in Serbian medical institutions, deciding the most important issue was not in preventing war or in protecting women (and men) against male violence but rather the 'murderous actions of Serbian women against their unborn children'. Patriarchal blaming of women for all the world's evils, coupled with simultaneous absolution of men for their sins changed the already weakened socialist-based gender regime. In its place was to arrive a new–old gendered regime of traditional men and women, or of desirable warrior masculinity and desirable subservient femininity. Promotion of conservative/hierarchical gender arrangements and the militarisation of a society seemed to have gone hand in hand, supporting and reinforcing each other.

The rise of ethnic nationalism in Serbia and other former Yugoslav republics suppressed even further the official doctrine (though not fully implemented) and practice (though not comprehensive and in places only 'skin deep') of gender partnership/equality that was promoted during 50 years of socialism. At the same time, even though both women and men associated themselves with nation-states and nationalism, the use of direct violence remained a male prerogative. In other words, when a 'narcissistic injury and rage' (Barash & Webel 2002, p.120) was activated during those years, and when in the pursuit of vengeful justice great violence was selfrighteously employed, it was not expected that this was to be employed by either him or her (2002). Such expectations were almost exclusively directed towards men. Not surprisingly, the actual enactment of direct violence was almost exclusively in men's hands. It was this gender who, in the territory of former Yugoslavia between 1991 and 2000, engaged in the age-old practice of asserting alpha male status by taking the life of another. These masculinity battles were waged on the official battlefronts as well as among the civilian population, they were waged during official political meetings as well as during various practices of everyday living, and they were waged via use of 'milder' (ethnocentrism) as well as extreme forms (torture, murder) of violence.

Parallel to this, wars in the former Yugoslavia further reduced women to beyond being 'innocent victims' of collateral damage. Women also became conscious military targets, over whose bodies masculinity battles were waged. Violation of 'other women' became a means of male communication, signifying dominance of one group of men over another group of men. This also means, as feminist theorists have repeatedly argued, that women were not seen as humans or persons in their own right, but were objectified and reified as mere bodies belonging to the other group of male warriors. So no matter what their education, level of income or socio-economic background prior to the war, almost all women had their status, which could have shielded them from patriarchal oppression, automatically removed during wars. In those, like in many other wars, all the gains women had previously made towards achieving equality in their society almost completely disappeared.

The perceived orientation towards peacefulness among women should therefore come as no surprise. It would be a logical conclusion reached by most women, based on their knowledge and experiences if they were aware of a common gender dynamics during wars. Given that feminists have frequently investigated the gender dynamics involved in violence and during wars, it also comes as no surprise that the majority of feminist theorists and activists have most often taken a strong anti-militaristic, antiwar, nonviolent and peace-oriented political stance. Such a position is, of course, based on *informed choice* and logic and has nothing to do with the innate peacefulness of women. Rather, it could be better understood as being a result of having access to alternative lenses with which to view the world. In this particular instance, that lens was of feminist epistemology and theory, which has since been used by feminists, pro-feminists and even non-feminists in order to resist the pressure of the dominant (patriarchal, nationalistic) ideology. As the standpoint epistemological position asserts, once alternative worldviews based on the 'situated knowledge' group based experiences (Haraway 1988) of marginalised social groups are articulated they can become a resource for a 'double viewing' of perceived reality. These alternative worldviews can, and have been, used by various social groups since, and have thus provided a long-standing viable alternative to various forms of violence stemming from patriarchy.

The same feminist lens can still assist in sharpening the focus on specific ways in which gender continues to be implicated in the making of wars and violence. This 'seeing' is critical if we wish for an alternative future. Despite all the relativism and caution resulting from challenges thrown at the violent-men/peaceful-women hypothesis, the empirical facts relating to the gendered nature of violence remain pretty consistent. In situations of both individual homicide as well as mass killings/torture in wars, direct violence is still committed most frequently by men. The unspeakable and horrific crimes against women during wars on the territory of the former Yugoslavia were in almost all instances committed by men. The horrific crimes against men were also in almost all instances committed by men. Such gender dynamics have, of course, not only been limited to the former Yugoslavia. Men being perpetrators of direct violence in wars (genocide) as well as in times of official peace (homicide) has been a constant theme throughout much of written history. Globally, a vast majority of empirical studies confirms the view that, somehow, 'violence and being a man seem to go hand in hand' (UNESCAP 2003 quoted in Warters 2010, pp.659–60). This is because:

> Compared with women, men, especially young men, are overwhelmingly involved in all types of violence. It is mostly men who commit acts of personal violence – against women and girls, as well as towards other men and boys. Men are also most often implicated in other types of organized or institutional violence as victims and perpetrators of violence. Around the world ... militaries consist of only men or mostly men. Men fight more than women – in wars, in the home, schoolyard, and on the street. It is primarily men who are drafted into jihadist, nationalist or separatist movements or who perpetrate acts of terrorism. In general, men use weapons more than women, and are imprisoned and murdered more than women. It is also a fact that, in general, men control more resources and wield more power than women (2010).

So whether it is gang wars, crime wars, wars on drugs, civil or religious wars, war on terror and other inter-state wars, gender wise there seems to be one common denominator: men. This, of course, does not mean that all women are peaceful and all men violent. But the figures do show that violence is somehow connected with the 'practice of masculinity' (social and cultural practices of prevalent male behaviour) even though there is very little evidence based on current research to support the claim that violence is predicated on 'maleness' (biological characteristics, being of male physiology).

Going back to the data, the UN Economic Commission for Europe's (2012) figures for 42 countries (mostly EU, north American and some former USSR countries) show that men's share of criminal convictions in the period between 2005 and 2010 average at around 87 per cent, the lowest figure sitting at 74.7 per cent (United Kingdom in 2010) and the highest at 95.9 per cent (Armenia in 2007). Further, of people in Western societies who have been convicted of killing, men have consistently made up around 90 per cent of the numbers. If violence in wars was added, 'to say that 95% of direct violence is committed by men, is probably an understatement' (Galtung 1996, p.41). In this context, some features of the statistics on homicide appear to be 'incontrovertible ... men commit murder much more frequently than women ... and the ratio of men killing women to women killing men is about 8 to 1' (Walklate 2004, p.132). 'More than 90 percent of the violent, brutal, sadistic type of crime ... comes from the young, mostly male, but increasingly joined by the female' (Nisbet 1982, p.228). But despite this slight increase in homicidal female behaviour, 'the vast majority of violent acts across the world, past and present, are committed by men' (Edwards 2006, p.44). As Edwards points out, 'From pub brawls to building bombs, and from forced prison buggery to battered wives, the problem seems to be men: men swearing, men punching, men kicking, men smashing, men bashing, men destroying things, other men, women, themselves, even the world.' Further, 'the universal gendering of war' means that 'in war, the fighters are usually all male' (Goldstein 2001, p.10). At the turn of millennium, Goldstein continues, the gendering of war in the interstate system remains 'stark':

> About 23 million soldiers serve in today's uniformed standing armies, of whom about 97% are male (somewhat over 500,000 are women). In only six of the world's nearly 200 states do women make up more than 5 percent of the armed forces. And most of these women in military forces worldwide occupy traditional women's roles such as typists and nurses. Designated *combat* forces in the world's state armies today include several million soldiers (the exact number depending on definitions of combat), of whom 99.9 percent are male ... In UN peacekeeping forces, women (mostly nurses) made up less than 0.1 percent in 1957–89 and still less than 2 percent when UN peacekeeping peaked in the early 1990s (2001, pp.10–11).

Since the early 1990s the number of women in UN peacekeeping forces has grown, but remains marginal. As of 2012, out of 'approximately 125,000 peacekeepers, women constitute 4% of military personnel and 10% of police personnel in UN Peacekeeping missions. Women also account for approximately 30% of international civilian staff' (UN, 2012). Further, despite women's increasing participation in world armies (for example, the 2005 Human Security Report informs us that women's inclusion among government armed service personnel remains between 5 per cent and 15 per cent in 'many countries', up to 30 per cent in some guerrilla and terrorist groups and that girls constitute up to 40 per cent of child soldiers around the world [Human Security Centre 2005, p.111]), Goldstein's comprehensive historical account on *War and Gender* found only one society – Dahomey Kingdom, from the sixteenth to nineteenth centuries – with a 'large-scale female combat unit that functioned over a long period as part of a standing army' (Goldstein 2001, p.60). When they *do* participate in combat women make 'fine soldiers', continues Goldstein, but still:

> Overall, the war system works to push women away from killing roles except in the most dire emergencies such as when defending their homes and children. This does not necessarily protect women participants from harm. Women have faced great danger on the battlefield ... [but] [w]hat these women do *not* share with the men around them is *the task of aggressive killing* (2001, p.127, second italics added).

Given such long-standing expectations, it is not surprising that current evidence from both pre-history as well as from written history equally points to only a 'handful of known cases in which women have participated in combat in substantial numbers' (2001, p.22). 'The world's military and ethnographic museums' writes Glen Paige, confirm previously described gender patterns given that they offer:

> ...scant evidence that women, half of humankind, have been major combat killers. Granted that women kill, that some have fought in wars and revolutions, that in some societies women and even children have engaged in ritual torture and murder of defeated enemies, and that women are being recruited for killing in several modern armies. But most women have not been warriors or military killers (Paige 2009, p.39).

In summary, all the available historical and statistical data shows that humans of male gender, or 'men', 'are by far the principal perpetrators of rape, war, torture, incest, sexual abuse, sexualized murder, and genocide' (Glass 2012). More than '90% of criminal and war violence is committed by men, making gender a major factor of war-peace' (Galtung 2009). This data also finally puts to rest the violence as part of 'human nature' hypothesis, because, at best, it could be claimed that it is part of 'male nature'. Even though 'human nature' arguments still abound and inform certain politics and behaviours, with the benefit of a feminist lens, we can now see clearly gender dynamics of violence, even though explanations of this dynamic remain varied. We can also see clearly now how views on the natural human propensity for violence arose from certain naturalised views on gender relationships, which assumed that, firstly, men and maleness represented the norm, the essence of 'human experience', and, secondly, that it is men who should be proprietors of the public sphere, including politics, diplomacy and the waging of wars. If, on the other hand, women were considered to be 'half of humankind' and then it was their behaviour that was observed, discourses about violence somehow being rooted in 'human nature' would have simply been impossible. That is, given the overwhelming evidence that shows that physical violence is mostly carried out by those members of the human species who are physiologically male, violence may be at best considered to be a 'male social pathology' (Barker 2005, p.3).

But where exactly is this 'male social pathology' coming from? How could it be best understood and then, obviously, addressed? Is it sufficient to say that men are not violent 'by nature' but it is our societies and cultures that make them so? Or, do we need a somewhat more sophisticated analysis?

As already touched on in Chapter 1 (in the section on raising children and worldview), gender (in)equality and the privileging of males/maleness in patriarchy correlates somewhat with the degree of war and violence within society overall. This correlation may help explain the widespread expectation that men will engage in tasks of aggressive killing and the rarity of women in combat. This is mostly because 'a society would have to be an outlier from the general pattern to have women warriors ... [as] relatively peaceful societies would not need them and highly sexist societies would not tolerate them' (Goldstein 2001, p.399). In other words, relatively peaceful societies with strong gender equity have greater focus on peaceful conflict resolution (and thus do not need so many soldiers), whilst masculinised, patriarchal and warrior societies' social structure is dependent on a justwarrior/beautiful-soul dichotomy. In this later instance the place for beautiful souls is, of course, at home, and not on the battlefield.

The only scenario, therefore, in which we would see large number of women in combat, for an extended period of time, would be in societies that are highly militarised/warrior-like, but with great(er) gender equity. This scenario has been rare in history, although it has existed. For example, a phenomenon that links egalitarian gender order and high level of collective acts of violence is *temporary gender equality.* Temporary gender equality refers to the situation when gender equality may not be on the agenda in other (more peaceful) times but is evoked in desperate times, when a society needs to mobilise women for 'men's work'. Such temporary 'gender equality' – for purposes of militarily defending society – was previously elicited by a number of socialist, postcolonial and nationalist movements. But as soon as the 'larger' goals were achieved, these societies and movements would once again demilitarise all women but not all men. A similar scenario of 'high(er) gender equality + high(er) militarisation' is increasingly coming into existence within Western societies: the goals of liberal feminism (inclusion of women in the existing public sphere) have been appropriated by militarised societies (wherein the overall framework remains patriarchal, traditional masculinity based, competitive and violence-inducing). The percentage of women in Western militaries has shown 'a marked upward trend in recent years' (Cockburn 2010, p.106). For example, in the period between 1973 and 2008 women's participation in the US Army increased from '2 per cent to around 20 per cent' (2010, pp.106–107). Since the official policy male-only drafting was removed in 2010–11, after nearly two centuries, the Serbian military has also opened its doors to women. That same year, of 127 cadets promoted into the rank of officers, 19 were women (Vojska Srbije 2012).

These developments seem to be, paradoxically, a consequence of the continual militarisation of one society (United States) and a consequence of the demilitarisation of another (Serbia). Both are, nevertheless, arising from a creation of a professional army and related to the absence of drafted men. Despite being somewhat paradoxical, such developments should not come as a surprise. In the context of (even diverse) patriarchal societies, where maleness and masculinity are more highly valued, so are the activities traditionally associated with them, such as military service. The 'push' for women to masculinise and militarise themselves, either via social militarism or via direct participation in the military and combat, is, therefore, much stronger, and much better financially rewarded, than is the 'push' for men to demilitarise, engage more within the private sphere of family or 'feminise' themselves in any way. In fact, men who do so, who embrace traditional 'feminine' qualities of care, nurturing and peaceful conflict resolution are often ridiculed or belittled by the wider patriarchal society. From bullying in the schoolyards to fights in male prisons, one theme is constant: the worst insults men have thrown at other men are those marking them 'as impotent and emasculated, a coward, wimp, eunuch, boy, homosexual, or woman, a man who has "no balls"' (Gilligan 2009). This fits within the general historical pattern in patriarchal societies, where direct violence resulting in severe injury or death has been used against homosexual as well as effeminate men to punish them for masculinity transgressions. Similar insults have historically been thrown at men refusing to fight in wars, and they too were often violently punished.

Not only are these newer trends (masculinisation–militarisation) of women and constant themes such as the ban on perceived feminisation of men extremely detrimental for peace, they are also as far as one can be from feminist eutopia. This eutopia has been expressed via a vision for the preferable future and an improved society where dominance, existing social hierarchies and their maintenance via violent means are weakened. So the militarisation of women seems the result of yet another exceptionally 'smart' patriarchal strategy helping this system survive. In other words, the phenomenon of the 'military as an equal opportunity employer' is not exactly the positive and progressive change the majority of twentieth-century feminists had in mind. Nonetheless, even this negative change can help further understand how patriarchy and militarisation interlink and support each other.

Interlinking these two systems reveal why and how 'masculinity wars' continue to take place. For example, feminist theorists have highlighted the ways in which the global distribution of power remains firmly in the hands of what Mary Daly called 'The Planetary Men's Association' (1978, p.326). In such a world, 'dominated by men, the world of men is [also], by definition, a world of power' (Kaufman, 1994, p.142). Ever since the eighteenth and nineteenth centuries, when authors such as Mary Wollstonecraft, Bertha von Suttner, Rosa Luxemburg or Emma Goldman pointed out the 'continuum of violence running from domestic violence to war' (Weber 2006), or between private and public tyranny, this private/public connection has remained a cornerstone of feminist theorising. Second-wave radical feminism, in particular, exposed male violence against women and children within the sanctity of family, and demanded such violence be seen as not a private but a public and political issue. From Virginia Woolf's vision of a feminist and transnational society of 'Outsiders' – rejecting the whole patriarchal sex-gender system and its links with violence, via the efforts of second-wave radical feminism – the movement for which one of the main goals was to oppose war and violence, visions of futures societies living in peace have remained an important feature of feminist eutopia. Further, in the area of international politics/political theory, theorists such as Cynthia Enloe, V. Spike Peterson, Jan Jindy Pettman, Joy Damousi, Marilyn Lake, J Ann Tickner, Carole Pateman, Sara Ruddick, Christine Sylvester, Rebecca Grant, Kathleen Newland and others have challenged the alleged gender neutrality of war and political decision-making. Implicit as well as explicit in their work is a view that genuine peace should not be defined merely in negative terms as the absence of war, 'where order is imposed from outside by domination' (Warren & Cady 1994, p.5). Rather, peace is seen as a process of building 'life-affirming, self-determined, environmentally sustainable ends [which] are sought and accomplished through coalitionary, interactive, cooperative means' (1994).

In a nutshell, most of them proposed that the creation of sustainable peace could not be achieved without fundamental social changes, including those relating to changes of patriarchal gender regimes. Further, peace theorists such as Elise Boulding, Birgit Brock-Utne and Betty Reardon have also been influential in expanding the robust 'masculine' field of international politics to include peace education or to investigate ways in which 'the roots of militarism, violence, and other forms of peacelessness, [lie] within our own families, neighborhoods, schools, churches' (Alger 1996, p. x). This has resulted in the assertion that it is critically important to simultaneously transform *both* 'sexism and the war system' (Reardon 2000).

Given the huge social disparities that result from the uneven distribution of power between genders, it is 'hard to imagine' that 'a structure of inequality on this scale' (Connell 2005, p.83) could be maintained without violence. To study violence and its alternatives also means to study power, including, or perhaps especially, gender-based power arrangements. This is because, despite twentieth-century efforts to transform this reality of the world, globally patriarchy – albeit in its many specific and concrete manifestations – continues to massively influence the (uneven) distribution of power and privileges. For example, the 2010 *Global Index of Women's Power*[4] shows that, globally, improvements in gender equality over the last century are due largely to the closing of health and education gender gaps (96 per cent and 93 per cent of the gap closed, respectively). At the same time, the gender gap with regard to economic participation remains wide (only 59 per cent closed globally). The gap is the widest as far as political empowerment is concerned (only 18 per cent has been closed). Men are thus, globally, still 'vastly more likely to control a major block of capital as chief executive of a major corporation, or as direct owner' and are 'ten times more likely than women to hold office as a member of parliament' (Connell 2005, p.82). This is despite the fact that women and men work on average about the same number of hours in the year, at least in the wealthy countries (2005), however, the difference in economic and political power is based on how much of that work gets paid and is done in the public sphere. In spite of all the talk about allegedly achieved gender equity in post-feminist times, and in spite of the higher percentage of women in the military in some countries, a global gender order where 'men dominate women ... is a structural fact, independent of whether men as individuals love or hate women, or believe in equality or abjection, and independent of whether women are currently pursuing change' (2005, p.82). Most importantly, it is due to such a social context, rather than the link between women and peace per se, that peacemaking is seen as somehow inferior to the real business of doing politics (through war and violence).

Within this overall global social context it is thus crucially important to analyse more than just the 'sexual division of war', that is 'who does what' in war (Cockburn 2010, p.105). It is perhaps more crucial to examine the interconnection between war 'shaping the gender relations of a given society, while in turn [seeing how] a certain gender order may be ... predisposing a society to war' (2010). In other words, if we are to better understand individual and collective violence and, alternatively, possibilities for peace, the connection between gender relationships and power has to be further investigated. This also means recognising that 'gender is an integral, not an accidental, feature of the worldwide structure of diplomatic, military and economic relations' (Parpart & Zalewski 2008, p. viii). Crucially, this recognition no longer means limiting 'the examination of gender in politics to an investigation of women only, as much contemporary research has tended to do' (Nagel 2005, p.397). Equating 'human nature' with men, and 'gender' with women, are both remnants of pre-feminist thinking. Rather, we must 'think about gender in terms of power relations [and] as with any structure of power and inequality (such as race and class), it becomes necessary to study the powerful (men!)' (Messerschmidt 2005, p.197). In other words, if 'nation states are gendered institutions, as much recent [feminist] scholarship asserts' (Nagel 2005), not studying men, maleness and masculinity means missing 'a major, perhaps *the* major, way in which gender shapes politics'.

This study could be done by investigating 'men and their interests, their notions of manliness, and the articulation of masculine micro (everyday) and macro (political cultures)' (2005, p.397). As previously mentioned, gender order based on huge power imbalances cannot avoid constituting men as 'an interest group concerned with defence, and women as an interest group concerned with change' (Connell 2005, p.82), so it is perhaps not surprising that a significant number of male theorists of masculinities wishing to transform violent social arrangements have chosen to critically engage with feminism. This has resulted in a major shift from identifying a 'women question' within the social sciences of the nineteenth and twentieth centuries to investigating the 'man question' (Parpart & Zalewski 2008, p. viii) at the beginning of the twenty-first. Analysis of notions of manhood and masculinity, their practices and their links with violence/peace, has thus recently become a new focus in gender-based analysis, and is increasingly used for understanding peace–conflict–violence dynamics.

So who were those men that caused Zoran's déjà vu and how could their behaviour best be understood? More specifically, what made some men turn into promoters and perpetrators of horrific acts of violence – in my country of origin in the 1990s, as well as in other places and times? How and why were some of them transformed from relatively 'benevolent' individuals in times of peace, to personifications of monstrosity in times of war? Where did they come from and what were the gender-based mechanisms that supported their violent behaviour? Most importantly, can current gender research assist in finding some of the best ways to minimise the impact of men behaving violently in our societies and cultures, and, alternatively, to maximise the impact of peacemaking and nonviolent masculinities?

In: Slobodan's train ride

Slobodan-Boba Vlahović was born in 1949 and like many boys in his post-war generation he was given a name that meant 'being free' (*slobodan).* Freedom within SFRY was premised on doing the right thing politically, which would include following the official communist party line and the general mores of the time. Being the son of a highly ranked communist politician, Veljko, may have given Slobodan credibility and yet, like everybody else, he too was expected to not rock the boat. All his life he remained apolitical, disciplined in his work and family life, and followed the general privileges and expectations awarded to his gender. This included serving in the army and learning how to obey authorities. Within socialist Yugoslavia, the authorities had a habit of randomly asking men and women for legitimation documents, and to this day, carrying an identification document, called a *lična karta* ('identity card', also known as *osobna iskaznica),* has remained an obligation of each and every person who is 16 years of age or over living within the former Yugoslav territory.

On Sunday, 27 February 1993, when the authorities asked him to provide his identification card, my uncle

Slobodan initially did not think much of it. This was, of course, not the first time he had been asked to provide his identification card. This was also not the first time that he had been sitting in the number 671 train that operated from Belgrade to Bar as he often travelled from Serbia to Montenegro to visit his paternal relatives and do business. But it was the first time he witnessed a process in which the showing of identification cards led to the torture and death of some of his fellow passengers.

Slobodan and other passengers were identified twice, the first time immediately after the train left Belgrade by the train conductor and the Yugoslav police. Against the normal custom, though, the conductor wrote passenger's names on their tickets with the justification of looking for people engaged in smuggling. During the second identification it became clear that something was not right. When Slobodan looked up at the men asking for the identification cards he realised that some of them were members of a paramilitary group rather than the official Yugoslav policemen.

The train he was in had been, up to this point, travelling through the territory of the then Federal Republic of Yugoslavia (1992–2003), but a brief section of the train ride passed through newly independent Bosnia and Herzegovina, or, more specifically, through the Republika Srpska – the Serbian controlled part of Bosnia. During the train's ninekilometre passage through Republika Srpska, it – again not following the usual pattern – stopped at the Štrpci station, located between the stations of Zlatibor and Priboj (both in the Federate Republic of Yugoslavia at the time, now both in Serbia). A group of armed men boarded the train and, together with other men in uniform already on the train, demanded the identification cards of all travellers. After 'identification' they took 19 or 20 men, aged between 16 and 60, from the train without much protest by them or by other travellers. As if to confirm Hannah Arendt's 'banality of evil' concept once again, the eeriest thing about the incident Slobodan witnessed was that everything happened in ominous silence. There was no major strife and the whole process took no longer than half an hour. Afterwards, the train continued on its route, as if nothing untoward had happened, reaching the next station in about ten minutes. The train was not stopped there for any immediate investigation into the incident. Yugoslav (consisting of Serbian and Montenegrin) authorities, for their part, did not try to establish what had happened.

The event did not make it into the news for four days, and even then it was reported as most likely a 'staged incident' to 'invent the alleged endangering of Muslims', 'create strife' and forward a certain 'political agenda'. Rumours subsequently went around that the men who were taken from the train were armed, deserters from the Bosnian army or otherwise 'guilty' on some other unspecified grounds. It took over a decade for the case to become more widely released to the public, predominantly courtesy of new digital technologies, the men's families, initiatives from the Islamic and Bosniak communities in Serbia as well as initiatives by various peace/human rights organisations.

We now know that those kidnapped men were identified in the 'train of death' as non-Serbs, solely based on their names. Out of possibly 20 men taken from the train, 19 are no longer publically 'nameless'. The kidnapped and murdered train passengers were Adem Alomerović (59 years old), Ismet Babačić (30), Fehim Bakija (43), Tomo Buzov (retiree, age unknown), Rasim Ćorić (40), Sead Đečević (16), Muhedin Hanić (27), Rifet Husović (26), Nijazim Kajević (30), Esad Kapetanović (19), Ilijaz Ličina (43), Fikret Memetović (40), Safet Preljević (22), Jusuf Rastoder (45), Šećo Softić (48), Džafer Topuzović (55), Favzija Zeković (54), Zvezdan Zuličić (23) and Hail Zupčević (49). Most of them were either students or employees within institutions in Montenegro and Serbia, one was a citizen of Bosnia and Herzegovina and all the others of the Federal Republic of Yugoslavia (Serbia and Montenegro). We have since heard of the frantic attempts by their families to find out where these men were and what had happened to them after they failed to reach their destinations. Some of their family members spent years contacting every single institution and political entity that they could think of, in both Serbia/Montenegro as well as in Republika Srpska, usually to be dismissed, even humiliated.

Days after their 'disappearance' some of the family members travelled to Republika Srpska trying to negotiate their release. In the end, however, those family members lost their teenage sons and nephews; others lost brothers, husbands and fathers, often the sole breadwinners in the family. But instead of providing support, on at least one occasion the organisation they worked for fired them for 'not showing up to work'. The state, for its part, gave no compensation to the families who were left without any means of support. In at least one instance, a woman whose husband disappeared was told by an official from a Serbian government agency to go and 'ask Alija [Izetbegović, president of Bosnia and Herzegovina] for help'.

We now know the men were abducted by a paramilitary group called *Osvetnici* (Avengers). Presumably this group of Serbian Bosnian men was taking revenge for some unspecified crimes against their fellow Serbs. We also know now that the paramilitary unit's members 'took the abducted citizens to the village of Prelovo near Višegrad, robbed them of their money, jewellery and other valuable possessions and physically abused them in a primary school's gym' (*Tanjug* 2012). The abducted train passengers were then 'tied up with wire and taken by a truck to the garage of a burned-down house close to the banks of the river Drina where they were murdered' (2012). We have also heard that at least one of those men was 'finished' by having his throat slit, after he attempted escape and was shot and wounded in this attempt. Most died from gun wounds; all were tortured. We have since found out that the commander of the Avengers paramilitary unit at the time was Milan Lukić, who was sentenced to life imprisonment for this and other crimes by the International Criminal Tribunal for the former Yugoslavia (ICTY). The only individual convicted for his role in the crime in Serbia-Montenegro was Nebojša Ranisavljević. He was sentenced to 15 years' imprisonment by the FRY Higher Court in the town of Bijelo Polje (in northern Montenegro) on 9 September 2002 (2012). At that trial firm evidence that linked the Avengers with other military and government bodies in Serbia and FR Yugoslavia was supplied (Humanitarian Law Center 2005).

Evidence pointed out that as early as the beginning of February 1993 official memos were sent by Yugoslav Rail to Serbian and Yugoslav authorities warning about plans and even reporting some previous attempts to kidnap train passengers. However, not only did these warnings fall on deaf ears, but discussions took place in some police units about the 'legitimacy' of Republica Srpska officials to mobilise 'deserters' and others. To this day, no representative of any state organisation has been held accountable for the murders. To this day, no significant financial compensation has been offered to the families; a number of them are especially outraged that such compensation has been given to families of a number of Hague (ICTY) prisoners. Of the 19 men taken from the train, only three bodies have been found and identified. The failure of national officials to properly investigate the crime remains a significant but marginalised political issue in Serbia. My uncle Slobodan Boba Vlahović can no longer testify as a witness. He died in 1995 from a heart attack, at 46 years of age.

Out: Men as violence subjects and objects

Behind these actions, behind the drafting, kidnapping and taking of men, there were very concrete actors. To start with, they included the political decision-makers, certain types of (mostly) men who sit 'at the helms of national governments and movements around the world' (Nagel 2005, p. 397), and who create the framework within which such actions take place. They articulate the influential ideologies and dominate the ruling structures of nations and states (2005), they make decisions to start waging war and they give direct orders for the collection of 'cannon fodder'. They also give direct and indirect orders for certain groups of men to be 'taken out', imprisoned or killed. These decision-makers (including many 'fathers of nations') are further supported by the military men, those who are required to embody the figure of the hero that remains 'central to the Western cultural imagery of the masculine' (Connell 2005, p.213). Of all the sites where masculinities are 'constructed, reproduced, and deployed,' argues David Morgan, 'those associated with war and the military are some of the most direct' (1994, p.165). Military-based activity represents 'the traditional way in which the nation is built and strengthened, whether through conquest, defense, or warfare' (Reeser 2010, p.173). As such, it has 'historically ... been an all-male institution' that served as both a coming-of-age tradition for boys as well as the means of making the nation more masculine (2010). And 'despite far-reaching political, social, and technological changes' Morgan argues:

> the warrior still seems to be a key symbol of masculinity. In statues, heroic paintings, comic books, and popular films the gendered connotations are inescapable. The stance, the facial expressions, and the weapons clearly connote aggression, courage, a capacity for violence, and, sometimes, a willingness for sacrifice. The uniform absorbs individualities into a generalized and timeless masculinity while also connoting a control of emotion and a subordination to a larger rationality (Morgan 1994, p.165).

The 'Avengers' from the train, despite being from a paramilitary formation, also wore uniforms, which, in their view, gave them legitimacy. In their delusional and perhaps even semi-conscious state of mind, they too believed themselves to be the embodiment of the historical role of 'Serbian hero'. To this day, one can find books and posters in Serbia defending Serbian heroes imprisoned by the ICTY. Sadly, this type of logic remains behind the reverence of other nation-state heroes as well – despite their brutality towards heroes from the other side as well as against unarmed civilians. Even more unfortunate is the continuing support that militarised and patriarchal societies give them. Their actions, unpunished and even rewarded by the 'men on top', or political decision-makers, enable the continuation of cycle of violence.

Both these groups of men, the actors, are further supported by discourses that sprung from 'masculinized memory, masculinized humiliation and masculinized hope' (Enloe 1990, p.45). In this context, the presence of women in politics, especially given that they are almost always in the minority, does not significantly change the overall highly masculinised political culture. Time and time again research has shown that individual women who find themselves in highly masculinised environments most often adopt the already existing dominant thinking and behaviour. The nation-state, for example, is commonly imagined as masculine, and this is the case not only when women's actual participation is non-existent. Rather, its frames of reference are most often also masculine, including the central notion of 'citizenship'. For example, terms such as 'honor, patriotism, cowardice, bravery, and duty are hard to distinguish as either nationalistic or masculine because they seem so thoroughly tied both to the nation and to manhood' (Dudink et al. 2007, p. xi). There is also another range of 'gendered-masculinized' requirements for citizenship, like 'independence', 'rationality', [and] respectability' (2007). Further, as mentioned in the previous chapter, most nation-states imagine their origins via the 'masculinist birth' of being born 'on the killing fields' (Lake 1992), wherein their rightful place within a community of nations was forcefully asserted. In other words, 'though women might breed a population, giving birth to babies, only men, it seemed, could give birth to the political entity, the imperishable community, of the nation' (Lake 1992, p.307). At times, this masculinist birth is presented as the ultimate masculine utopia. Such a utopia is envisioned by some as the 'masculine allure of adventure' wherein some men may experience their enlistment in wars with 'anticipation and excitement, [with a] sense of embarking on a great adventure, [desiring] not to be "left behind", or "left out" of the grand question that the war represents' (Nagel 2005, p.402). This is also true for some politicians, who, like Slobodan Milošević or Martin Špegelj, connect such grandiose and traditional–patriarchal masculinist fantasies with the survival of nationhood.

At the individual–group level, those two groups of main actors that enact violence – decision-makers and those executing their explicit and implicit orders – both embody or attempt to embody a particular type of masculinity that RW Connell has termed 'hegemonic'. Hegemonic masculinities are vastly interested in maintaining the 'dividend' that they receive from patriarchy in terms of 'honour, prestige and the right to command [as well as gain] a material dividend' (Connell 2005, p.82). Connell terms this masculinity 'hegemonic' because 'at any given time, one form of masculinity rather than others is culturally exalted' (2005, p.77). In a patriarchal–warrior-like society, such hegemonic masculinity will be similarly constructed. In explaining what this hegemonic masculinity is in contemporary Western/global patriarchal society, Connell argues it 'can be defined as the configuration of gender practice which embodies the currently accepted answer to the problem of the legitimacy of patriarchy, which guarantees (or is taken to guarantee) the dominant position of men and the subordination of women'. It is not the case that 'the most visible bearers of hegemonic masculinity are always the most powerful people'. Still, hegemony is 'likely to be established only if there is some correspondence between cultural ideal and institutional power, collective if not individual' (2005). For example:

> the top levels of business, the military and government provide a fairly convincing *corporate* display of masculinity, still very little shaken by feminist women or dissenting men. It is the successful claim to authority, more than direct violence, that is the mark of hegemony (though violence often underpins or supports authority) (2005).

Men embodying hegemonic masculinity, within a context of patriarchal, violence-based society, do not seek to dominate and subordinate women only. They also aspire to dominate other, 'subaltern' men or 'dissenting', 'alternative' masculinities. In other words, the hegemonic masculinity of dominance requires both other 'lower' masculinities as well as women (real and symbolic femininity) to exist as its opposites. Such a construction of hegemonic masculinity also requires discourses on 'real men' and desirable manhood, which are, in the context of patriarchal societies, most often defined by stereotypical psychological traits of machismo. A 'real man' then is a cool guy, a tough guy as well as often *the* guy who solves problems through violence. Within 'the culture of violence called patriarchy' (Gilligan 2001, p.62) the notion of hegemonic masculinity is therefore 'literally defined as involving the expectation, even the requirement, of violence' (2001). In this context, negotiation and nonviolent conflict resolution have often been equated with weakness and passivity, both seen as 'feminine qualities'. 'Real men' of androcracy (Eisler 1987, 1997) thus do not negotiate; they fight. They do not mediate; they serve justice. They do not compromise; they use violence to assert righteousness.[5]

Even though hegemonic masculinity or the ideal of hegemonic masculinity is not 'normal in the statistical sense' (Connell & Messerschmidt 2005, p.832), given that only a minority of men might enact it, it certainly is normative within the context of a dominator (Eisler

2000), patriarchal society. Such a society is characterised by the existence of highly asymmetrical gender roles, further reinforced by the 'differential social psychology of men and women' (Gilligan 2001, p.58). Such differential social psychology requests of men that they possess psychological traits such as mental endurance, bravery, the valuing of high social achievement, respect for authority, self-control and low empathy and sensitivity to other people (Brock-Utne 2010, p.210). These 'normative masculinities' (Mosse 1996) are expected to embody 'western male codes of honor', which focus on a number of 'manly' virtues which include (Nagel 2005, p.400): 'willpower, honor, courage, discipline, competitiveness, quiet strength, stoicism, sangfroid, persistence, adventurousness, independence, sexual virility tempered with restraint, and dignity'. These virtues also reflect masculine ideals such as 'liberty, equality, and fraternity' (2005). Women, on the other hand, are requested to exhibit 'feminine' qualities such as 'tenderness, intimacy, nurturance, passivity, dependency, forgiveness, and the capacity to feel anything, psychical or emotional, including pain, fear, depression, love, compassion, vulnerability, sadness' (Gilligan 2001, p.63). If such qualities are detected in men, for example vulnerability, they do not serve as a determent against violence. Rather, the logic behind hegemonic masculinity development requires such vulnerability in men to be obliterated, and the easiest way to achieve this is via the killing of men that embody, or are perceived to embody, it.

Sadly, the range of emotions allowed for men who act out hegemonic–androcratic[6] masculinity to exhibit and feel is narrow, limited mostly to anger and its variants such as rage and hate. In both broader Western as well in Serbian and Yugoslavian cultural contexts, hegemonic–androcratic masculinities are allowed public expression of certain feelings (such as feeling confident, annoyed, aggravated, frustrated, cranky, impatient, irritated, angry, detached) while suppressing others, or hiding them within the private sphere of the family (such as feeling affectionate, compassionate, loving, afraid, worried, sad, vulnerable, helpless). In such a context many men are psychologically already prepared to enact violence any time their 'honour' is in question, or any time that they may perceive themselves (and those they are expected to 'protect') as vulnerable.

As already mentioned, vulnerability is particularly 'dangerous' for hegemonic, normative or 'real' masculinities of androcracy/dominator society. This is because 'perpetrating violence remains perceived as "masculine", [while] suffering violence tends to have a "feminising" or emasculating effect' (Edwards 2006, p.61). In both situations of wanting to maintain power or of fearing loss of power, contemporary hegemonic–androcratic masculinities commonly resort to violence. That is, violence comes as a result of wanting to re-affirm hegemonic masculinity that may be under threat or is perceived to be under threat. Without finding 'lesser' men whose violation is to re-affirm acting out of hegemonic masculinity, the latter form of masculinity could not exist. And it is by that very act of violation that violent masculinity practices are further enhanced.

Hegemonic–androcratic masculinity therefore continuously requires both 'subservient masculinities and women [to] exist as its counterpart' (Cook-Huffman 2010, p.214). In other words, 'as the hegemonic ideal was being created, it was created against a screen of "others" whose masculinity was thus problematized and devalued' (Kimmel 2005, p.415). In situations of differential power distribution between men, those who embody 'power over' approaches within patriarchal society, that is, those who embody hegemonic masculinity, seek ways to dominate other men, 'weaker' masculinities. These subaltern masculinities are usually minorities of other men: those belonging to other cultural, religious or ethnic groups, or sexual minorities (for example, gay men). Asserting masculinity against effeminate homosexual men is especially important and in this process 'words such as "wimp", "sissy", "girl" and "gay" are frequently used interchangeably to confirm hegemonic masculinity as exclusively heterosexual' (Swain 2005, p.222).

The masculinities of 'other' men are often problematised by either being perceived as 'weak and effeminate' or by being seen as 'hypermasculine, violent and uncontrolled' (Kimmel 2005, p.415). Such construction allows for the problematisation of masculinity of men from different (cultural, ethnic, religious, class, racial) groups, as either 'too much' (threats) or 'not enough' (wimps). What results from this are masculinity wars from which there is no escape for *any* man. Men embodying or wishing to embody hegemonic–androcratic masculinity cannot escape them because their very identity would be threatened. 'Other men' cannot escape them by either manifesting hegemonic masculinity (threats, and participation in masculinity wars as subjects) or by not manifesting it (wimps, and participation in masculinity wars as objects). In either case, they are a legitimate target. The connection between patriarchy and other systems of domination and violence are obvious. What is also clear is that, within a patriarchal–militarised social system, although 'masculinity wars' are inevitable, different groups of men engage in them for different reasons. For some men, masculinity wars – wars in general – are a means of (re)establishing a 'reasonable and right–righteous masculinity' (as in maintaining their power of a dominant group), for others, masculinity wars are evoked as a '*resource* for successfully accomplishing masculine identity particularly when, as it were, all else fails' (Messerschmidt quoted in Edwards 2006, p.6) – that is, the liberation of colonised men, men from marginalised social, cultural and religious groups. For yet another group of men, their engagement in masculinity wars is premised on their efforts to live up to certain models of manhood (Barker 2005); that is, young men participating in gang wars. Commonly, hegemonic–androcratic masculinities from one group fight hegemonic–androcratic masculinities from another group, drawing all other masculinities as well as femininities into their ludicrous wars. Because they are the ones who carry violent means of coercion, from knives and guns to nuclear weapons, it is their will that, presumably, must be obeyed. So a great number of lives are sacrificed on the altar of their holy masculinity wars, where there is often little logic as to who perishes and who lives, despite the efforts by hegemonic-masculinities-in-the-form-of-political-decision-makers who try to convince us otherwise.

Further, in some situations young men are literally 'dying to prove that they are "real men" (Barker 2005). They do so by engaging in gang wars or risky activities. Many men are similarly conscripted into the military and into the war, based on those real-men discourses. Even if they are not too keen, in situations where doing of manhood is equated with doing of state-organised violence, participating in such violence is often the only option available to them, the only way they know how to perform their masculine identity. Thus it could be argued that some forms or practices of masculinity 'may *constitute* violence in themselves' (Edwards 2006, p.61). These may include forms of masculine identity such as:

> Hardness, insensitivity to pain and an unflinching willingness to inflict it when deemed necessary ... seen as vital to many forms of heroism. Practices,

> contexts and outcomes range from minor and mundane including the stigma on crying, suffering in silence and the promotion of the stiff upper lip, to the major and life-threatening such as training for war and military combat (2006).

Such expectations within patriarchal/militarised societies may, to a large degree, explain the differential use of violence by men as compared to women. That is, patriarchal society relegates women to a private sphere and honours them not by their engagement with violence, which is reserved for men, but by their 'chastity outside marriage, and fidelity (and fertility) within marriage' (Gilligan 2001, p.60). Therefore, within 'the culture of violence called patriarchy' (2001, p.62) the role of 'violence–objects' and subjects is assigned to men, wherein men are expected to turn themselves and other men into such subjects–objects during wars or while competing for resources and power in general. The role assigned to women, on the other hand, is that of 'sex-objects' (2001) as well as the role of beauty objects (Wolf 1991). The stronger the patriarchy, the more resilient this template. Such differential social psychology for men and women demands that men use violence not only for 'competition' but also in order to undo 'shame' (Gilligan 2001). At the same time, exactly the opposite is true for women:

> ...women are shamed not for being too submissive, dependent, unaggressive, and sexually

> inactive or impotent, as men are, but rather, for exactly the opposite traits: being too rebellious, independent, aggressive, and sexually active. Thus, if a woman responds to being shamed by becoming aggressive or violent, that may only lead to more shame rather than, as for men, to less (Gilligan 2001, p.58).

Warrior societies of course, feed into such hegemonic notions of femininity and masculinity, and androcratic masculinities that are intimately interlinked with violence. When nations are imagined (Anderson 1991), they are also imagined as communities of desirable masculinities and femininities. In this process violence commonly:

> becomes a way for men to accomplish masculinity and to maintain positions of privilege within the hierarchy. Masculine identity is often so closely linked to violence that violence may be the glue that holds communities of young males together. Acts of violence serve to both create the male self and to valorize the masculine ideal (Cook-Huffman 2010, p.214).

The notion of hegemonic–androcratic masculinity is important for peace and conflict studies because it recognises that both a plurality of masculinities as well as the hierarchy of masculinities exist, hierarchy that is often asserted and maintained via direct and structural violence (Connell & Messerschmidt 2005, p.832). And while violence in dominator societies may be exercised 'against young men during rites of passage into manhood ... the mark of male maturity.. is most often a demonstration of one's capacity to exercise violence against others' (McInturff 2010, p.223). This plurality and hierarchy of masculinities, as well as understanding of actions needed for the maintenance of hegemonic–androcratic types, further explains the paradox of violence most often being a male prerogative, with the simultaneous reality that not all men are violent, and that even those that are violent are only violent in specific situations. Further, such conceptualisation of masculinity allows for seeing the victimisation and vulnerability of men themselves, something that has also only very recently become a (more) common place in peace and conflict theorising.

This new theorising has enabled us to see that when violence is exercised in wars, most victims of men are men. Until recently this was hidden from public view, because the winners of masculinity battles have focused on their hero status not their victimhood while trying to achieve it. The template of heroism is so strong that even when wars are lost, defeat is constructed in terms of heroism (for example, the Serbian loss at Kosovo in the fourteenth century, the Serbian defeat by NATO forces in 1999). 'We survived and we defended the country,' said Milošević after (by all rational accounts) a devastating defeat by NATO, echoing the formulation of many others before and presaging those who come after him. As always, he proclaimed, Serbian people were brave and proud, and their great victory over NATO (led by him) meant that the territorial integrity and sovereignty of Serbia (including Kosovo being part of it) could never again be questioned.

Unlike women whose victimhood in wars is presented as such, and most commonly appropriated for nationalistic agendas, victimhood of men is most often repackaged as heroism. The reality of men as victims of war, however, is stark. Sadly, these victims of male gender are commonly young–younger men, or those of combat age. It is them the hegemonic–androcratic masculinities of decision makers love to sacrifice, so that their ambitions for power or territory are finally satisfied.

In: Dying to be men

Like my Uncle Slobodan, I too witnessed the identification process that was to take some men to war and death. During the 1990s, Serbian men were needed as cannon fodder, which has been a traditional role in wars for centuries for men from lower classes and for younger men. The majority of men from Serbia, some 15 per cent of the male population that participated in the wars on Yugoslav territory in the period between 1991 and 1999 was drafted. Very few, overall, volunteered to go to war. Most of my friends did not want to go to war, and so several managed to go overseas and even more went into hiding. But this option was only possible for some men, men who did not have families to take care of and jobs to go to, who were financially supported by parents and had somewhere to hide, most often in other people's homes (of friends and relatives). Police and the army regularly visited the homes and workplaces of those men marked for drafting – one of my friends had nine visitations to his home in a week. Further, police and the military were fetching men from trains, buses and streets, and even from cafés and pubs. Most men could not hide outside of Serbia either, because neighbouring countries closed their borders and the 'civilised West' would not issue them visas. If they were to fight others they would take the role of murderers and aggressors. If they were to fight their own government, they would take the role of traitors. Wherever they turned, there was no escaping participation in war, one way or another.

I was in a café when an evening of pleasant socialising ended with the removal of several young men who were taken into the night by two heavily armed policemen. The café was located on the 23 October Boulevard, a street I had lived in for 15 years, a street named in honour of the day in 1944 when my hometown of Novi Sad was liberated from the Axis occupation. That night the policemen came with the intention of 'liberating' a certain group of men from their civilian status. They walked in and while one just stood there in the middle of the café with his legs slightly spread and his hands tucked over his weapon-carrying belt, the other demanded that the music be turned off. They also asked all of us to show them our identification cards. In dead silence, the process of identifying us was carried out. Without any words, a couple of young men were shown the exit door with a slight movement of the head and eyes, as if saying 'Let's go'. Those men did not ask where they were going, for they knew. All of us sitting there also knew.

Once the police left the café so did most of the patrons. The music was turned back on, but it was much lower and hardly anybody was in the mood for partying, socialising or celebrating any longer. This was a solemn occasion when, we later found out, a couple of young men who left Croatia because they did not want to have to choose between their Serbian (ethnic) and Croatian (citizenship) identity, and who did not consider it their 'masculine duty' to have to do so, were sent back there to fight somebody else's war. Once caught, deemed capable and drafted by the military, they had very little choice but to be part of the army and try not to get killed – by killing others.

Never before were the nation–states' and androcratic decision-makers' sacrificial practices of sending young men to death more visible to me then when I visited my grandmother Zora in 2000, a year after the hegemonic–androcratic masculinities of the 'civilised' and 'rational' punished overly aggressive Serbian masculinities who waged civil wars in the former

Yugoslavia (Slovenia, Croatia, Bosnia and Herzegovina) and Serbia (Kosovo). In 1999, NATO intervened on the territory of Serbia and Montenegro. That year a man who had promised to 'his Serbian people' after his Gazimestan speech in 1989 that no one will be 'allowed to beat you' decided to draft yet another group of young Serbian men from my grandmother's town of Kruševac (and elsewhere) and send them to defend Kosovo. Shot from across a hundred of kilometres radius, the bombs dispatched by NATO were directed towards legitimate 'military targets'. And in those military targets, young men from Kruševac and elsewhere, armed with guns and rifles, sat waiting for the command to take down the foreign enemy, the occupier. Those young men in their early twenties sat and waited, obeying their state, their army and their president, waiting patiently for a chance to show their own patriotism and loyalty, as well as to 're-affirm their manhood'. They never got that chance.

No enemy soldier (from NATO) died during the three months of bombing of Serbia (including Vojvodina and Kosovo) and Montenegro. No Serbian politician who made decisions that saw those young men sent to almost certain death died. On the other hand, countless young draftees, some volunteers – hardly any volunteered for this war, compared to the wars in Croatia and Bosnia – as well as thousands of civilians in Serbia and Montenegro of all nationalities did die. The families of the killed organised the funerals and the wakes, informing communities of the events through the local paper. Pages upon pages of local papers were filled with obituaries, mostly photos of young men, the years of their birth and death under those photos, with occasional poetic outpourings of grief in a couple of sentences and with the critical information of where and when the funeral was to take place.

Out: Men's expendable lives

This lack of real or perceived choice is what inspired a number of theorists to argue that despite men being predominant violence subjects the right terminology for men in regards to violence is, in fact, that of being 'violence objects'. This is because the patriarchal mindset considers each capable male over a certain age a soldier, a potential warrior, irrespective of a particular man's inclinations, level of military training or even (in)ability to use weaponry effectively or access it. Patriarchal societies assign the role of fighting in wars to men and most commonly they are 'not given any choice about the matter':

> if they refuse to treat other men as objects of violence, and thereby simultaneously become objects of those men's violence, they will be shamed and insulted (called cowards) and then turned into objects of their own army's violence. 'Deserters' have traditionally been shot. And just as men are shamed for refusing to treat other men and themselves as violence-objects, they are

> honored for being willing to do so (Gilligan 2001, p.59).

'Killing the enemy in warfare is violent', but is not only simply expected of men, it is also the 'grounds for being awarded a medal' (DeKeseredy & Schwartz 2005, p.355). The patriarchal mindset that is internalised by both sexes also sees it as somehow 'more "appropriate" to kill a man than to kill a woman' (2005), which is yet another reason for Gilligan's use of the term 'violence-objects' for men. This argument is further expanded by Kathleen Barry:

> I first began to think about dehumanization of men ... when something struck me as oddly wrong about the reports of civilian casualties as 'the loss of innocent life' ... That term 'innocent lives' nagged me until I finally asked myself, 'If we agree that it is wrong to kill civilians in war, then there must be others who *can* be killed. Our language, even that which we use to expose killing civilians, condones killing. That is, we, as societies, states, countries, peoples, conspire to agree that it is all right to kill some people, those whose lives are not innocent. Who are these people?' Men in combat (2010, p.6).

Within the overall paradigm of war, therefore, 'it is acceptable, if regrettable, inevitable and unavoidable that men will be killed in combat – on every side' (2010). Even international humanitarian law has forsaken men, argues Barry. For example, 'Article 3.1 of the 1949 United Nations Genève Convention indirectly, yet nevertheless decisively, holds that only those persons taking no active part in the hostilities ... shall in all circumstance be treated humanely' (2010, p.8). Turning this around means that those engaged in hostilities are excluded from protection of their right to live or from being treated humanely, which also means that 'the Geneva Conventions actually violate the Universal Declaration of Human Rights of 1948, which guarantees that "everyone has the right to life, liberty and security of persons"' (2010, p.9). Men in combat thus know that they are killable, legally, making them our 'expendable lives' (2010, pp.7–8). If our androcratic societies make them be so inconsequential, no wonder such awareness, even at the subconscious level, makes them repay us not only by 'heroism' but by monstrosity as well.

This expendability of violence-objects – that is, of men, or more precisely men of combat age – makes them 'the most vulnerable and consistently targeted population group' for violence, 'through time and around the world today' (Jones 2006, p.201). Bosniak men taken from trains and buses in Serbia and Bosniak men in Srebrenica who were summarily executed just because they were [other] men were not the only ones vulnerable and victimised. Such male vulnerability is a global and long-standing historical phenomenon. It is men who 'bear the brunt of armed conflict', argue the authors behind the 2005

Human Security Report (Human Security Centre 2005, p.110). 'Both in uniform and out, men have been, and continue to be, killed, wounded and tortured in far greater numbers than women' (2005). Despite difference in ratios that are time and place specific, data still consistently shows that most of the victims of war and violence are of male gender. Men of 15 to 55 years of age are 'nearly universally perceived as the group posing the greatest danger to conquering force' (Jones 2006, p.201) and are therefore killed due to 'part revenge and part bleak strategic logic: killing battle-age males minimises future threats to the victors' (Human Security Centre 2005, p.111). This group of men is also most likely to 'have the repressive apparatus of the state directed against them' as there is:

> a broad spectrum of the forms of state and sub state violence to which men and boys are disproportionately vulnerable ... [which includes] police and death-squad killings and 'disappearances'; gender-selective roundups, torture, and 'filtration'; vigilante violence, incarceration without trial; and violence against gays (Jones 2006, p.202).

In some parts of the world, for example in countries such as 'Jamaica, Brazil, Colombia and some parts of sub-Saharan Africa, young men's mortality rates are higher than in countries with declared wars' (Barker 2005, p.1). Young men aged between 15 and 25:

> die at rates far higher than their female counterparts, and at rates higher than men of any other age group ... Worldwide, [their] leading cause of death ... are traffic accidents and homicide – both directly related to how boys and men are socialized (2005).

'Why the worry about young men', asks Gary Barker before giving data that justifies such worry:

> In India and other parts of South Asia, there have been numerous studies and reports on 'missing women and girls' ... In parts of Latin America, while on a much smaller scale, there are 'missing young men'. In Brazil, for example, the 2000 census confirmed that there were nearly 200,000 fewer men than women in the age range 15–29 because of higher rates of mortality through accidents, homicide and suicide among young men ... By the year 2050, Brazil will have 6 million fewer men than women, principally because of violence (2005, p.1).

Observations about most men's reluctance to go to war and engage in acts of collective violence could also serve to justify the terminological shift from men as violence subjects to men as violence objects. From the Serbian saying *'Rado ide Srbin u vojnike, dva ga vuku a trojica tuku!'* 'Gladly a Serb enlists (to be a soldier), two (men) are dragging him and three are beating him!' to peace scholars' observations that it is the principal task of men's military training to overcome 'the average individual's deep-seated resistance to killing' (Paige 2009, p.39), there is a recurrent theme of most men's reluctance to engage in violence. 'Contrary to the idea that war thrills men, expresses innate masculinity, or gives men a fulfilling occupation', writes Goldstein, 'all evidence indicates that war is something that societies impose on men, who most often need to be dragged kicking and screaming into it, constantly brainwashed and disciplined once there, and rewarded and honored afterwards' (Goldstein 2001, p.253). This is not only the case in so-called peaceful societies, for which Goldstein finds very little evidence. While his point about the rare existence of peaceful societies throughout history could be easily disputed via Douglas Fry's 'Seven Ways to Make Peaceful Societies Disappear' (2004), the point Goldstein makes about non-peaceful societies is highly valid: 'even the most warlike peoples must be "persistently nagged into committing acts of inhumanity" ... "it takes a major effort to make aggressive warriors out of tribal [male] children" [even] ... in warlike societies' (2001, p.253).

Some mechanisms of turning Yugoslav and Serbian men (and women) in general into violence subjects and objects have been described in previous chapters (notions of selective remembering and the politics of victimhood; social militarism; collective violence pedagogy; colonisation, imperialism and 'balkanism', nationalism). In addition to these discourses, and almost indistinguishable from them, is the androcratic discourse on maleness and manhood. All the previous discourses are critical in creating a war/violence culture, but the issue of gender is crucial. Even though gender does not stand alone in determining one's identity and behaviour but rather exists in 'a complex relationship with other identity markers, including age, race, religion, ethnicity, language group, caste, class and sexuality, which can exacerbate inequality and vulnerability to violence or mitigate them' (McInturff 2010, p.223), gender still 'profoundly affects the likelihood that an individual will participate in a violent act, or be the subject of a violent act' (2010, p.222).

Gender also has an impact in determining the type of violence to which a particular individual will be subjected (2010). At the group level, it influences the rationale and the meaning behind the enactment of acts of collective violence. In both homicides and genocides, men are disproportionate objects of violence *and* they are disproportionate subjects of it. This is not the result of a public sphere traditionally belonging to them, because violence takes place in the private sphere as well. And this is certainly not the result of men being more active, as women do as much if not more work, albeit their activities are usually unrecognised/unappreciated and not adequately rewarded financially and socially. In both these spheres, the link between the war system and the gendered system of patriarchy is indisputable via the particular social practice of hegemonic– androcratic masculinity. Without specifically raising and forcing men with the goal of satisfying the demands of this type of masculinity, we would not have a group constantly primed and prepared for the enactment of violence. As peace scholars have repeatedly shown, the waging of war is not the result of a random event, but of continual processes or sets of processes that finally lead to it. So if we had a different set of processes for the enactment of nonviolent masculinities (and femininities), we would also have different types of decision-makers and different type of 'security'. Further to this, without the patriarchal war system that turns men into both violence subjects and objects, via activation of a number of discourses that demands men embrace the task of aggressive killing, collective violence at a scale seen in wars would not be possible.

This connection is not straightforward though. That is, two systems are so intertwined in patriarchal societies that violence is strongly connected to questions of masculinity while simultaneously masculinity is predicated on violence (Edwards 2006, p.60). There is a 'reverse causality' between war and gender (Goldstein 2001, p.411), and 'neither sexism nor the war system can be overcome independently from the other' (Reardon 2000, p.252). In other words: 'war will not be unmade without remaking masculinity. That is an imperative, if we are to have peace' (Barry 2010, p.10). But as each war most often remasculinises society and forces men into roles of violence subjects–objects, without challenging the war system that reinforces patriarchal (or androcratic–hegemonic) masculinity, manhood defined in this way will continue to be a major factor of war–violence.

To return to the questions raised earlier, it seems that we know exactly where the men who enacted the violence previously described came from. They came from patriarchal systems and worldviews that define desirable masculinity in terms of its connection with violence. For many men who live in patriarchal social systems and worldviews, violence too often becomes 'the only perceived available technique of expressing and validating masculinity' (DeKeseredy & Schwartz 2005, p.362). It is the only way for them to validate their own identity/sense of self and of their belonging to the broader (ethnic, national) group. Because the link between androcratic– hegemonic masculinity and violence is both assumptive as well as widely held, it has the 'quality of appearing to be "natural"' (Nagel 2005, p.400). But similarly to the doing of peace – via the presence of social actions that promote positive peace and structural justice – the doing of gender also denotes a process. Doing of gender means the enactment of femininities and masculinities – rather than simply accepting a state (of being a natural or real woman/man). This new focus on the *performativity* of gender (Butler 1990) has by now become critical to our understanding of how hegemonic as well as alternative masculinities and femininities are created.

Most importantly, precisely because gender is in contemporary gender theory understood as something we *do* rather than who we *are,* or, as a role that we perform and which is socially constructed, this assumes a possibility for change. Courtesy of peace, women's/feminist, some spiritual/religious and ecological social movements, alternative nonviolent masculinities (and femininities), which are marginalised, have already been imagined as well as practised. The nineteenth and twentieth centuries have seen scores of women challenge traditional notions of (subservient) femininity. Challenge to traditional notions of hegemonic–androcratic masculinity by both women and men is, however, in its embryonic stages. Thus, explicitly describing, practising and enhancing nonviolent masculinities, to paraphrase earlier points by Messerschmidt, Nagel and Galtung, may then be a major, perhaps *the major,* factor of nonviolence and peace. In other words, in analysing pathways to peace, this major factor should not be missed.

In: Mirna's voice

Mirna was born in 1969 in Belgrade, the daughter of my aunt Svetlana and her husband Izudin from Sarajevo. While she spent her early childhood years in Sarajevo, her parents' divorce brought her back to her birthtown. And so it was in Belgrade that her nearly decade-long involvement in politics – via street protests and nonviolent demonstrations against Milošević's regime – was born as well. She first took part in street demonstrations in 1991, on 9 March – just before the whole of Yugoslavia started to collapse – in demonstrations that were seeking the establishment of true democracy. These demonstrations arose as a protest against the editorial politics of Radio-Television Belgrade:

> I and many of us gathered there were opposing the descent into totalitarianism that we were strongly against. Given that we did not speak the same language as people obsessed with Milošević, and given that we could only hear their voices and not our views publicly broadcasted, we had to take it to the streets. Streets and city squares were the only places where we could find similarly minded people, where we could express our views. Streets and city squares gave us a voice. They were the only public spaces where you could show anybody that you were against what was going on in Serbian society and on Serbian television; to show anybody that you were against all that, that you were neither satisfied nor happy with what was happening.
>
> The first street gathering that I participated in was at Terazijska česma Square. Terazijska česma was a place of gathering on that day due to demonstrations at Trg Republike, a common place for prodemocracy protests to take place, being brutally supressed the day before. Yes, [I participated in] all the students' and citizens'

protests that were organised in the period between 1991 and 2000 in Belgrade. My last public protest took place on 5 October 2000, when Milošević was finally removed from power. The reasons why I participated in all those protests for nearly ten years were many. First, one could not tell if the system under Milošević's command had any kind of meaningful structure, the goals of that system, party and state were not apparent; you did not know if there would be war tomorrow or not, if you were to fight with your nearest neighbour or with the whole world – or not. And that horrible isolation from the rest of the world, negation of everything that was beyond the borders of the state in which you live was actually perceived as something 'normal' by the regime and its supporters.

But that was not normal to me. There was also a general feeling of imprisonment and that you were constantly being under threat. Imprisonment was also felt when you needed 700 papers (figuratively speaking) just to get a visa to travel, and you constantly had to provide some sort of justification to somebody as to who you were. Then, under that regime many people were hungry, our monthly salary was five German marks, shop shelves were empty, there was a war nearby, and masses of refugees everywhere. Most importantly we had no idea where all this was leading, what kind of future we were going towards. All of us, who opposed the regime, thus had to create an imaginary future, a desired future where we wanted to be, because nothing else was explicitly offered in any case, against which you could fight or complain. Of course, even in such a repressive regime you could find ways to inform yourself, if you wanted, and so we did find alternative ways to inform ourselves. The person who wants to know, always does know. You felt powerless as you were against all that was going on, so you looked for like-minded people, primarily in our immediate surrounding, amongst family and friends. We then joined protests because they were in line with our political stand; we wanted to show how many of us disagreed with the regime. Given that media was state controlled where else could you show such disagreement but on the streets? This is how it was.

The demonstrations of 1996 and1997 were different from those of 1991. I participated in both students' as well as citizen-based demonstrations then. Student-based protests were organised separately, because we did not want to be used for some other political purposes by the existing political parties. The main reason for these demonstrations of 1996–97 was the stealing of votes by Milošević's regime. By this theft, my voice and the voices of many others were also stolen. So, if a regime steals your voice – the only legitimate way in democratic societies to express your opinion towards those in power – then, what is left? If voting is our only means for nonviolently changing government, in democratic societies that has to be respected. The regime was saying that we, the students, were being manipulated, they were saying we should focus on our studies and not get politicised in this way. But if my voice is stolen through rigged elections, how else can I express my disagreement? Stealing caused feelings of disempowerment; personally, disempowerment frustrates me more than anything else, so what else is left but to take it to the streets?

The main drivers of the 1996–97 demonstrations were the need for recognition of the reality: the majority of the people wanted a change of government, but the elections were rigged. These mass demonstrations were but one organised protest in the continuum of demonstrations that took place between 1991 and 2000. They were the longest lasting (and very successful in my view) because even though Milošević was not removed from power then, people who led the demonstrations – such as Zoran Đinđić, Vesna Pešić and Vuk Drašković – were later elected to office. The president of Serbia at the time, Milan Milutinović, on the other hand, was later tried for war crimes by the ICTY.

Some people felt the demonstrations were not successful because there were so many years of protesting and nothing was changing; I do not see it that way. In the end, all our goals were met: the recognition of voting results and the democratic removal of Milošević from power: this finally happened in 2000.

The situation during those latest protests in 2000 was the most dangerous. The regime had used violence in the past. In the 1990s and in 2000 they used arrests, tanks, water cannon, police cars rushing into the mass of people, batons, tear gas, guns, armoured cars, anti-terrorist units – anything to maintain their power. In 2000 we knew they would be brutal, as they really felt their power slipping away. The 1999 NATO bombing made them even more radicalised and violent. Still, in those ten years I never worried about violence, whether I would be injured or not, because I never went there to 'pick a fight'. I was focused on the goal, I was focused on the expression of my political voice and I was focused on the future I wanted. Demonstrations were nonviolent as the thinking behind them was along these lines: If I do not want somebody to use repression against me then obviously I should not use violence myself. But even though we were not using violence, the police were.

I don't think gender dimension featured prominently, actually, I don't think it was at all significant. I mean, the police were all men, because it is men who normally work for the police. As for us demonstrators, we were 50/50. I don't think these policemen treated women and men demonstrators differently, because a number of women got badly beaten up as well. Leadership positions, however, even in these protest movements were mostly occupied by men. I think that reflects the overall political situation in Serbia, men in general take those type of positions in politics. After the goals of the protests were achieved, most women withdrew from participation in politics; they went back to their own lives. I myself was not interested at all in gaining any particular prominence, entering official politics or in openly exhibiting myself. My only motive was to show publicly my point of view, and to ask that election results be officially recognised. Most girls and women I knew had similar motivations, so, after our goals were reached, we felt no further need to continue with such intense political engagement. This was also the case with most men, only a handful actually, in the end perhaps only two, entered the official politics. But during Milošević's oppressive regime, the gender composition of demonstrators was quite balanced: we were all equally interested in what was happening. Perhaps, women were a little bit more persistent – when numbers started to wane in various demonstrations cycles, I think it was more women who were still there.

Out: Feminist eutopia – alternative peace-oriented masculinities and femininities

The peaceful and pro-peace demonstrations that Mirna participated in not only showed that different power is possible, their participants also modelled different, nonviolent, masculinities and, equally nonviolent, femininities. Both these groups transgressed the dominant view that revolutions or social change equals violence, and that the only way to remove violent dictators from power is through the only language that they understand (that is, violence). Both these groups transgressed the dominant expectations of their gender, which commonly exist within a context of patriarchal, warrior or violence-based societies. To start with, women protestors abandoned the requirement to remain passive, subservient and apolitical – and to do their peacemaking work within the constraints of the family. They reclaimed the public sphere as their own, and demanded a just and peace-oriented society. Men protestors, for their part, abandoned patriarchal requirement to link their masculinity with violence, especially when engaged in political battles. Unlike violent revolutionaries and warriors (military and paramilitary), who symbolically link the hegemonic masculine principle with violence, these male protestors embodied a different form of masculinity. And unlike the Serbian hypermasculine war volunteer and official army and police units, male street protestors engaged in partnership with women during those years of their joint political struggle.

Together they modelled gender equality through overall participation (women protesters made up between 44.9 and 49 per cent of the participants in the 1996–97 demonstrations) and commitment (both genders attended the protests in equal measure, in other words they were not heavily male or female dominated). While at the beginning some sexism did creep in, it later dissipated (Blagojević 1999). For example, the throwing of eggs, initially defined as evidence that the politicians who were opponents of Milošević's violent regime did 'not have balls', was later reinterpreted as a 'symbol of the birth of a new world which has to crack the shell in order to come out' (1999, p.122). Later props used during the protests (by male and female participants) included flowers, songs, parades, dress-ups, humorous skits, graffiti, street theatre, music performances, mock awards and elections, all aimed at delivering 'sophisticated and humorous political messages' (1999, p.115). Participants in the nonviolent youth movement *Otpor* (Resistance), aimed at overthrowing Slobodan Milošević in 2000, continued with this tradition, coming from the decade of protests in the 1990s. Their main symbol, a clenched fist, indicated unity and solidarity with the oppressed rather than the dominant, hegemonic group, as well as strength and defiance (Wikipedia 2010).

Serbian paramilitary guards (Milan Lukić, Željko Ražnatović Arkan, Vojislav Šešelj, 'Kapetan Dragan' and others), on the other hand, founded not only the explicitly named Avengers but also the 'Tigers', the 'White Eagles', the 'Scorpions', the 'Yellow Wasps' and the 'Wolves', all of which symbolically connect the hegemonic masculine principle with violence – piercing, penetrating, powerful, virulent and potentially lethal. Both their actions as well as such symbolism was to connect them with the hegemonic–androcratic form of masculinity. Similar to policemen 'legitimising' our identities in the café incident, these groups have shown their desire for dominating through their symbols, actions and even body language.

Serbian *Otporaši,* war resisters and nonviolent protestors walked and positioned their bodies differently. Their body language was not that of male dominance and hegemony (as in: chest pushed forward, arms held slightly away from the body to take up extra space, legs similarly spread and extended, walking with that unmistakeable swagger, a serious or frowning face) but was largely non-threatening (relaxed extremities and walk, taking as much space as the body really needs, softer facial expressions). Despite this, and despite the nonviolent nature of the protest, all protestors were occasionally attacked violently by carriers of hegemonic–androcratic masculinity.

As could be expected, given the earlier theoretical points in regards to 'differential psychology' for men and women, there was also a gendered difference in verbal attacks on men and women. These verbal attacks aimed to discredit protestors by challenging their masculinity (for men) or, alternatively, chastity (for women). So while both groups had to contend with accusations of being traitors, spies and 'foreign payees', it was only women whose chastity was called into question – the most commonly thrown gender specific accusations for them were those of whore and slut. On the other hand, men who refused violent ethnic nationalism and the role of hegemonic–androcratic masculinity, whether as war deserters, draft evaders and conscientious objectors or as street protestors, continuously had to come to terms with their masculinity being challenged. They had to resist attempts to construct their gender identity as inclusive of violent masculinity, which asks for fulfilment via participation in direct violence and wars. They had to come to terms with discourses that constructed them as 'cowards and lesser men, who hide "under their mother's skirt" or leave the homeland altogether ... who are "faggots" and "scumbags," people whom a real Serbian man has to cut out from his inner circle' (Milićević 2006, p.281). Occasionally they were also accused of being *pizd* e (cunts) (Forum B92 2009).

As Gilligan explains, this challenge to their masculinity makes perfect sense within the patriarchal worldview that constructs desirable femininities as chaste, and desirable masculinities as violence subjects–objects. In this process, the patriarchal worldview demands that the maleness/masculinity of the opponent be challenged, this being part of the overall masculinity wars. This logic is based on the dominant assumption that 'the reduction of masculinity equals insult by default' (Milojević 2003, p.33). And so those who embody nonviolent masculinities, in addition to resisting oppressive systems of power, must also resist attacks on their very own gender identity. They have to stay firm in their own definition of appropriate masculinity, of their own interpretations of what real men do, or do not do. Nonviolent protestors of the 1990s and 2000 did just that. Furthermore, they actively embraced traditional feminine principles of support, caring and empathy with others. Women protestors, on the other hand, embraced traditional masculine principles of autonomy, assertiveness and of having a public/political voice. Together, they succeeded in *Bringing Down a Dictator* (York 2002) and in giving birth to the embryonic peace-oriented civil society in Serbia. Simultaneously, they constructed and manifested new stories of gender.

Therefore, in addition to social practices that connect masculinity with violence, there always have been alternative, nonviolent ways to perform masculinity. These existed even in the most violent societies and environments. Definitions and understandings of masculinity in a number of peaceful societies, and various spiritual, political and religious communities, also provide ample historical evidence wherein the otherwise widespread 'performativity of masculinity = performativity of violence' link was either severed completely, or did not feature as prominently as it does in violent, patriarchal societies. Indeed, instead of hegemonic– androcratic or violent–patriarchal and domineering masculinity, their hegemonic (as in normative and socially prescribed/desired) masculinity is predominantly nonviolent.

To start with peaceful societies: the performativity of nonviolent masculinities in them (already touched upon in Chapter 1 in the section on raising children and worldview) is underpinned by spiritual, philosophical and cognitive templates that consider violence to be harmful, unnecessary and detrimental, rather than as a phenomenon arising from 'human nature' or 'male nature'. These nonviolent templates do not consider violence as unavoidable and even moral, and they reject the story about good violence and bad violence (Howell & Willis 1989; Bonta 1996; Boulding 2000; Eisler 2000; Kelleher 2010). Most importantly, in peaceful societies and other peace-oriented spiritual/religious and political communities, normative masculinity is not defined via the use or the right to use 'good' violence. Furthermore, in more gender egalitarian societies and communities, differentiation between masculinity and femininity is not imagined in hierarchical terms (Eisler 1987), even though there is gender differentiation of labour. Crucially, aggression and violence are not automatically connected with maleness; on the other hand, angry persons and warring neighbours are perceived in negative terms and as negative role models (Boulding 2000; Kelleher 2010). Both boys and girls are raised with values of nurturance, harmony, self-restraint, cooperation, sharing and generosity, fair and mutual exchange (that is, ceremonial gift giving). All these values are integrated within a worldview and cosmology that focuses on the interconnectedness of all life (Bonta 1996; Boulding 2000). Both historical as well as contemporary peace-oriented communities raise young men to 'care for other human beings, to be emotional and warm' (Brock-Utne 2010, p.209). They may define male power via different protective capabilities; and such different type of power may indeed incorporate what patriarchal societies consider feminine values of caring, gentleness and compassion.

The idea, asserted frequently in Western political theory, that men need to 'compete and that women are an important object of competition' is contradicted by evidence from at least four of the peaceful societies described by Howell and Willis (1989, p.12). When these, and other peaceful societies, are compared to patriarchal and violent ones, we can see even more clearly the connections between social definitions of masculinity and 'the propensity towards violence and sexual violence' (Hearn 2010):

> In societies where men were permitted to acknowledge fear, levels of violence were likely to be lower; in societies where masculine bravado, repression and denial of fear defined masculinity, and masculinity and femininity were highly differentiated, violence was likely to be higher. Themes linking with interpersonal and inter-societal violence included: most public interaction being between men, rather than between men and women, or among women; boys and girls systematically separated at early age; male economic activities and products of male labour prized over female's (2010).

This differentiation between females and males, including the sexual division of labour and sexual division of 'life giving/taking' (that is mothers/soldiers), is as natural as is violence resulting from human or male nature. In fact, 80 years of research into the gender-based psychological and character differences between males and females, in population studies by psychologists, has shown 'remarkable similarity' between these two groups (Connell 2009, p.60). Perhaps not surprisingly given the social construction of gender, it is when gender differences are potentiated, that they grow larger, but at times when they are minimised, they grow smaller (2009).

So not only has the idea of an innate character dichotomy between women and men been 'overwhelmingly, decisively refuted ... The broad psychological similarity of men and women as groups can be regarded, on the volume of evidence supporting it, as one of the best-established generalisations in all the human sciences' (2009, p.65). It is remarkable 'how similar the two sexes become, psychologically, when gender fades into the background' argue Michael Kimmel and Cordelia Fine: 'Love, tenderness, nurturance; competence, ambition, assertion – they are *human* qualities, and all human beings – both women and men – should have equal access to them' (Fine 2010, p.237).

These positive human qualities can be, and often are, then, equally shared among genders. All societies and cultures, including extreme dominator–patriarchal–violent cultures have had alternative ways of promoting peace-oriented masculinities. Given the noise hegemonic– violent masculinities create, the voices of alternative–peaceful masculinities are often lost. However, although society may function in many ways to 'promote male violence, there remain in any situation other means of expressing one's masculinity' (DeKeseredy & Schwartz 2005, p.356). Working in a context where violent masculinities are the norm (youth gangs, South America), Barker found there were still many young men who succeeded in staying out of gangs, and out of violence. They did so by finding another identity, or another masculinity 'hat', for example by excelling in 'sports, or music or [they] have some culturally relevant skill that allows them to feel secure in achieving a non-violent and more gender-equitable versions of manhood' (Barker 2005, p.147). These other skills could include being adept with computers, excelling in one or more academic subjects, being involved in a meaningful extracurricular activity or having mechanical abilities, which becomes their 'source of belonging, pride and self-esteem' (2005). As well, Barker found that young men with a strong religious conviction – and who found a sense of identity in their religion and a peer group with fellow members of the same religion – were 'also able to stay out of gangs with relative ease' (2005). In addition to having a special skill or a religious conviction, three other factors helped with the ability to differ and resist pressures to embody violent masculinity: some degree of metacognition, an alternative worldview and different masculine ethics.

Metacognition helped young men with 'self-reflective abilities, that is living a reflective life' (2005, p.148) and enabled them to question traditional views of manhood. Younger boys who were desperately trying to fit in, on the other hand, 'to be socially recognized and not to be seen as "geeks" or "wimps" often have [had] tremendous difficulty stepping back and questioning the versions of manhood that are forced upon them' (2005). But young men who were 'able to think about how they think', on the other hand:

> Showed a higher degree of awareness of their own emotional life, what Howard Gardner and others have called emotional intelligence ... They

> were able to see when they were losing control, and were able to identify and use coping or anger management strategies ... they were also aware of when they need to use those strategies ... a combination of coping or anger control strategies (2005).

Earlier, I highlighted the role of the alternative worldview and its importance for the creation of both alternative nonviolent masculinities and societies. Barker's research confirms this. More specifically, it confirms that in violence-based societies 'to change the behaviour, it is necessary to work with young men to question these [traditional, patriarchal] beliefs – to question the gender matrix – at the societal and individual level' (2005, p.154). This questioning is supplemented by assisting them in developing different 'masculine ethics of ... care, respect and empathy' (2005). Such ethics and worldview are instrumental in supporting alternative, nonviolent, adaptive and healthy characteristics of masculinity, within a broader context of a positive psychology perspective (Kiselica 2010, p.134). This positive psychology/positive masculinity model is radically different from the 'differential psychology' within patriarchal society that Gilligan (2001) has described. While providing an overview of the 'positive psychology/positive masculinity' model, Mark Kiselica highlights ten main pathways of possible intervention, or of strengthening the link between healthy masculinity and positive psychology. Some of those pathways include:

- male relational styles (that is, men and boys having fun and developing 'friendships and intimacy with each other through shared activities')
- male ways of caring (boys and men raised with the expectation of caring for and protecting their loved ones and friends)
- generative fatherhood (engagement in positive and engaged fathering)
- humanitarian service of fraternal organizations
- male heroism (the positive qualities of traditional masculinity through acts by heroic men which could include 'everyday heroes, such as hard working, devoted fathers') (2011, pp.133–38).

Even the traditional 'hero's journey' (Campbell 1949) could be (and is) used as a symbol for the development and enhancement of nonviolent rather than violent masculinities. As is already the practice in numerous peace education initiatives globally, these peace heroes may include local or international people, less or more famous peace personalities, activists or writers/philosophers, men or women, younger people or older people, those from within the same cultural group and those from another – pretty much anybody who actively works towards positive peace, using nonviolent methods.

Other examples of concrete initiatives to build nonviolent masculinities to strengthen peace include, 'Be a man – do not be a violator' clubs in a number of places, including in the former Yugoslavia. These clubs are working to redefine 'a real man' as, among other things, 'nonviolent, respectful of girls and sexually responsible' (Budi Muško 2011). As well, white ribbon campaigns are working globally to end violence by men against women. Often humorous, some white-ribbon campaigns asked men to *swear:* 'never to commit, excuse or remain silent about violence against women' (White Ribbon 2012). This later initiative is in stark contrast to white-feather campaigns in which traditional, violencesupporting femininities engaged in shaming men for their 'cowardice' in not going to war. Such social practices show the strength of the socially sanctioned enforcement of particular femininities and masculinities, as well as of the social construction of the violent-men/peaceful-women thesis. When they are socially and culturally encouraged to do so, women do engage in violence, as freedom fighters, and as perpetrators of structural/cultural/economic/psychological/epistemological violence. Further, women informed by nationalistic and patriotic narratives continue to play a substantial role in motivating men to perform violence against the other group on their behalf. Traditional patriarchal–hegemonic femininities, by accepting women's lower status in a society, by not challenging male political and economic dominance and by not challenging the overall warrior culture, play an important role in the maintenance of patriarchal/sexist and violent social systems.

Work towards peace therefore requires simultaneous transformation of both violent masculinities and violence supporting femininities. In other words, alternative, nonviolent masculinities need alternative, simultaneously nonviolent and empowered femininities. As men do their work on abandoning violent and hegemonic ways of expressing masculinity, they need support from other men as well as from women, in a similar way that generations of women needed support by progressive men to be able to finally express their public/political voice. This means the continuation of resistance to the patriarchal society and the worldview that devalues women by objectifying them, while simultaneously devaluing men by dehumanising them and turning them into subject–objects of violence.

This is important because traditional/patriarchal gender relations have consistently been 'both cause and consequence of war ... [and so] a logical implication is that the strategies of movements that seek to end militarization and war must include a transformation of gender relations' (Cockburn 2010, p.114). Contemporary masculinity studies have also shown that, unlike the positive-masculinity ethics and psychology described above, it is more traditional and unreconstructed models of masculinity that tend to 'correlate most strongly with patterns and practices of violence' (Edwards 2006, p.62). The practices or the performativity of such traditional, patriarchal, androcratic, dominant, domineering, normative (Mosse

1996) or hegemonic (Connell & Messerschmidt 2005) masculinities are not only detrimental to women and subservient or other masculinities. They are, as well, detrimental and repressive to hegemonic-androcratic men themselves, who are unable to develop 'full and complete personalities ... [but remain] just well trained thumping machines' (Edwards 2006, p.61). As such they remain subjects-objects of violence as well. Alternatively, what nearly two decades of systematic masculinity studies have shown is that although men may be 'encouraged to live up to the ideals of hegemonic masculinity and can be sanctioned for not doing so, violence is just one of many ways of "doing gender" in a culturally specific way' (DeKeseredy & Schwartz 2005, p.356).

In a similar fashion to feminism empowering generations of women to develop their voice beyond the limitations of traditional femininities, critical men's studies (Brod & Kaufman 1994; Polk 1994; Bowker 1998; Whitehead & Barrett 2001; Connell 2002, 2005, 2009; Ervø & Johansson 2003; Kimmel et al. 2004; Connell & Messerschmidt 2005; Higate & Hopton 2005; Seidler 2005; Edwards 2006; Anderson 2009) have recently opened up spaces for men wishing to express the belief that 'change is possible [and] that fewer men have to die or kill or injure others to prove their manhood' (Barker 2005, p.155). Such belief must be based on hope, because 'hope is the basic component of all change and vitality, of development' (2005). This hope is further based on men 'finding other and far less harmful ways of communication or expressing their feelings of anger, hurt or frustration' (Edwards 2006, p.62), as well as on creating 'cultures of gender and manhood in which young men are encouraged to express their frustration and personal pain in ways that do not include physical violence or substance abuse' (Barker 2005, p.155). Instead of simple acceptance of 'globalised visions of a hegemonic masculinity' (Seidler 2005, p.141), there is a need for 'spaces for reflection in which diverse cultural masculinities can be recognised'. This cannot be created by men alone. Rather, they 'need to be encouraged to engage in processes of transforming masculinities to help sustain more equal, loving and open relationships with partners and children as they struggle to realise new visions of gender and sexual justice' (2005). It is thus the responsibility of each and every person, of all genders, and each and every society, to encourage such spaces for the development of nonviolent masculinities, if we are to have longer-term and more solid peace.

The de-linking of men and violence, however, does not necessarily have to be done at the expense of de-linking of women (including mothers) and peace. As already discussed, the 'military represent[s] one of the major sites where direct links between hegemonic masculinities and men's bodies are forged' (Morgan 1994, p.168). However, this link would best be severed by the overall demilitarisation of societies and *not* by the militarisation of women. In other words, the true mechanism for gender equity is not in women's militarisation but in women's emancipation (Zajović 2009, p.27). Similarly, the true mechanism behind global human security is also not in men's militarisation but in their emancipation from being considered 'our expendable lives'. The true challenge to patriarchy as well as to violence, therefore, arises only when *both* empowered femininities and nonviolent masculinities jointly embrace a 'force more powerful': the power to live and let live.

CHAPTER 4

Living trauma, eupsychia: The political is personal

> [Peace] ... is strangely ephemeral. It is something like breathing; one only becomes acutely aware of its importance when one is choking (Simon 1980).

In: The dissolution of Jelena

My dear daughter, my beloved grandchildren,

Today is 6th April 1999 and the spring in Novi Sad is in full bloom. The city looks more beautiful than ever, or this is how it seems to me. Every evening we lower down the window shutters, open the windows and go to bed with a hope that nothing bad will happen tonight. We believe that residential buildings are not under threat. And so we sleep in our beds, in our pyjamas and with a bag next to our bed in which there are 'necessities', 'just in case'. However, they roar every night. The most difficult day was when the bridges were destroyed. The bridges that took us to the seaside, to the Fortress, to Belgrade and over which we used to return home happy. Novi Sad is wounded, it weeps and wails. I don't understand why they [NATO] are targeting Novi Sad? Sadly, without our bridges Novi Sad will never be the same. Great sadness is in us, and yet we still have everything. Food, water, electricity, radio, TV programs and a great hope that this madness will stop.

And now about us coming to visit you! There is war and we cannot travel. I have been given a war schedule and leaving my work would mean that I could no longer be able to come back into the country. I would also lose my job and for now there are no new job openings, everybody must stay at the jobs they had when the war began. I sincerely hope this will not last forever and that we will be able to visit you as soon as conditions change. Your sister is coping fantastically. The only bad thing is that she is unemployed at the moment. As far as my work is concerned, even though there are heaps of problems, the work actually helps me a lot. Given that the bridges have been destroyed I now have to cross the Danube over a scaffold; they are packed with people and shaky, but still I don't find that to be a problem. If I didn't work I believe I would most likely be extremely depressed. Psychologists advise us that we should work as much as possible, physically as well, to socialise and read, and this is exactly what we are doing. Your dad is angry all the time, still, he manages to sleep well. It is rather surprising that we all sleep well and a lot.

Hugs and kisses to you and the kids,

Love, Mum.

Dear Sis,

I just spoke to our parents, Dad says he is good and Mum asked me to help her with getting the needed documents from the Registry so that she could travel. She is very keen to come and visit you but disappointed that Dad no longer agrees to travel with her. His physical condition has deteriorated, but worse than that is that he no longer wishes to go to countries that were supportive of the NATO bombing. He keeps on saying: '19 powerful and wealthy nations against one small and impoverished country, where is justice in that?' But as there is nothing we could do about all that, unlike Dad, I don't think about it at all. Mum, on the other hand, is not coping well. She was much better during the bombing, seemed on the top of things. Now, she is frequently depressed, and I know her work is very stressful. They have received more refugee children but the Ministry is not paying for their living expenses because they are citizens of 'another country' now! Ministries of those 'other countries' are equally unconcerned. Some foreign donor agencies are helping, but that is sporadic and ad hoc, very stressful. Anyhow, I hope she will get some rest when she visits you.

Dear Sis,

I did not go to work today, nor yesterday. The reason: our Mum's new condition. For the Australian visa she had to go to the police so that she could get proof that she did not have a criminal record. But a new regulation was introduced that such data must be collected in one's place of birth, so technically she needs to send a request to Engels, Russia, where she was born. We are not even sure if they have any such record of those born in displacement camps during the Second World War, especially given that she spent only a couple of weeks there, and we doubt that she is registered in Moscow either. In any case, any such request for more information sent to Russia will take at least one to two months. Plus it is completely ridiculous given that she left Moscow when she was three years of age. But bureaucracy is relentless, and even though Mum tried to explain she had lived in Belgrade since she was three and in Novi Sad for the last twenty-five years they could not care less. Apparently they were also very rude to her. And so she went home, took some tablets and washed them down with spirits. Then, at three o'clock in the morning, Dad heard some noise, and found

Mum semi-conscious with a broken glass all over the room. She also cut herself at a number of places trying to collect the broken glass, then shook the carpet through the window and dropped it, then went out in the middle of the night trying to get it back, then fell and bruised herself, then Dad finally managed to put her back to bed, and pick up the broken glass and the carpet from the street. All this has obviously made his heart condition worse, so today he's been breathing with difficulty, but hopefully his medicines will help. This morning he called the medical centre to get some help for Mum but they don't do home visits and she won't go there. Her mental state has been getting progressively worse since last year's NATO bombing, well actually since the country collapsed and war started, and I think she's been using these tablets and alcohol before, but never this bad. Anyhow, I don't know what to do and I can see that Dad does not know either.

Love, Vesna

Out: Horizontal and vertical breakdowns

Violence is not merely killing another ... violence isn't merely organised butchery in the name of God, in the name of society or country. Violence

> is much more subtle, much deeper, and we are inquiring into the very depths of violence (Krishnamurti 1989).

'Everyone has a breaking point,' my colleague Heather Millhouse says. She has worked in the area of peace and conflict for decades, and she's seen the negative impact violence has had on people's mental health many times. The 1999 NATO intervention in the former FR Yugoslavia (Serbia and Montenegro) was a breaking point for my mother, Jelena.

For 57 years Jelena had coped with life as best she could. Her birth was in a barracks for people displaced from Moscow due to Operation Barbarossa – the invasion of the Soviet Union by the Axis powers in 1941 – and she grew up with the unhealed trauma of her mother Mira and grandmother Zinka who experienced the disappearance of Mirko, their father and husband, respectively. Jelena also suffered the unspoken but ever-present trauma her adoptive father Veljko carried from the Spanish Civil War and had fantasies about what her life would have been like if she had been raised by her biological father, Vasiliy. Then she had coped with the ever-present but hardly spoken about trauma her husband, Zoran, carried. She also had broken sleep patterns all her life, which a Belgrade psychiatrist diagnosed as a consequence from Second World War air raids when, as a child, she was regularly being woken up and taken to shelter in her infancy. During times of peace, or since her

1945 arrival in Belgrade as a three-year-old, up until 1991 when the war in Yugoslavia started, she not only coped with life but also thrived at times.

Jelena Milojević (maiden surname Vlahović, surname at birth Skrobova) completed her schooling and gained a university degree, built her career in the government's social services, raised a family and engaged in politics. She was a classic example of a socialist 'superwoman', both a hardworking professional as well as a responsible housekeeper and mother, with a cherry on top: her political involvement in the communist party. Like her grandmother Zinka, she was also a recipient of numerous awards for her professional work and political engagement:

> for her dedication to our society and for her personal example; for leading improvements in the social care of children, especially children without parental care as well as of the elderly; for contributing towards socialist self-determination, brotherhood and unity, equity, accord and community in the SFRJ; for demonstrating high level of moral, character and general human qualities, for which she earned respect from her associates and the broader community.

She rose to the post of Minister for Social Service in the government of the then autonomous province of Vojvodina, and was a president of the Socialist Alliance of Working People of Yugoslavia (SSRNJ) from 1989 to 1990. SSRNJ was 'the largest and most influential mass organization in SFRY from August 1945 through 1990 – before its dissolution, its membership was thirteen million, [which included] most of the adult population of the country' (Library of Congress 1990). SSRNJ was dissolved courtesy of Serbian political leadership, more specifically of the Serbian Social Party (SPS) under the leadership of Slobodan Milošević. As proudly stated by his successor, the current president of SPS Ivica Dačić, during the celebration of 20 years since the dissolution of SSRNJ:

> SSRNJ was a backward organisation which had to be abolished. They were so backward that they did not even know how to use all the buildings they had, the equipment, furniture and membership dues that were accumulated from years of difficult labour and the contributions of the whole of the former country. Then we arrived and put all that into the service of people. This is why today is an important day in the history of new Serbia, where something like this [organisation] must not be repeated ever again (Dačić 2010).

The year SSRNJ was dissolved, Jelena was working as a member of the Executive Council of Vojvodina (Serbia's northern province), whose chairman was Radoman Božović, one of Milošević's trusted men. Božović rose to power after the so-called yoghurt revolution in Vojvodina. This was the orchestrated removal by Milošević of 'power hungry', 'autonomists' and 'armchairers' – in other words, the political leadership that was still resisting his absolutism. The yoghurt revolution was part of a broader 'antibureaucratic revolution': 'a series of mass protests against governments of the Yugoslav republics and autonomous provinces in 1988 and 1989' (Wikipedia 2012). These events led to the 'resignations of leaders in SAP Kosovo, SAP Vojvodina and SR Montenegro, who were replaced by politicians close to Slobodan Milošević' (2012). In the name of this antibureaucratic revolution, as well as in the name of restoring 'Serbian rights and pride' (Jenkins & Sofos 1996, p.247):

> Milošević used the 'moral panic' which had emerged in Serbia and Montenegro over the sensitive issue of the alleged 'Albanisation of Kosovo' to justify the need for constitutional reform. He thus initiated a purge of civil servants, industry managers, journalists and university staff who might pose obstacles to his reforms or were likely to be disloyal, introduced a new Serbian constitution, and effectively abolished the autonomous status of Kosovo and Vojvodina (1996).

It was these revolutions, Milošević later boasted, that signalled the beginning of the end of socialism all over eastern Europe. In reality, the emergence of street democracy, under which Jelena and many other undesirables were 'purged', signalled the beginning of 'a new form of authoritarianism, competing nationalisms and the break-up of Yugoslavia' (Vladisavljević 2008). Some in the Yugoslav press not under Milošević's control as well as the international press 'began to compare Milošević's campaign of local putsches through rallies and marches to the campaigns of Mussolini and Hitler' (Glaurdić 2011, p.33). His purges, although in a much milder form, also had elements reminiscent of Stalin's, in which Jelena's grandfather Mirko, among others, perished. These early warnings – of impending doom – went unaddressed, despite the certainty by some actors of what was to come. For example, 'a CIA report asserted that in case of success of overthrowing the Montenegrin leadership, Milošević would turn to Bosnia-Herzegovina and Macedonia, and with coups in those republics "would produce a Serbian-led national regime dominated by Milošević"'(2011). 'In no other conflict has there been so many early warnings and so little preventive diplomacy,' wrote Jan Oberg (1999). He continued:

> Kosovo's catastrophe was among the most predictable of all. It is intellectual nonsense that 'everything else has been tried and NATO bombings was the only option left ... the response of the NATO powers to the Bosnian crisis was [also] ad hoc and largely mismanaged (1999).

In 1992, the article 'Preventing War in Kosovo' by the Transnational Foundation for Peace and Future Research stated:

> It is a fragile calm we see today in Kosovo. There is still a political time and space for preventive diplomacy. The conflict holds very powerful and destructive potentials and will not go away. It will explode if nothing is done very soon ... The international community bears responsibility for not stimulating or using military actions but, instead, helping identify peaceful solutions with peaceful means before it is too late (TFF 1992).

US Intelligence, as reported in November 1990 in the *New York Times,* predicted as well that 'Federated Yugoslavia will break apart, most probably in the next 18 months, and that civil-war in that multi-national Balkan [sic] country is highly likely' (quoted in Gallagher 2003, p.37). But, apparently, the international community could 'only observe how the imminent catastrophe, *which all Yugoslav experts* were predicting, unfolded' (Bennett 1995, p.181, italics added). So, the logical conclusion is that, given that the experts and intelligence services of the world's major powers and presumably their political leadership knew in advance about the imminent catastrophe (Woodword 2008, p.411; Rogel 2004, p.77), they decided not to put (low-cost) preventative measures in place and then later involved themselves militarily (at extreme cost) to put an end to the war in the former Yugoslavia. This military intervention was then intended to put an end to the most atrocious violent conflict in post-Second World War Europe, conflict that apparently 'shocked the world'. 'As a widely predicted outcome,' argued Halpern and Kideckel however, 'the descent of Yugoslavia into the civil war qualifies for [Barbara] Tuchman's definition of folly' (2000, p.40). Tuchman's long-term historical study into why predictions of disasters failed to prevent catastrophes from happening largely link these follies to the rejection of reason (2000). For events to qualify as folly, Tuchman says the:

> acts have to be clearly contrary to the self-interest of the organization or group pursuing them; conducted over a period of time, not just in a single burst of irrational behaviour; conducted by a number of individuals, not just one deranged maniac; and, importantly, there have to be people alive at the time who pointed out correctly why the act in question was folly (no 20/20 hindsight allowed) (summarised by Hourvitz 2010).

Sadly, very few significant preventative initiatives took place. Efforts by NGOs notwithstanding, what we were left with were reactive, pastoriented approaches wherein old-style diplomacy was used, ad hoc and sporadically. What we were also left with were the violent methods various groups utilised in order to minimise the dystopia of violence and war by employing the very same methods it demanded that others abandon. This is because the realities of militarism, imperialism and nationalism, as discussed in Chapter 2, are so naturalised that they have become givens; they have become the only realities and it is within these givens and realities that any action must take place. Action within the frameworks of this holy trinity is defined: 'doing something' equates with military intervention and violent conflict resolution. Too often, however, the issue of doing something is raised only once the mechanisms of violent conflict and full-blown war are already fully set in place. Pacifistic approaches are then left with the almost impossible task of proving that they alone would work when the folly has taken over and the rationality of approaches upon which pacifist ways rest are undermined by nationalistic and militaristic hysteria. In the meantime, militarism, imperialism and nationalism are tolerated as 'the way of the world'. Once mobilisation for war takes place, however, people 'resist war at their peril' (Young 2010, p.51). In periods of national mobilisation for war, pacifism is the antithesis of the 'mores of the time' and 'hyper patriotic anti-"pacifist" responses are common' (2010). In other words, bellicose and nationalistic frenzy becomes the rule of the day, encouraging people to act violently and irrationally, often even against their own interests.

The best time for nonviolent intervention, of course, is before full-scale violence takes place. The best time for both pacifistic as well as perhaps even militaristic (that is, deployment of preventative UN peacekeeping forces) humanism in the case of former Yugoslavia was therefore in the period between 1989 and 1991, to coincide with the proclamations of independence by Slovenia and Croatia, for example, or as soon as the first shots were fired in 1991, *not* in 1995 and 1999. But we have very few diplomatic mechanisms in place for these and similar situations that require preventative peacekeeping (protecting all citizens, and especially minorities) to arrest the development of large-scale violence: a global political system built on nation-state sovereignty as well as on state's right to use weapons remains paramount. The best method for interventions would have been through nonviolent efforts to keep, make and build peace. So unfortunately, while many of these nonviolent approaches were attempted by various groups and individuals, in the former Yugoslavia and globally, they were swallowed and silenced by social militarism and shortterm thinking. Initiatives to save the country from ruin – for example, those proposed and attempted by (SFR) Yugoslav Prime Minister Ante Marković – were frequently rejected by the international community as 'too costly'. Not only that, argues Metta Spencer, 'the financial aid package' and the 'economic therapy' designed by western financial and political organisations actually contributed to the deepening of the crisis and 'crippling of the [Yugoslav] federal system':

> State revenues which should have gone as transfer payment to the republics and autonomous provinces were instead funnelled towards servicing Belgrade's debt with the Paris and London clubs. The republics were largely left to their own

> devices, thereby exacerbating the process of political fracturing. In one fell swoop, the reformers had engineered the demise of the federal fiscal structure and mortally wounded its federal political institutions. The IMF-induced budgetary crises created an economic 'fait accompli' which in part paved the way for Croatia's and Slovenia's formal secession in June 1991 (Spencer 2000, p.167).

It is rather ironic that the money that was not there for a peaceful transition of SFRY into democratic and market-oriented Western-style democracy, was there many times over for the waging of war, both by local as well as international players. It is also paradoxical that violence was seen as a legitimate answer to the Yugoslav crisis that was partially fuelled by the collapse of its 'federal fiscal structure' (2000), given how much wars always cost. In the end, the economic cost of the 1990s wars for Yugoslav people was, at the very least, billions and billions of dollars. The economic pauperisation of the Yugoslav population, from which most of the new states are still struggling to recover, dramatically unravelled during the war. This included the collapse of the monetary and fiscal system in Serbia and Montenegro in 1993 and 1994 – the year I left the country – due to hyperinflation, which was one of the highest ever recorded. Towards the end of 1993, for example, our wallets were filled with 500 billion dinar (500,000,000,000) banknotes, the highest nominal value ever recorded in the history of the national currency. The prices of all goods skyrocketed overnight regularly. Only the cash economy worked and personal cheques and credit cards were no longer accepted. What this meant was that an increasing number of people struggled to simply survive.

The middle class I belonged to shrank quickly. The value of our salaries halved in a matter of hours. People went straight from their workplaces (if they were lucky enough to still be employed given the unemployment rate ended up around 60 per cent towards the end of the 1990s) with their incomes as banks collapsed directly to the markets and shops. Delaying a visit to the market by a couple of hours would cost half a salary. Our family friend, a gynaecologist and director of a maternity hospital, was too busy to go for a couple of days. Eventually, for his monthly income, he managed to buy a bar of soap (see Milojević 2001, 2004). Finding products that hadn't yet increased in price became a sort of national sport. I recall going to a couple of stores and literally grabbing products from the side of the shelf that shop assistants had not yet managed to tag with the new price. My salary at the university that year was approximately 50DEM (approximately $50) per fortnight, so money was tight. I remember having to return a tub of yoghurt to the shelf because neither my mother, who worked as a senior manager, nor I, a university teaching assistant, had enough money between us to make the purchase. I also remember being paid in chicken meat and laundry detergent, courtesy of the workers' union. This pay was perhaps more substantial than my great-grandmother Zinka's reward under Stalin's regime (the additional '100 grams of sugar and half a kilogram of flour' for her 'outstanding' work efforts), and yet strangely similar.

During the last few years I permanently resided in FR Yugoslavia (Serbia and Montenegro), inflation was running at 60 per cent per day '...in only four years, Yugoslavia's gross domestic product (GDP) slid by 60 percent (GDP in 1989 was about $3,300US, by 1993 it was $1,250US)' (Cohen 2002, pp.161–62). Although these figures may sound dramatic, they were 'nothing compared to the real drama of the period leading up to January 1994, which was hyperinflation':

> While the monthly rate remained relatively 'low' until the beginning of 1993 it began to edge over the 200 per cent per month level in February of that year. By July it was creeping over 400 per cent, in August it reached 1,880 per cent. At an annualised rate that is 363,000,000,000,000,000 per cent, or in plain English 363 quadrillion per cent. This was but a fraction of what it was to become ... From August 1993 until the next January, Serbia lived through times recalling Germany's ill-fated Weimar Republic. When the November inflationary rate hit 20,190 per cent *Vreme* spoke of an 'inflationary Tsunami' ... There were no words then for the final figure some six weeks later, which was a monthly rate of

> 313,563,558 per cent. At an annualised rate this is 851, 000,000,000,000,000,000,000,000,000,000,000, 000,000,000,000,000,000,000,000,000,000,000,000, 000,000,000 per cent.
>
> The largest bank note issued during the period of hyperinflation had a face value of 50,000,000,000 dinars and was virtually worthless two weeks after its introduction (Judah 2000, pp.267–68).

All this happened in the part of the SFRY that had not officially participated in the war and was at the time not directly hit by bombings and shelling, although the situation was to a significant degree a result of its (in)direct involvement in wars in Slovenia, Croatia and Bosnia and Herzegovina. The situation in Bosnia and Herzegovina was, of course, much worse, as the magnitude of physical violence there paralleled that of economic collapse:

> the war in Bosnia left more than half of Bosnia's 4.3 million citizens displaced, up to a quarter of a million people dead, between $15 billion and $20 billion worth of infrastructure in rubble, industrial production sliced to less than 10 per cent of pre-war levels, and as much as 80 per cent of agricultural equipment destroyed (Ramet 2005, p.186).

Further to how much war cost the local people, the 'resolution' of conflict via NATO's military interventions cost those countries as well. NATO's 1999 military involvement alone was estimated to have cost US$100 million for the first 24 hours, and US$10–30 million per day after that, with the total cost of the 'campaign' falling between US$2 and $4 billion (Bieber & Daskalovski 2003, p.116). 'Constructive' use of those billions, for the alleged 'better and more peaceful futures', created further damage to the local economy, which will be felt for decades to come. The cost of the widespread damage to the Yugoslav industrial and transport infrastructure by NATO bombing, for example, was estimated between US$30 and 100 billion (Daianu & Veremēs 2001, p.177).

The insidious cost of all modern wars also manifests via toxic fumes, harmful and hazardous substances carried in short-and long-lived air pollution, the destruction of natural habitat, pollution of water and soil, leftover bombs and bullets, chemical waste and general military trash. In addition to the immediate consequences caused primarily by 'explosions, fires and the release of toxic substances into the environment, the long-term consequences are of greater importance owing to contamination of the environment by slowly decomposing chemicals' (Martinović-Vitanović & Kalafatić 2009, p.255). Leftover toxins continue to injure and kill hundreds of thousands of people, although the exact numbers are almost impossible to ascertain. What we do know is that during the bombing of Yugoslavia by NATO, 'chemical, petrochemical, petroleum and other industrial facilities and storage areas filled with hazardous and harmful substances were targeted in a planned and deliberate manner, resulting in the release of thousands of tons of hazardous matter into the environment [which] ... caused ecological damage of enormous proportions' (2009, p.254). At one stage, for example, the level of toxic substances in Pančevo, where one of the Serbian oil refineries is located, was reported to be 7000 to 10,600 times above the recognised safe limit (for carcinogenic vinyl chlorine monomer).

Watching from a distance, courtesy of modern global media, I could see images of the black cloud from another purposely hit industrial facility – a refinery in Novi Sad – engulfing my hometown, with my parents, sister, and friends still living in it. These strikes impacted not only the FR Yugoslavia (Serbia and Montenegro) but also other countries in the region, such as countries downstream of the Danube (Romania, Bulgaria). The NATO bombing of Yugoslavia was no 'humanitarian intervention' but rather a humanitarian and an ecological disaster brought upon by 'chemical warfare' that resulted in an 'ecological catastrophe' (2009). What would be a disaster upsetting almost everyone in peaceful times – one that the majority would do their best to prevent – becomes a legitimate action during times of war. During those times, even the 'rational' and 'civilised' world calmly and deliberately engaged in actions that caused devastating consequences – consciously creating an ecological catastrophe.

This is true of all modern warfare, and so making the shift towards a sustainable and ecological civilisation is next to impossible unless militarism is not arrested. For example, another 'humanitarian' intervention, protecting the world from terrorism, or in other words the ongoing Iraq catastrophe had, by 2010, resulted in more than 60 per cent of Iraq's water supply being polluted, 25 million landmines being left unexploded, bombdamaged factories continuing to release various unsafe chemical toxins into the environment, forests in the north and palm groves in the south being flattened to remove hiding places of insurgents, land being saturated with unexploded bombs, chemical waste, rubble and trash and unknown quantities of radioactive dust from depleted uranium being released into the environment (Castleden & Wareham 2010, pp.26–27). Further:

> War's toxic legacy is seen in multiple other sites around the globe. One of the worst examples is Vietnam, where dioxin from the approximately eighty million litres of Agent Orange sprayed over the environment between 1962 and 1971 continues to take a heavy toll. Large areas of the country are still contaminated and the Vietnamese government estimates that hundreds of thousands of children have been born with birth defects as a result.... The world's most destructive weapons, nuclear weapons, have left a radioactive legacy

> wherever they have been [used], developed and tested ... (2010).

In summary, 'war destroys countries' environments, not just their people' (Othman quoted in 2010, p.26). 'War and its effects have led to changes in the social, economic and environmental fabric. It will take centuries to restore the natural environment' (2010) of countries where modern wars have been waged. However, this environmental cost of war, like the psychological cost of war, is rarely taken into account, despite the world's militaries – fighting wars in our names, on our behalf and with our money – being direct contributors to the current environmental degradation as well as to climate change. Militaries deplete finite resources – their weapons and vehicles are all energy intensive, their tools such as bombing, explosions and fire all emit enormous amounts of carbon and, last but not least, they are the biggest purchasers of oil in the world (2010).

At an individual level, the psychological effects of wars for most people are also massive. In my mother's case, the (not-inevitable but largely avoidable) events of 1988–91, led to her complete withdrawal from politics, because of her disagreement with the philosophy and methods used by Milošević and people loyal to him. The philosophy and ideology she personally subscribed to had by then largely been abandoned, in her own country as well as almost globally. All opposition to the regime was discredited by the din of the regime's controlled media as either belonging to the 'reactionary remnants of the old regime' or being the actions by the 'fifth column of foreign payees'. Not much sympathy was forthcoming from other places either, as she, like so many others, was boxed in as 'an aggressor' (a Serbian), and as such deserving of punishment.

All these events led to much more than one woman's personal drama. Jelena's slow and painful dissolution paralleled the collapse of a whole country (SFRY): 'It is as if my life counted for nothing. Everything I believed in, everything I worked for and everything I aspired to now means nothing.' Everything SFRY officially stood for, all the positive values such as equality of the people, social justice, brotherhood and unity, multiculturalism, internationalism, self-alignment and self-reliance, was thrown out with the bath water of socialist-communist totalitarianism and economic mismanagement. From being a respected professional and politician, Jelena became persona non grata almost overnight. Simultaneously, from a country admired by some as a 'rising star of communism' (Norris 2008, p.133), due to its relatively liberal government policies and the apparent lack of dissent, SFRY quickly became the worst of them all. Jelena's own multicultural and multiethnic background was no longer seen as an asset but a liability. In a similar manner to the way voluntarily mixing diverse ethnicities had to be separated militarily (Hayden 1996, p.788), people like Jelena had to violently separate parts of their own cultural-ethnic identity: 'I no longer know who I am,' she and many others agonised. Not knowing who they were or where they were coming from posed difficulties for many in finding a path towards a new desired future.

'War creates an endless aftermath of anguish and devastation,' writes Leila Levinson. 'All participants are casualties, and through them, so, too, are their families' (2011). This is true of both interstate wars as well as of political battles waged within totalitarian regimes. Jelena's husband, and my father, Zoran, was also punished by the new (Milošević's) regime. A specialist dental prosthetist and not politically involved, he was denounced in the media for some alleged, largely unspecified, transgressions at work. Our phone was bugged. Jelena's every move was watched, or so it seemed. Yugoslav republics that she considered part of her own country, including her ancestral land of Slovenia and places she travelled to frequently for work and leisure (Croatia and Bosnia and Herzegovina), places where she had relatives and friends, were brutalised by a series of civil wars. She was no longer sure of her identity and belonging within this new–old country, as the only other publically offered alternative at the time in Serbia was Serbian nationalism.

What finally broke this one woman's spirit was when bombs fell on the town she lived in as part of NATO's 'humanitarian war'. Together with others living on the territory of Serbia and Montenegro, who actively encouraged or passively approved the rise of Serbian nationalism and its role in wars in SFRY, Jelena and many others like her who dissented or disagreed with the regime, were also to be 'disciplined'. This punishment included the violent bombing of places wherein hundreds of thousands of refugees from other Yugoslav republics had relocated. The punishment even included the killing of those that NATO was apparently protecting. While the 'precise death toll from the NATO–Yugoslav hostilities over Kosovo remains uncertain and controversial':

> many thousands of military personnel and civilians were killed and injured. As many as 11,000 Kosovar Albanians may have been killed in over 100 massacres (some estimates range from 5,000 to 10,000). Serbian civilian dead have been estimated at between 1,500 and 2,000, and perhaps another 5,000 people were wounded by the bombing (Cohen 2002, p.280).

Like Lenard Cohen, Aleksandar Pavković also argued that the 1999 aggression by NATO not only killed scores of those that the intervention was supposed to protect but was instrumental in the creation of new injustices:

> The war took the heaviest toll on those whom NATO sought to protect: early estimates suggest that many more Kosovo Albanians, both KLA fighters and civilians, were killed in the war than [other] Yugoslav soldiers or civilians. Nonetheless,

> NATO troops entering Kosovo were joyously greeted by Kosovo Albanians as liberators. The KLA fighters, free at last to take control of the cities and the countryside, started to kill Kosovo Serbs as well as Kosovo Albanians whom they regarded as Serb collaborators. As many Kosovo Albanian refugees followed the advancing NATO forces from Macedonia into Kosovo, so the Serbs from Kosovo, together with their clergy, were following the withdrawing Yugoslav military units into Serbia. As before, the liberation for one national group meant enforced exile for another (Pavković 2000, p.197).

To this day, this 'resolved' conflict continues; so does Jelena's despair. 'There is nothing left to look forward to,' she concluded before emotionally checking out of her life. 'My whole world is gone.' The world that was gone took away her two younger brothers in the process, permanently and irrevocably. Together with the other 300,000 to 500,000 people who left Serbia during the last 20 years alone, it also took her first-born daughter some 14,000 kilometres away, creating yet another grievance from which she was not able to recover.

In: Surviving peace, 1 traumatised survivors breathe

After the beginning of the war I ended up as a refugee in a foreign country. For the first four years I did not experience any problems. And then, 'suddenly', when I had already managed to learn a foreign language and had started to go to school in order to gain the same education I had in our country, and when you would think I could now relax ... BAM! It was like life stopped! I was afraid to go out into the street by myself, I was afraid to stay alone at home, I couldn't tolerate people around me, noise, not even strong light. I felt I was woven from extremely sensitive nerves, which at the smallest stimulus would make me feel as if I were about to explode ... as if everything and anything could destroy me. Heart palpitations, a feeling as if I am to faint, knees shaking, and a sensation that some invisible hand was rising from my stomach towards my throat and wanted to strangle me. Horror!

I am 20 years old and have a huge problem. Since June, that is, the last five months, I have been struggling with [feelings of] suffocation. It started all of a sudden. I visited every possible doctor and they all told me I was healthy and that all that was happening was related to 'nervousness'. But, I don't really believe them. If it is as they are saying it would have been over by now. Especially since they told me nothing is wrong. A doctor gave me medicine but there is no change, no improvement. I still choke, can't fill my lungs. I choke during the day and throughout the night. Sometimes it is weaker, sometimes it is stronger, but it is always there, it never completely goes away. Breathing is tiresome, because I have to fight and strain for every breath. I don't know what to do. I wonder if this will ever stop. I am afraid that choking will one day increase to such a level that I will indeed suffocate, but no one will be able to help me, since no one really knows what is wrong with me. Is it possible that nothing is wrong with me? How is it possible that somebody is choking for five months, but nothing is wrong with her? And how can I cure myself? How can this stop? Thanks in advance.[2]

I am 42 years old and for the last fifteen years I have been dragging myself to visit psychiatrists. I changed quite a number of them, drunk a whole pharmacy of antidepressants and other medications, and all that was in vain. I get better for a few months and then all is the same again. Panic, suffocation, exhaustion ... True hell.

What is three and half years of war compared to these last fifteen years after the war ... nothing ... if somebody is suffering it is an illness caused by suspicious privatisation, the increase in prices, poverty, the futile search for work, while simultaneously seeing that the riches of those people who profited from war are growing day after day.[3]

Every day patients arrive at medical clinics complaining of a feeling of suffocation, lack of air and feelings of tightening in their throats. These difficulties are often accompanied by dizziness, the feeling of being in a daze, and an increased heart rate. These symptoms could appear occasionally or last throughout day and night. The patients are commonly frightened because they are scared of suffocating. Such a lack of air is very uncomfortable and each doctor should take those symptoms of their patients seriously. As always, it is helpful for doctors to have sufficient time to talk to patients and conduct a thorough clinical examination, including ordering further tests. With these results doctors can make a diagnosis and choose an appropriate specialist. The most common causes of suffocation seen in our clinics are: presence of a foreign object that restricts breathing, pneumothorax, heart weaknesses, acute and chronic illnesses of the respiratory organs, thyroid gland disorders, tumours, anaemia, digestive disorders as well as psychological illnesses (neurosis, depression or psychosis).[4]

About seven to eight months ago it all started: heart palpitations, dizziness, weakness, pain at the back of my head and neck, laborious breathing, tiredness, nausea ... In such situations I start to panic (normal reaction?). Then it all starts growing into an immense fear: what am I going to do when it happens again? It happened many times. Each and every change bothers me: too many people, noise, and sometimes it happens even without any apparent reason. I saw a doctor and he concluded I was depressed and told me not to do night shifts any more. But what can I do? I live and work in a foreign country and the night shift work that I've been doing for more than a year is my only choice for income generation at the moment. I work at night and during the day I take care of our son, because my wife goes to work then. The doctor gave me anti-depressant and told me to change my lifestyle, but how can I? The medication that the doctor gave me made me feel even worse so I now take sedatives on my own accord. One night I ended up in the hospital's Emergency Ward. They told me that everything is fine but that I have a condition called hyperventilation. They gave me sedatives that I take when I feel extremely unwell. I understand that this may sound to some people like a harmless problem; but trust me this is not so. It is horrible when these attacks happen, and lately they are happening very often. Life here is very expensive, and seeing doctors is

> neither simple nor cheap. The worst is that the company that gives me night shifts does not show any understanding for my difficulties. I am aware that no problem has an instant solution but if somebody could give me good advice I would be so thankful. Simply put, I only wish to function in a normal way.[5]

Out: Concentric cycles and ripple effects

> 'Humpty Dumpty had experienced a dissolution of a country through a war,
>
> Humpty Dumpty was not the same as before,
>
> All the king's horses and all the king's men, couldn't put Humpty together again.'

Can one go back and function in 'a normal way' after the massive traumas and dislocations that all wars and all situations of life-threatening violence inevitably bring with them? What happens to people who were impacted by them, once these events are over? What occurs to those left behind, those who are still dealing with the consequences, even after a particular war or a totalitarian regime fades from our collective consciousness and is replaced with the global media's focus on yet another one? A non-Yugoslav person who built his academic career partially on his analysis of and writing about the Yugoslav wars of the 1990s told me that he has since 'moved away' from the topic. As much as I both admire and detest his nonchalant attitude, my main question is: will I ever be able to do the same?

Twenty years after the dissolution of my birth country through war and violence I think of such events in terms of 'horizontal and vertical' breakdowns, (Kuzmanović 2004). What I studied within official histories in school and at the university, what I read in numerous academic books and policy papers, what I heard through local and global media – about wars that have clear beginnings and ends, rather limited sets of causes and immediate consequences in terms of human deaths and economic costs – no longer makes sense. I now think of wars in terms of a continuum of multitude sets of causes and consequences, in terms of choices made by key players to engage in violence among numerous alternatives, and in terms of a continuum of practices enacted on a daily basis. I now see wars and other acts of collective violence as largely avoidable occurrences that nonetheless are premised on long-standing social structures (such as militarism and patriarchy) that are a result of long-term applications of concrete (individual and collective) actions. In other words, wars and intergroup conflicts are neither inevitable nor based on 'primordial hatreds', and certainly they are not 'givens'. Rather, they are results of a sequence of choices and violent actions, which can, at any given time, be replaced by another sequence of alternative, nonviolent actions.

Every side in the wars that took place in the 1990s claimed to wage a 'just war' for the protection of (our own) people. I find these categories extremely problematic. It is, of course, possible to ascertain who engages in a particular aggressive act, how and when (for example, the siege of Sarajevo, massacre in Srebrenica, Operation Storm [*Oluja*] in Croatia, NATO bombings), it is also possible to ascertain which side is more brutal, aggressive and dishonest in negotiations (that is, Serbian regime under Milošević, the Republika Srpska political leadership under Karadžić). But to see reality the way most nation-state discourses continue to present it ('we – all good', 'them – all bad') has become unacceptable to me, as it is both deceitful and dangerous.

It has also become much more obvious that the effects of wars do not stop when collective violence does, but continue for many more years, decades, even generations. The 'horizontal and vertical breakdowns' are about the human (lives, wellbeing), economic and environmental costs of war, as well as long-term social, cultural and psychological costs. Negative impacts of war (and violent political uprisings/suppression) on people run in concentric circles. The first circle includes people who die in wars; the one I witnessed develop before leaving the country in the end permanently took away the lives of between 150,000 and 260,000 people. Those witnessed by my parents, grandparents and great-grandparents – events described previously – took millions to their deaths: the first and second Balkan wars saw 220,000 dead (140,000 killed directly, 80,000 from diseases related to war); First World War, 20 million; Stalin's 1936–37 Purges, 13 million; 1936–39 Spanish Civil War, 600,000; Second World War, 55 million. It is unknown to me how many casualties, whether directly or through the yet unknown consequences of nuclear testing and fallouts, the so-called Cold War (mid 1940s to early 1990s) created. But we do know that millions died in the Cold War superpowers' proxy wars around the globe, most notably in Southeast Asia and countries such as Vietnam and Korea.

The second circle includes those who are injured or have family members, close community members and friends and relatives die in those events they are witnessing. This circle also includes those who witness atrocities and survive attacks on their lives (that is, survive bombing, fallouts from fighting, attempts to murder, etc.). And it includes those who are forced to leave their homes and their lives behind due to violence and/or social collapse. During the 1990s Yugoslav wars, between 3.7 and 4 million people were displaced or became refugees. Globally, the number of people forcibly uprooted by conflict and persecution in 2008 stood at 42 million (UNHCR 2009). By the end of 2010 the figure had grown to 43.7 million people worldwide, which is 'the highest number in the past 15 years' (UNHCR 2010).

The third circle comprises the direct descendants and children born in communities significantly impacted via the first and second circle. The cultural and psychological impacts of 'anguish and devastation' (Levinson 2011) experienced by their families and communities and its transfer onto subsequent generations have now been well recorded by scholarly research (such as the compilation by Danieli [1998]).

The fourth circle includes those who come into contact with people who belong to the first three circles. Historically these were people in the countries where refugees and immigrants settled, and who lived in relative peace for longer periods of time. Today, due to globalisation and ease of travel, human contact has vastly intensified and so have contacts between communities that experienced longer periods of peace and newly traumatised people and groups.

The fifth, hypothetical, circle would include those who neither died, nor were injured, nor had ancestors or close community members witness wars and other acts of collective violence (revolutions, colonisations). Given the sheer magnitude of collective violence that took place in the twentieth century and the intensification of human connectedness, I believe the whole of humanity is to be located in the first four circles – including even those who are not aware of how war and other acts of collective violence have impacted upon them.

This impact of wars and other acts of collective violence is multi-fold and by and large negative, painful and traumatic for most of those involved. Certainly, not everyone is impacted in the same way. Genetics, personality, gender, worldview, religion and religiosity, environmental circumstances, cultural and social factors all play a role. Some people are, of course, more resilient than others. Subjective experience of the event also plays a crucial role. This is because the objective exposure to a threatening event may be insufficient for a psychological trauma to develop; rather, it is also necessary that the person exposed feels 'fear, helplessness, or horror' (Laufer & Solomon 2006, p.430). Further, a previous exposure to trauma as well as 'more severe and longer exposure to traumatic events may lead to more posttraumatic stress' (Gavrilović et al. 2002, p.257). But even though it may manifest in various ways and with different intensity among different people, research clearly shows the existence of long-term traumatic consequences for most people who experience massive social collapse and/or collective acts of violence. For example, studies focused on youth populations in conflict areas 'as far apart as Ireland, Rwanda, the Middle East, and former Yugoslavia' (Laufer & Solomon 2006, p.429) have repeatedly implicated exposure to war and political violence in a range of pathological effects and behaviour problems among children and adolescents. These studies have pointed to resultant pathologies such as somatic problems; attention, memory, and learning difficulties; nightmares and sleep issues; depression and anxiety disorders; and behavioural problems, such as disobedience, violence, and risk taking (2006, pp.429–30).

Running in overlapping cycles are the human, economic, social-cultural, psychological and environmental impacts of wars. While the first two factors were traditionally counted within dominant discourses on war, and socio-cultural structures sometimes analysed, consideration of the psychological and environmental cost of war is a fairly recent endeavour. As far as the former is concerned, concentrated scientific research was prompted only by the advent of psychoanalysis and the events of the First World War. That war in particular spurred a:

> significant interest in war trauma and war-related neurosis. Concepts such as shell shock and war neurosis originated in this period, but even after many years of studies of trauma and psychological dysfunction, the question was raised as to whether trauma reactions in war were expressions of bad will and of immoral character (Sveaass 2012, p.1,133).

While 'significant knowledge about trauma and rehabilitation' was developed in this period, insights were in general not translated into other areas of society and interest in the topic in general waned, only to be resurrected in the aftermath of the Second World War (2012). Post-Second World War attention was expanded beyond shell-shocked soldiers, and so the trauma of civilians, especially the trauma of concentration camp survivors, was investigated (Frankl 1946; Eitinger 1964: Eitinger & Strøm 1973). The period of Cold War further 'encouraged research and interest in the trauma of fear, in particular in the intensive process of international armament and the imminent threat of nuclear war' (Sveaass 2012, p.1133). The effects of this were studied in both children and adults, who expressed concerns about 'having shorter life expectancies, stress reactions, and bad dreams' (2012). Studies since then have focused on post-war displacements, involuntary migration and its impact and severe trauma among US Vietnam war veterans, all leading to a 'new diagnostic category' of post-traumatic stress disorder, which was included in the DSM-III in 1982 (2012, p.1134). These studies have all unequivocally concluded that:

> War [as] the multifaceted threat to human existence ... exposes people to the health-damaging psychological, physical, chemical, biological, and mechanical stressors. The war has a deep and devastating social and economic impact on the population involved, thus producing additional and lasting repression ... War integrates the deprivation of basic existential needs and of all human rights and values; it eliminates emotional comfort; it causes irreversible material and kin losses, physical exhaustion, and

> psychological breakdowns; and it makes futile all everyday routines (Flögel et al. 2010, p.468).

Because the first response to stress – to try to escape – is not usually possible during wars due to the multitude of stressors and the impossibility of avoiding them, what results is a substitution of one stressor for another (2010). This is why the full display of adapted survival mechanisms takes place in those who are experiencing war stress. These include 'changes in behavior, hormonal impairments, neurological disorders, metabolic changes, genetic shifts, and all kinds of diseases' (2010). In summary, 'Stress-induced consequences, depending on the severity and the duration of the exposure to the stress experience', include 'PTSD, interrupted pregnancies, susceptibility to malignant diseases, cardiovascular insults, suppressed immune response, hormonal disorders, and all types of emotional instabilities or psychological impairments' (2010). These impairments may then result in 'suicide, homicide, and other types of violence' (2010).

Despite the indisputability of such devastating consequences for survivors, there are historical and social reasons why long-standing trauma from war was not previously accounted for. To start with, discounting trauma and its long-term consequences, not acknowledging the magnitude of its existence and the ripple effects that may come of it, is crucially important for modern warrior societies. Without this discounting, it would be hard to put forward arguments that military intervention will be made up of 'surgical strikes' that 'result in minimum collateral damage', or that intervention will be 'quick', and 'over by the spring'. It would also be impossible to put forward arguments that say a military intervention is necessary for securing long-term benefits for people, that wars give us freedom and are necessary to protect our way of life, our culture and our identity. If the reality of long-term devastation is taken into account so would the reality that the world's militaries kill humans and their spirits, destroy plants, animals and ecosystems, and contribute to long-term environmental degradation as well as social and economic collapse. Rarely is the connection made to any of these beyond the physical killing of humans. This is so even when it comes down to the economic cost of war. For example, few make the link between the United States' expenditures of around US$1 trillion (Belasco 2009) in less than a decade on the war against terror and the economic troubles that triggered the Global Financial Crisis (GFC) in 2008.[6] Rather, discourses about wars somehow being good for economic growth are often heard (that is, economic benefits from the production and selling of weapons, rebuilding of infrastructure after war revamping the economy, etc.). The severing of the links between short-term actions and long-term consequences is, however, necessary if the militarised system developed by androcratic societies is to continue. In other words, the delusion of limited negative impact and potential longerterm benefits is necessary if we are to have military activities in the first place. Such longer-term benefits are, however, counted predominantly in terms of potential political gains (more power and territory) and not seen in the broader context, making the rationale behind the waging of wars still seem somehow logical.

Perhaps this is because androcratic societies and worldviews do not motivate their members/bearers to look far ahead, either vertically or horizontally, or beyond the first concentric cycle. Another reason behind military and political shortsightedness is the fact that long-term consequences are not something military personnel or politicians need to be concerned about too much in their line of work. Politicians need to worry about the next election cycle (three, four or seven years ahead), and the military needs to worry mostly about current and subsequent military action. It is, on the other hand, those in so-called caring industries that deal with the long-term consequences of wars and violence in their daily work. Incidentally, people employed in caring industries, or who participate in the informal and unpaid 'love economy', are mostly of female gender. Incidentally, those employed in high-level political and military positions are mostly of male gender. To put this differently, an actor of violence, such as a soldier, is the responsibility of politicians (who deploy him) and of the military (who train him and run day-to-day logistics). A wounded, incapacitated or psychologically damaged ex-soldier, on the other hand, is the responsibility of his family or of the welfare sector (through veterans' pensions and benefits, etc.), unless he is left completely to his own devices. Similar division exists where the protection of the civilian population is concerned. The former (politicians and the military) deal with 'glory', the latter with consequences of those 'glorious' battles – the devastating impact they have on civilians, soldiers, the economy and the environment.

It seems that humans almost always end up seeing what we look for, and we look for what concerns us, what is relevant to us in our life and work. Historically, the building and maintaining of nations were almost exclusively based on the glory paradigm and these glorious histories were, as the old adage goes, written by the victors. So hegemonic–androcratic masculinities discount the realm of emotions, in a similar manner to the way that they discount peace, designating to it labels of 'weak' and 'feminine', and thus, consequently, irrelevant. Further, the psychological costs of wars and violence are also often discounted because they are hard to count and measure. Disagreements about exact human losses and damage to the economy are magnified many times over when it comes to this specific topic. Still, new research focus now makes it possible to more accurately ascertain the psychological effects of wars, on both civilians and combat veterans.

Research confirms that, throughout the world, constant worry, anxiety and depressive disorders are rampant in traumatised populations during social collapse and war (WHO 2005). Studies have consistently shown negative long-term effects of war on mental health and have directly linked 'exposure to prolonged war-related traumatic events ... with high prevalence rates of mental disorders' (Sabes-Figuera et al. 2012, p.1). Community studies in war-torn areas have shown the 'enormous increase of mental disorders (total: over 60 per cent, neurotic disorder: over 40 per cent, psychotic disorders: about 20 per cent' (WHO 2005, p.98).

Studies focused on the former Yugoslavia have confirmed the detrimental effects of social collapse and war on the general population. In Serbia in 2000 it was found that, of the respondents, 80 per cent were afraid of civil war and 70 per cent of hunger (Kuzmanović 2004). That same year half of respondents stated that they experienced 'chronic exhaustion, tension and worrying' (2004). In Bosnia and Herzegovina, a study by Dahl et al. (1998) found that 71 per cent of women who had survived the most severe kinds of trauma (concentration camps or other kinds of detention) had six or more symptoms on the Post-traumatic Symptom Scale (PTSS-10) (quoted in WHO 2005, p.98). As could be expected, the worse the trauma the worse the detrimental effects. A study based on interviews with displaced women from Srebrenica, showed a very strong presence of symptoms of PTSD (82 per cent), depression (80 per cent), anxiety (76 per cent) and weakened social function (72 per cent) (2000, p.25). Goldstein et al. found that 94 per cent of Bosnian children interviewed met DSM-IV diagnostic criteria for post-traumatic stress disorder (Bell et. al. 1997). Another study, which assessed 791 children who were aged six to sixteen years during the 1994 siege in Sarajevo, found that 41 per cent had significant PTSD symptoms (Altwood et. al. 2002). A further study confirmed 'the additive effect of trauma exposure on trauma reactions' among children (Smith et. al. 2002). This study also linked PTSD to levels of exposure as well as to maternal reactions to trauma. In Croatia, shortly after war broke out in 1991, an estimated 1 million people were exposed to war trauma (Pivac et al. 2007, p.48). A study by Mollica and colleagues in 1999, in which 534 adults from a refugee camp were interviewed, showed that approximately 39.2 per cent met DSM-IV diagnostic criteria for depression and 26.3 per cent for PTSD (quoted in WHO 2005, p.151). In 2000 Kozarić-Kovačić and colleagues found among the 350 displaced men and women interviewed, the following rates of PTSD: 50.3 per cent men, 36 per cent women; alcohol dependence: 60.5 per cent men, 8.1 per cent women; and comorbid alcohol dependence and PTSD: 69.6 per cent men, 11.7 per cent women (quoted in WHO 2005, p.151).

Studies have also shown that these detrimental effects are long lasting. For example, for several years following the Yugoslav wars (Bosnia- Herzegovina, Croatia, Kosovo, the Republic of Macedonia, and

Serbia) prevalence rates for post-traumatic stress disorder ranged from 10.6 per cent to 35.4 per cent (depending on region), mood disorders ranged from 12.1 per cent to 47.6 per cent and other anxiety disorders ranged from 15.6 per cent to 41.8 per cent (Priebe et al. 2010). A similar study in Kosovo, eight years after the 1999 war, showed that 11.9 per cent of participants met the diagnostic criteria for PTSD, while the prevalence of depressive disorder (MDE, major depressive episode) was 30.6 per cent (Eytan & Gex-Fabry 2011). Findings, based on research conducted in 2005–2006, showed the following prevalence of mood disorders: 35.9 per cent in Serbia, 25.9 per cent in Croatia, 12.1 per cent in FYR Macedonia, 22.7 per cent in Bosnia and Herzegovina and 47.6 per cent in Kosovo. Post-traumatic stress disorder ranged from 10.6 per cent (Macedonia) to 35.3 per cent in Bosnia and Herzegovina. Other anxiety disorders were also high, for example 20.7 per cent in Serbia and 23.6 per cent in Kosovo (Sabes-Figuera et al. 2012).

Sadly, those who left the country often faired even worse than the population that remained. Using the same methods to compare refugees with those who stayed in the area of conflict, one study found that postmigration stressors or post-migration risk factors such as separation from family, feelings of not being accepted in the host country, having a temporary residency status, being unemployed, difficulties in obtaining a work permit or work in their own profession, financial difficulties, inadequate accommodation, lack of proficiency in the host country's language, difficulties in accessing medical care, and so on, were all associated with higher rates of both mood and anxiety disorders (Bogic et al. 2012, p.6). All in all, the prevalence of mental disorders among refugees from the Yugoslav war who were long-settled in Germany, Italy and the United Kingdom were as follows: '54.9% had at least one of the studies' DSM-IV disorders ... rates of anxiety disorders were 43.7% and of mood disorders 43.4%' (2012, p.3). The study by Sabes-Figuera had similar findings: 45.1 per cent of the studies' ex-Yugoslav population in the United Kingdom had a mood disorder, and the rates for Germany were even higher (57.4 per cent) while in Italy the rate was slightly lower (30 per cent) than the average psychological impact of war in a study (31.7 per cent) which compared this impact across eight countries (United Kingdom, Germany, Italy, Serbia, Croatia, FYR Macedonia, BiH, Kosovo) (2012, p.3). The reasons behind the differences in the figures are numerous and beyond the scope of this chapter. The main point is that a range of psychological and other medical disorders developed years after the violent conflict on the territory of the former Yugoslavia was officially over.

Long-term effects of the 1990s wars and social collapses continue, if judged, for example, by the exponential growth of the use of sedatives in Serbia. Between 1996 and 2006 sedatives were the most sold medicines in Serbia (Radivojević 2006). In 2009 alone, pharmacies sold 10 million boxes of sedatives (population 7 million), 800,000 more than in 2008 (Mišković 2010). During the first three months of 2012, compared to the first three months of 2011, an additional 2.3 million boxes of sedatives were sold. For just one brand of medication (bromazepam), doctors issued nearly three million scripts (Popović & Davidov-Kesar 2011). In addition to sedatives the most common 'method for relaxation' in Serbia is alcohol (Mitrović quoted in Radivojević 2006). In 2012, 40 per cent of people in Serbia were reported as drinking alcohol every day (B92 2012). Only 10 per cent of children below the age of 16 have not yet tried an alcoholic beverage. The other drug commonly used for stress reduction, nicotine, is the only one that is decreasing in use. In 2000, over 40 per cent of the adult population smoked but this had dropped to 33.6 per cent by 2006, and remained around 34 per cent in year 2009 (Blic online 2009). This decrease is attributed to recently introduced policies that penalise smoking in public places, as well as to anti-smoking public information campaigns.

Research also shows that overall suicide rates decreased during the war but then increased afterwards. For example, in a 2002 Croatia-based study by Bosnar and colleagues (quoted in WHO 2005, p.151) the suicide rate increased from 16.2 during the war to 19.1 per cent afterward. The study compared the pre-war, mid-war and post-war period, and the increase it recorded was higher among men in general and among those below 40 years of age in particular. The lowest rate of suicide overall was during war, and such a situation was witnessed in Serbia as well. Research by Doroški confirmed that the lowest rate of suicide in Serbia was in 1999, during NATO bombing (2012). He explains this as people's reaction to drastic danger, which 'forces people to use their last atoms of strength for mere survival'. However, as is the case in many post-conflict societies, after these events the rate of mental disorders, including suicide, dramatically rises as reactive, anxious and depressive conditions 'wake up'. Further, while some of these disorders may be suppressed during times of extreme danger and latent during social stability, it is during chronic conflict and disharmony that they manifest (2012). During those times *existential* or *whole life* crises are common and potentially very damaging to a person, as my mother and many others experienced.

Whole life crises refers to 'a relatively intense and often dramatic state of discrepancy in which the whole functioning of a person, the life choices that person has made, the beliefs upon which they have constituted their lives, are disputed ... a change that is not impartial and occasional but more or less whole and substantial...' (Vlajković quoted in Beara 2011b). They lead to disruptions of 'fundamental schemas about the self, others, and the future' (Tedeschi 1999, p.319). They can also set in motion 'distressing and sometimes dysfunctional patterns of thinking' (Tedeschi & Calhoun 2004, p.2). An existential or whole life crisis is not an event, although it may be a consequence of a single event, but a process that lasts (Vlajković et al. 2000, p.11). In situations of social collapse there may be myriad such single events, some of which may be more and some less traumatic. Among the most traumatic, of course, are loss of a child, parent, spouse/partner and other family members as well as experiencing direct threats to one's own life (bombing, shelling, being shot at, physically injured, tortured or psychically abused). Leaving one's home, belongings and friends, and subsequently losing identity, professional status and an economic means of survival, all of which accompany wars and social collapse, are also very stressful and traumatic. Daily stressors, such as waiting in queues to receive humanitarian aid, spending days in refugee camps, and facing various administrative obstacles (documents, visas), while of less intensity, may add up and reinforce damage to already fragile emotional states (2000). Major traumatic events most commonly create a low tolerance for frustration. This has been well documented among war veterans (Beara 2011a, 2011b; Špirić 2008). Situations when a veteran 'snaps' after a relatively minor incident are common. Self-harm by refugees has also been recorded as well as an increase of conflict within families (Vlajković et al. 2000).

That the waging of wars is not in 'our nature' but rather a psychosocial pathology is confirmed by the negative effects on those who are supposed to be the most resilient: combatants. Soldiers are psychologically primed and militarily trained to engage in combat, they are also engaged in direct actions and are given more power, including the right to exert power through the use of weapons. And yet, a significant number of soldiers develop psychological disorders, during, and especially after, wars. During the 1991–1995 war in Croatia around 10,000 war veterans developed PTSD, which constitutes a 15 per cent prevalence (2000). It is currently estimated that between 1500 and 2000 Croatian war veterans have committed suicide since the end of war in Croatia (Pavković 2012), the state that officially *won* the war. Croatian war veterans also die on average 20 years sooner than the rest of the population, most commonly from heart attacks and strokes, as well as cancer, and are usually between 50 and 60 years of age (Lovrić 2011). Their families – wives and children – are also negatively impacted (2011).

In Bosnia and Herzegovina alone, over 4000 war veterans committed suicide after the war had ended (Frontal.rs 2012). Figures for Serbia are still unknown, 'but every veteran knows somebody who has committed suicide' (Beara & Miljanović 2012). In Croatia suicide among war veterans is a taboo topic and reasons behind suicide are trivialised (Pavković 2012). Psychologists working with war veterans, however, have identified mechanisms of post-war maladjustment. During the lasting process of war, most soldiers develop 'adaptive behaviour' characterised by violence, distrust and emotional numbness (Beara 2011a). This violence does not stop when the war does. Rather, due to 'the combination of hard conflict, low frustration tolerance, and medicament-alcohol cocktails' (2011a) impulsive reactions and further violent episodes often follow. Post war, a cycle of violence continues as 'the traumatized veteran is tense, impatient ... reacts impulsively and aggressively to insignificant causes ... shows numerous anxiety symptoms, has difficulties in feeling and showing love ... perceives the future to be grim' (2011a). Difficulties with finding suitable employment and establishing or maintaining quality relationships with others are common. Among the frequent neurotic conditions Beara and Miljanović enumerate, first and foremost are panic disturbances, and then various kinds of phobias, anxiousdepressive disturbances in everyday functioning, learning deadlock, inefficiency at work, hypochondria or sexual disturbances and similar:

> Sudden fear is connected with some physical symptoms in most cases. When one notices instability, insecurity, heart beating, *breathlessness,* arm and leg numbness, he starts to catastrophise his symptoms and to practically create his own problems. He feels that something ugly is going to happen, and that this could finish tragically.

> Fear of death or fear of insanity appears. People cannot find themselves; they do not know what is happening ... They ask themselves how it is that they can no longer go out of the house, get on the bus, make contacts as they used to. They walk with fear, trying to find escape from that situation, to take control over their life, but they can barely control *themselves.* After some time, they start thinking of themselves and of other people as being worthless (Beara & Miljanović 2012, italics added).

So even 'tough soldiers' have trouble breathing sometimes, even they, at times, somatise their fear.

This is not limited to the situation in the former Yugoslavia, however. In the first 155 days of 2012, there were 154 US military suicides, or nearly one every day (Thomson 2012). This is 18 per cent above 2011's corresponding toll (2012). Such a persistent rise in the suicide rate continues despite 'numerous recommendations from the Army and [Department of Defense] task forces ... [and] has frustrated all in the military' (2012). The obvious solution to this phenomenon, however, seems to escape them.

To conclude, the long-ranging consequences to mental and emotional as well as physical health, in addition to the human, economic and ecological cost of war, have been immense in the Yugoslav wars, as they are in every war. All these psychological and physical disturbances not only result in continuous inner psychological tension but can also lead to a host of other health problems as well as to homicides and suicides. Research findings highlight ongoing 'devastating effects of wars for the communities that experience them, [which] ... last long after the conflict is ended' (Sabes-Figuera et al. 2012, p.5). The full range of psychological effects is most commonly visible after the times in which the pure survival instinct is active (Doroški 2012; Kuzmanović 2004). It was especially after the worst in a series of traumatic events was over that 'posttraumatic depression arrived to claim its toll, because all energy has been exhausted' (Kuzmanović 2004). Chronic fear and depression mostly break people later, after the complete personality structure is broken down 'horizontally and vertically' (2004). 'We should not delude ourselves. It will take the next 50 years to cure the traumas we have now' conclude psychologists Beara and Miljanović (2012). This, sadly, may be an understatement.

In: Dear Diary

It has been recommended to me that I put down on paper some of the troubling experiences, including recurrent disturbing dreams, that I've had over the years. So here they are. The first upsetting recurrent dream I remember occurred with reasonable frequency when I was a child. It is hard to tell now how many times I had it or what were the circumstances I found myself in days prior to the re-appearance of the dream, for it was so long ago. But I do indeed remember it vividly because it was always the same; it occurred over a span of a number of years, possibly over a decade, and was usually very frightening. I was always in a group of people and we were trying to escape into the woods from some unspecified danger, lurking behind the trees. But in the middle of the woods there was a clearing and a small hill elevation where we would be exposed. Nonetheless that was the fastest way towards perceived safety and thus we would run towards the clearing, hoping to hide between the trees past that small and open elevation. I would usually see some people get to the place of safety when suddenly I would hear a burst from the machine gun, and feel bullets entering my back and into my lungs. The bullets would always enter at exactly the same spot, between my waist and neck. They always felt warm. There was no pain in my dreams, nor when I would consequently wake up, sweaty and gasping for air. The dream always felt so real that I would be compelled to touch my back, which never felt painful or chafed. The area where the bullets entered my back in my dream, however, always felt warmer than the rest of my body.

To this day I do not know the exact origin of this dream. I also don't know whether it was this dream or something else that made me convinced that I would die young. Despite my rather robust health in childhood, during my early teens I even placed a bet that I wouldn't live past 17! And despite all the empirical and rational evidence to the contrary this feeling of not reaching the average life expectancy followed me since I knew about myself. During my teenage years the dream about being shot was replaced by another recurrent one whose origin is easier to establish. Growing up in 1970s and 1980s Europe also meant growing up in the atmosphere of the Cold War and the implicit threat of nuclear arms. The litany of information presented to us during those times went along the following lines: Soviet and American nuclear arsenals together are fast approaching the figure of some 50,000 nuclear warheads, with the 'total explosive power of about 15 billion tons of TNT, or three tons of TNT for every man, woman and child on Earth, which is 750 times all the explosives ever used in war' (Barnaby 1988, p.136). 'This destructive power is equivalent to approximately 1,250,000 Hiroshimas' (1988). Which meant that 'in a large-scale nuclear war, no nation would remain unscathed. The north, on which most warheads would land, would be utterly destroyed. Civilization would, within hours, be blasted back to the dark ages' (1988).

Such precise information was expressed visually in another series of my recurrent dreams: a quick vision of a loud explosion, heat and strong streams of air that would obliterate all in their path. In the end it would be just me still standing, with a total silence and darkness, and with a vast nothingness around me. And then I too would disintegrate into the void.

Waking up from this dream was not much fun either, as the whole universe would feel simultaneously alien and hostile. The dream intensified after the Chernobyl accident in 1986 but settled down in a few years. Then, guns returned. The new gun-related recurrent dream was this time easy to connect with a real life event I experienced. On the 27th of May 1992 the 'breadline massacre', in which some 20 people were killed while waiting in a queue to purchase this food item, occurred in Sarajevo. A few days later I was in Belgrade, having a meeting over a coffee with a colleague in Vuka Karadžića Street, near the Faculty of Philosophy from which we had recently graduated. I hadn't finished my coffee that day. The cup broke, the glass shattered and the liquid spilled when suddenly, after a loud bang, everybody jumped from their chairs and onto the ground. It all happened so quickly that I still have no idea whether I jumped onto the ground myself, following the behaviour of the others, or whether somebody pulled me down. All I know was that suddenly I was pressed face down, breathing in the dust and filth from this inner-city Belgrade street. I remember the loud noise too, the shooting of guns and people's screams. 'So this is it', I thought, 'the war has finally arrived' in Belgrade, too.

Completely frozen, I was scared to look up and scared not to look up, I was suspended in time and space, confused as to where a safe exit might be. Once I started feeling my body again I realised I could move after all. I finally looked up and saw a young man, possibly my age or younger, kneeling on the window sill and shooting from there, fortunately not in my direction. Who he was shooting at, and who was shooting back at him, and where those other shots were coming from I had no idea. Was he perhaps suddenly going to change his direction and shoot at me and the other café-goers? Or not? I was completely ignorant of which way this event would turn in the end. All I knew at the time was that I felt so powerless, looking at this man who had the power and the means to take my life on a whim. After what seemed a long time indeed, but probably lasted only ten or so minutes in real, 'clock' time, a couple of people in front of me got up and ran inside a store within a nearby building, a mere few metres away. I did the same. I was safe, 'not a scratch'. Except that this event triggered another series of repetitive dreams in which clean-shaven young men dressed in black kept on threatening me with guns and shooting in my direction. The dreams did not subside once I left the country in 1994 and arrived in Australia. In fact, they intensified. Particularly puzzling was the appearance of men with knives. That dream, too, was always the same: men with knives would enter our home, threaten me or my children; in desperation I would grab their knives by the edge with my bare hands; the intruders, however, would burst into laughter, even if I stabbed them with their own knives after a fight. They were invincible, and I ... I was totally and utterly powerless.

Out: Past and present traumas

> We have encountered numerous children of survivors and [perpetrators] who have attempted to repair their parents' lives by eliciting testimonies or writing down the parents' histories. Many are journalists or therapists, engaged in professions that valorize the spoken word, knowing, and the telling of stories (i.e., the witnessed narrative) as ways to impact on others and/or heal (Auerhahn & Laub 1998, p.37).

Living trauma, the title of this chapter, refers to the experienced reality in which trauma has to be carried by survivors in their everyday lives after an actual traumatic experience, or a series of traumatic experiences, caused by violence. The title also implies that trauma continues to live, semi-independently, finding various ways to express itself irrespective of survivors' desires. That is, the most commonly used strategies in dealing with trauma are those of suppression, of 'moving on' or 'getting on with one's life'. Wanting to forget and run away is also widespread. I have met a number of ex-Yugoslavs who migrated to Australia because 'it was the furthest we could go away' from the place of traumatisation. Further, a desire to 'protect the children' and not to tell them about traumatic events of the past is prevalent. Most of these mechanisms were present in both my maternal and paternal families, as they are in the majority of others.

What results, however, is a 'conspiracy of silence' (Danieli 1998, 2010a), a psychological defence mechanism aimed at the prevention of intrusive traumatic memories and emotions and at the continuation of life-family cycles as if 'nothing had happened'. Further, survivors are often faced with the following dilemma: acknowledging the damage done may be seen as the ultimate victory by the perpetrators of violence; not acknowledging it, on the other hand, may seem as the ultimate betrayal of the victims who perished (Danieli 1998). Conflicted with this, and told to 'let bygones be bygones' (1998, p.4), survivors often elect to not talk about their experiences. Researchers investigating this found, however, that this strategy does exactly the opposite: conspiracies of silence are 'the most prevalent and effective mechanism for the transmission of trauma on all dimensions' (Danieli 2010b, p.66). This is because:

> Like paper [silence] ... is a very thin and flimsy protection that rips easily ... it has proved detrimental to the survivors' familial and sociocultural reintegration by intensifying their already profound sense of isolation, loneliness, and mistrust of society.[7] This has further impeded the possibility of their intrapsychic integration and healing, and made mourning their massive losses impossible ... Both intrapsychically

> and interpersonally protective, silence is profoundly destructive, for it attests to the person's, family's, society's, community's, and nation's inability to integrate the trauma (2010b).

Furthermore, children are left without rational explanations as to why certain practices and adaptive mechanisms were developed – such as the already mentioned mistrust of society or hyper-vigilance – and unable to investigate whether these strategies remain significant for the hereand-now that they inhabit. Rather, new generations are presented with worldviews and behaviours as well as subconscious messages that reinforce the trauma-related cognitive template, for example, that the world is a dangerous place or that others should never be trusted. This template can subsequently influence the enhancement of worldviews and behaviours that may contribute to the cycles of self-fulfilling prophecies taking place. Much of what has happened in the Yugoslav wars of the 1990s, and why and how these things happened, can be attributed to earlier violent events of the twentieth and previous centuries. Much of what is happening in various current conflicts worldwide can also be attributed to earlier violent events. Manipulating unresolved traumas, getting people to overreact to minor threats and (merely potential) dangers, seems to be one of the easiest strategies that hegemonic-androcratic 'leaders of the people' can use to maintain their own power and influence. If there is a conspiracy of silence around trauma because of violence done in the past, communities cannot find 'words to narrate the trauma story and create a meaningful dialogue around it' (2010b). Crucially, this practice comes to be 'at the core of dynamics that may lead to symptomatology in the second generation' (2010b) and even beyond.

If not dealt with consciously and constructively, traumatic experiences may come back to claim their toll with interest. Moreover, depending on the frequency, magnitude and sheer horror that is witnessed, there is only so much that can be suppressed. One day, inevitably, suppressed thoughts and feelings resurface, sometimes even in subsequent generations, with trauma begging for transcendence. It is especially important to recognise this in light of most practices within post-conflict societies where the suppression-expression trauma continuum is always politically moderated. These practices of selective remembrance and selective representation of trauma/victimhood in the context of the former Yugoslavia were discussed in Chapter 2.

Of course, the suppressed narratives, politically unacceptable during socialist/communist Yugoslavia, did not simply 'go away'. Rather, passed on both directly as well as subconsciously, they were transmitted to subsequent generations. The pain of our ancestors became our own. In the absence of alternative peace-and-nonviolence-based cognitive templates, the fertile ground for 'narcissistic injury and rage' was created. Supported by the dominant discourses of social militarism, ethno-centrism and nationalism, as well as of patriarchy, violence grew well in that soil, fertilising it further with more of the same dung.

Intergenerational trauma transmission is critically important to the field of peace and conflict studies. As argued by Johan Galtung, a desire to welcome the dark prognosis of a trauma is 'important in explaining Iraq/Saddam Hussein, and Yugoslavia/Slobodan Milošević, in terms of their political behaviour' (2000, p.162). To this we could add other protracted conflicts, such as the Israeli–Palestinian, or the United States/Western world response to the September 11 attacks. Glory is best, concludes Galtung, but 'trauma is a good second best' (2000). That is, political leaders often tap into society's unresolved (or immediate) collective traumas, finding easy scapegoats for social, political and economic difficulties in others. It helps if that other was already unjust towards us in the past, or is somehow constructed as a historical or contemporary enemy.

Given most official nation-state histories, the arguments that propose these divisions are extremely easy to find. In this context revenge is infinitely easier than an investigation into one's own contributing role in the conflict. While victims were/are real, and should be acknowledged, it is the politics of victimhood or CGT (Chosenness–Glory–Trauma) syndrome (Galtung 2002, p.23) that continues to plague our 'deep cultures'. Past–present traumas, therefore, too often continue to influence repetition of violence, creating self-fulfilling prophecies, in turn, wherein *we* die because *we* must in order to survive! Parallel to this *they* also must die for *us* to live, protect our freedoms, way of life and prosperity. Yet another fertile soil is created in such a way – in this particular instance, sprouting (overtly or covertly) genocidal politics and actions.

Given these dynamics it comes as no surprise that nationalistic Bosnian Serbs referred to Bosniaks (Bosnian Muslims) as *balije* and Turks, the latter term evoking and using the colonisation (and brutalisation) of Slavs by Ottoman Turks in the medieval period, for the political purposes of the 1990s. Other periods of traumatisation, specifically those of the Second World War, were also remembered and used for the political purposes of the day. Croats were referred to as Ustashe and fascists by the nationalistic Serbs, and traumatisation of Serbs in Jasenovac concentration camp during the Second World War in particular became a new hot topic. Nationalistic Croats for their part referred to Serbs as Chetniks or Gypsies – implying that they were a lower race. Additionally, it is a historical fact that the father of the indicted war criminal (first Yugoslav then) Serbian general Ratko Mladić was killed by Croatian Ustashe in 1945. A number of texts bring evidence from interviews with Mladić that not knowing his father because of his murder was indeed a defining factor in his life, influencing his political choices and military actions (Halberstam 2003, p.295; Rogel 2004, p.129). Another trauma, the suicide of his daughter Ana in 1994, was reported to have had a profound detrimental influence on him and on his military 'tactics' a year before the Srebrenica massacre took place (Mastilović Jasnić 2011; Stojaković 2011). In interviews and conversations Mladić claimed she too was murdered (Bulatović 2006).

Put together, the experiences of the previous traumatisation of some of the key players of the 1990s Yugoslav conflicts on, for example, the 'Serbian side' are striking. Radovan Karadžić's father 'fought with the Chetniks against the wartime Nazi occupation and against Tito's Partisans, the rival communist resistance movement, and later served a prison sentence under the Tito regime for these activities' (Day et al. 2002, p.295). The architects of the Serbian totalitarian state, Slobodan Milošević and his wife Mirjana Marković (an important political figure at the time in her own right) both came from families in which violence, suicide and homicide (during and after the Second World War) impacted them. According to her own account Mirjana was 'born in a forest' in 1942 as enemy forces were closing in on the partisans (Djukić & Dubinksy 2001, p.4). That same year her mother was 'shot as a traitor to the party ... apparently for having given names of Communists to the enemy under interrogation and torture' (Bringa 2004, p.182). She seemed to have further suffered from the abandonment by her father, and was subsequently raised by her maternal grandparents.

Another indicted war criminal, Vojislav Šešelj, was born in eastern Herzegovina, an area of the former Yugoslavia extremely brutalised during the Second World War. In addition to this he was later imprisoned, and most likely tortured, during the socialist rule in Yugoslavia (he was arrested for conspiring to overthrow the regime in 1984). A number of Serbian psychologists have publically described Šešelj as a sociopath, or even a psychopath who finds pleasure in 'shocking and taunting those he comes into contact with' (Rogel 2004, p.138). A leader of Serbian paramilitary formations that committed horrendous acts of violence in Bosnia and Herzegovina, Željko Ražnatović – (also known as 'Arkan'), reported being brutalised by his father, a Yugoslav army colonel, as a child. What is more, he received military-type training when working for the Yugoslav secret police, presumably with the mission 'of liquidating Croat Ustasha elements living abroad' (2004, p.135).

Yet another leader of Serbian paramilitary formations, Dragan Vasiljković, alias 'Kapetan Dragan', was reported to have spent his early years in a Belgrade home for abandoned children, before being reunited with his mother and siblings and migrating to Australia (Popović 2009). His biography was purposefully kept obscure for the purposes of myth making during the years of war; it was claimed that he had been a prominent member of the French Foreign Legion. It has since emerged that he apparently had numerous run-ins with the law as a minor and had received military training in Australia. While it did not train Vasiljković, the French Foreign Legion had provided training for yet another subsequent agent of political violence, Milorad Ulemek Luković, who also grew up in the family of a Yugoslav army officer. From the early 1990s Luković participated in a paramilitary unit, the Tigers, as well as in the special Serbian police force called the Red Berets. The latter unit was reputed to have been involved in wars in Bosnia and Kosovo as well as being implicated in orchestrating acts of terror in Serbia. Luković, alias 'Legija', is currently serving a 40-year sentence for the murders of prominent Serbian politicians, including Milošević's mentor Ivan Stambolić, and Serbia's first democratically elected leader after Milošević's removal from power, Zoran Đinđić. Military training and/or homicide of family members have been a recurrent theme among some other prominent players from the other side as well. For example, nationalist leader of Croatia from 1990–99, Franjo Tuđman, a general in the former Yugoslavia's army, also had members of his immediate family murdered during or after the Second World War (brother, father, stepmother).

To what degree these biographies influenced these people's propensity towards violent resolution of conflict, whether consciously or unconsciously, is not possible to fully ascertain. The larger question remains of what motivates some to choose the path of transcendence (Galtung et al. 2002), while others choose to re-create traumas. Nonetheless, put together, certain patterns do emerge in these biographies, and these patterns further support the theoretical insights discussed in previous chapters (that is, those relating to the raising of children, dominant worldviews within androcracies, the roles of militarism in general, and social militarism in particular, and the role of patriarchy). Previous trauma, however, does not only impact individuals, argues Danieli; even a whole society can behave as if it has PTSD (2010b). Psychological mechanisms of defence have both personal as well as societal dimensions. 'The most malignant component of the transmission is the raw, unintegrated effect that has never been processed in the parents' generation and, consequently, becomes internalized in their children in another place and time' (2010b, p.76). Further, it is a characteristic of intergenerational trauma transference that multiple traumas and stressors can become compounded over time:

> A trauma in one generation can be 'added to' traumas experienced in another generation. One implication of this additive quality of intergenerational trauma is that the 'healing sands of time' may, in fact, not be a dependable solution, and instead the traumatic experience might actually increase over time as additional events are added to what comes to be seen as an unending traumatic onslaught (Campbell & Evans-Campbell 2011, p.7).

And so 'events that appear slight and non-consequential to an outsider may in fact be imbued with much greater meaning by those suffering from the effects of intergenerational trauma' (2011).

The ripple effect of traumas that have resulted from historical acts of violence can be seen in both their internalised and externalised versions. Internalisation of trauma, as seen in the previous section, leads to a host of mental and other health disorders. Externalisation of trauma, on the other hand, leads to a host of violent behaviours, towards other individuals (homicide), other groups (genocide) or even towards the self (suicide). Most commonly, internalisation and externalisation of trauma are mediated by other social factors, for example by gender, which was discussed in the previous chapter. Furthermore, the same person may express trauma via internalisation (depression, anxiety, PTSD, physical illness) in one social setting and externalise it in another (usually towards those more vulnerable than the self). Such a situation is common among war veterans who perpetrate domestic violence. They frequently exhibit a combination of anxiety and PTSD symptoms coupled with 'extremely low frustration tolerance, alcohol and medication abuse, and perceptions of his own wife's behaviours as being humiliating and disrespectful' (Beara 2011a). This combination then leads to situations of physical violence and abuse against their wives, children and other family members, which in itself may start yet another cycle of violence and traumatisation for subsequent generations.

An understanding of the mechanisms of trauma transference, and the impact and consequences of these mechanisms is therefore critically important to understanding many conflicts as well as the dynamics of post-conflict societies. Hopefully, by better understanding this mechanism, better preventative and healing strategies can also be promoted. A summary of current research findings, as far as transgenerational trauma transference is concerned, is now possible, despite this being a recent area of research.

Scientific inquiry into the systematic impact of trauma on populations that experience it firsthand is but a hundred years old. Inquiry into the impact of trauma on the second and third generation is even more recent. The first book on 'traumatic stress that examines multigenerational effects of trauma across various victim/survivor populations around the world from multidimensional, multidisciplinary perspectives' (Danieli 1998, p.1) was edited by Yael Danieli and published in 1998. But even though intergenerational transmission of trauma is a relatively recent focus within the field of psychology (Danieli 2010b, p.65), as well as in peace studies, trauma's impact has been transmitted across generations throughout history. Trauma has been 'alluded to, written about, and examined in both oral and written histories, in all societies, cultures, and religions' (2010b). This new focus is important not only for individuals concerned but even for immediate post-conflict communities as well. Indeed, it is crucially important for the investigation into long-term prevention of the (re) creation of violence and the maintenance of, an often fragile, peace.

Initially, from the 1960s onwards, research was primarily directed towards second generations of victims, such as the children of Holocaust survivors. By now studies have been done on this as well as on the second and third generations of other groups, such as children of the survivors of other wars, asylum seekers, internally displaced people/refugees, indigenous peoples, children of Vietnam war veterans, children of atomic bomb survivors (Hibakusha Nisei), and on Sansei – children of Japanese-Americans interned by the US government during the Second World War. More recently (for example, Staub 2000, 2003; Hatzfeld et al. 2006; Hatzfeld 2006; Lev-Wiesel 2007), research into the role of previous trauma as a precursor for the perpetration of violence has also sprouted. In both cases multigenerational legacies of being victimised are preserved in 'story-telling, songs, and family patterns' (Reyes et al. 2008, p.297). This transfer takes place through both silence and underdisclosure as well as (age-inappropriate) over-disclosure[8] (Danieli 2010b). Other identified psychological mechanisms include 'identification-observation, modelling, and emulation [such as survivors' propensity for hypervigilance], and isomorphic re-enactment' (2010b, p.76). In this last mechanism 'the survivor's trauma experience is created in the offspring, perhaps unconsciously, but forcefully, transmitting the parent's worldview' (2010b). Carrying the pain via inter-generational transference, without acknowledging and recognising it, then results not only in negative feelings (such as feelings of powerlessness, isolation, loneliness, contradictory feelings, bitterness, emotional distance, mistrust of society and others) but also in violence (towards self and towards others). Having such thoughts and feelings and expressing behaviours in line with traumatic beliefs/worldview can be acute/chronic/lifelong and even passed on from generation to generation. In this latest instance, especially if there is a 'conspiracy of silence', later generations may feel the pain but struggle with identifying the sources of that pain (2010b).

Terms currently used for the transmission of trauma to subsequent generations are 'historical trauma', 'multigenerational transference', 'sequential traumatisation' and 'intergenerational PTSD'. These different terms, however, all refer to the same phenomenon: effects of harm, such as violence, or the suffering and pain of injustice, that have not been resolved and that have been transmitted from one generation to the next (Connors 2007). Historical trauma can then be defined as:

> trauma inflicted upon a group of people that share a specific group identity or affiliation, such as

> ethnicity, nationality, or religious [and ideological] affiliation. Such traumas may be temporally limited within a single generation, such as a war or devastating natural disaster, or, more commonly, they may occur over several generations as several discrete events come to be seen by the victims as linked into a single continuous traumatic experience (Campbell & Evans-Campbell 2011, pp.8–9).

The kinds of events that are typically experienced as traumatic are diverse. They include human-made and natural disasters, as well as collective and individual acts of violence. In general, however, several characteristics that make an event a traumatic one can be identified:

> First, they are often carried out intentionally by outsiders ... Second, either alone or in concert, they are profoundly destructive and generate high levels of distress. Such destruction can include the loss of human life, but also the destruction or desecration of highly valued or sacred objects, practices, and environments. Third, they tend to be highly collective, in that many, if not all, members of a community experience them as traumatic or later suffer from their effects. And fourth, their legacy is carried forward over generations and can have negative impacts on the physical, mental, social, and spiritual wellbeing

> of individuals, families, and communities well into the future (2011).

'Catastrophe is about to strike', the so-called vulnerability life trap psychologists have identified (Young & Klosko 1994), frequently develops among people who experience traumas. The worry that accompanies this mindset most commonly focuses on four types of vulnerability: health and illness, danger, poverty and losing control (1994, p.187). For example, if one is focused on danger, there is an exaggerated concern for one's own personal safety and the safety of loved ones (and, it seems, for the safety of any group an individual identifies with) and the world is seen as fraught with threats to one's life and wellbeing at every turn (1994, p.188). Others, who had previously experienced poverty in extreme circumstances, such as, for example, the Great Depression of the 1930s, may develop a 'depression mentality' that makes them always worried about money, afraid they will end up without a basic means of survival (1994, p.189). There is a consensus among psychologists that the origins of the vulnerability mindset can stem from personal experiences but also from a parental encounter with a serious traumatic event (or events) in which their life was under threat (1994). The messages that they come to embody, then – for example, that the world is (above all) dangerous – get transferred to subsequent generations in myriad little ways (such as habits) as well as through the dominant philosophy about life. This has been well documented in the case of children of Holocaust survivors, but perhaps not so well documented in the former Yugoslavia. In fact, despite all the stories about violence and animosities between groups, most attention was given to the external events, not the emotional landscape of the collective and not to how these events impacted on real people.

Research reported in Danieli (1998, 2010a, 2010b), Sullivan and Tifft (2006), Wilson and Tang (2010), Reyes et al. (2009), Campbell and Evans-Campbell (2011), Brave Heart (2007) and others, however, confirms the existence of such multigenerational, collective, historical and cumulative 'psychic wounding'. This wounding has both psychological as well as physiological effects. Children of Holocaust survivors in particular, but also others such as, for example, children of Vietnam war veterans, show a particular neurobiology (seen in measured cortisol levels) that may make them both psychologically and biologically more vulnerable to stress and trauma than control subjects (Danieli 2010b, p.70). The somewhat controversial field of transgenerational epigenetics confirms this intergenerational transmission of previous generations' lived experiences into the biology of subsequent ones. Most commonly quoted is the Överkalix study, which showed the influence of grandparents' exposure to isolation and famine on the health and longevity of their grandchildren (Haslberger & Greßler 2010, pp.67–83). Long-term detrimental effects were seen in the second generation of

Japanese-Americans interned during the Second World War (Nagata 1998, p.125). More than twice as many Sansei (third-generation Japanese-Americans) 'whose fathers were in camp died before the age of 60, compared to Sansei whose fathers were not interned' (1998, p.134).

Shorter life span has been confirmed in later generations of colonised indigenous people. While the reasons behind this may be multiple (that is, inadequate healthcare and continuous marginalisation in a society), nevertheless, in Australia in 1998, the life span for an Aboriginal woman was '20 years less, and for an Aboriginal man, 18 years less than for whites' (Raphael et al. 1998, p.336). It may not be surprising then, that those experiencing PTSD, and their descendants, report having a sense of a *foreshortened future.* Among children, that manifests as a 'pessimistic attitude about the future – a belief that one's life can end at any moment, and that therefore the future can be neither anticipated nor planned for' (Fletcher 2003, p.349). Adults who perceive foreshortened futures are 'often depressed or suffering from posttraumatic stress syndrome' (Beitman et al. 2005, p.67). They see 'no or very low or limited future possibilities':

> The individual feels no control over their future and perceives no opportunities to activate goals. No matter what is done, there is a sense of futility in influencing any positive outcome; the future seems an imperceptible void. Individuals affected

> in this manner lack plans, expectations, and hopes, and do not expect themselves or loved ones to live long, productive lives (2005, pp.66–67).

Parallel to this, a sense of 'fixity' develops – a feeling of being 'frozen in time', continuing 'static living in the traumatic rupture'. Exposure to trauma causes a rupture as well as possible regression and a state of being stuck (Danieli 2010b, p.68) in the free flow of life. Further:

> The fixity may render the individual vulnerable, particularly to further trauma/ruptures, throughout the life cycle. It may also render immediate reactions to trauma (e.g., acute stress disorder), *chronic,* and in the extreme become life-long ... *posttrauma/victimization adaptional styles ...* when survival strategies generalize to a way of life and become an integral part of one's personality, repertoire of defence, or character armour (2010b).

The past, in that sense, becomes the present, and the expectation follows that the future will bring 'more of the same'. Alternatively, new threatening impulses are perceived as signifiers of 'back to the past' scenarios – a potential threat to the immediate future as well as to longer-term survival. Overreaction to a comparatively minor stimulus may occur, followed by 'pre-emptive' defence. 'Pre-emptive' defence by one group is, logically, perceived as aggression by the group against which such defence is put into action. The cycle of violence continues. To outsiders such actions seem 'irrational', which further confirms the view of the victimised that others cannot possibly understand because they haven't gone through the same experiences. Feelings of isolation, loneliness, mistrust of society and others, especially foreigners, coupled with feelings of powerlessness and continued suffering as a group of people thus gets reinforced. These effects impact families and subsequent generations of previously traumatised groups of people – when violence has occurred on a massive scale these processes affect whole communities, societies, and nations (2010b). In other words, 'shared or collective trauma can lead not only to individual symptomologies but also, and much less well-understood, to collective symptomologies, as well as to collective interventions centered in the society as a whole' (Campbell & Evans-Campbell 2010, p.8).

The consequences of previous trauma can therefore be interfamilial (such as psychological and biological) or extrafamilial (socio-political and cultural). And beyond their psychosocial implications, multigenerational effects of trauma may also carry 'legal (that is, issues of compensation and restitution) and political (wars and cycles of violence, ethnic and racial strife) implications' (Danieli 2010b, p.70). Fortunately, research has also shown that heterogeneous responses to trauma, as well as diverse ways of coping, exist. Most importantly, some people who have lived through trauma have reported emotional and spiritual growth after experiencing a traumatic event (Aia et al., 2007).

Courtesy of the latest psychological research, the most successful methods of trauma recovery have also been identified. These occurrences can give hope to people living trauma. Some people who are experiencing trauma have managed to develop higher order cognitive schemas (cognitive templates and worldviews) that may serve as a more appropriate defence against violence in the future. These occurrences can give hope to societies that experience, have experienced or may experience wars and mass violence. Indeed, post-traumatic growth has also occurred at the societal level throughout history. One notable example is that of the Indian emperor Ashoka's kingdom of the third century bce, which transitioned from a warrior society towards a society based on philanthropy and nonviolence. It was the trauma of the battle of Kalinga, which left some 100,000 dead on the battlefield, coupled with his discovery of Buddhism and its doctrine of nonviolence (*Ahimsa),* that apparently made Ashoka drastically change the course of his politics. An early European warrior society, the Vikings, as well, transitioned into 'the most peaceful region in Europe, Scandinavia' (Boulding 2000, p.24). More recently, Japan's transition from chronic warfare and a highly militarised society with imperial ambitions to a society with largely pacifistic orientation has also taken place. Further, during the twentieth century a number of eastern European societies transitioned into more peaceful democracies and open societies. Globally, societies re-oriented from drastic practices of colonisation, imperialism and war-initiated looting towards trade as a means to acquire material goods and increase material wellbeing for their citizens.

All of these transitions occurred in the aftermath of massive-scale traumas, none more horrific than the bombing of Japan with nuclear weapons. Therefore, there is 'evidence of positive developments within many social systems in the aftermath of violence' (Tedeschi 1999, p.330). Once a decision to not re-create traumas in the future takes place at the collective level, and an alternative peace promoting worldview is accepted, the transition towards a more peaceful society becomes possible and indeed doable. Yet for that to occur, an individual and collective self-awareness of many subtle forms of violence as well as awareness of the alternatives to violence are crucial.

In: Welcome to Australia

'You are not coming here to live, are you?' were the welcoming words of the Australian immigration officer in 1994. My visa read 'temporary *residency* visa', subclass 418. I had no intention of challenging him. 'Oh, no, I am here to join my husband while he *temporarily* works here.' For my part, I also had zero intention of staying in Australia permanently. Eighteen years later all I can think about are the ominous words of one of my uncles prior to my departure: 'Nothing is as permanent as temporary solutions!' Still, when the immigration officer asked me whether I could confirm that I was 'not coming here to live' and after I agreed that that indeed was the case, I couldn't help but wonder what the point of my two-year residency visa was. Residence is, in most dictionaries, defined as 'the place in which one lives' or 'the act of dwelling in a place'. The immigration officer must have known that so what did the question really mean?

Equally puzzling were repeated invitations to undergo X-rays once I was in Australia, even after thorough medical checks (including X-rays) all came out clear prior to my temporary visa being issued in Belgrade. X-rays never showed any abnormalities and yet it seems I was on some special list of potentially contagious foreigners who may or may not pose a threat to Australia's public health. Even after these were cleared during the first two-year period of 'temporary' living, further tests were ordered repeatedly because of bureaucratic procedures (temporary visa renewals). I was X-rayed even when pregnant with my first child: 'Do not worry, the radiation from X-rays is less than what you get from the sun.' As a precaution, however, 'wear this apron'. After Chernobyl, I was not sure if I could trust the authorities, political or medical. Free-floating distress was impossible to ignore though, even as my concerns were dismissed as baseless. In any case, for years there was this feeling in the air, occasionally verified by a letter that would arrive in the mail, that I was on some sort of a watch list, and that there were suspicions that I was potentially passing unspecified contagious diseases on to the locals. At the same time, my husband, who obviously lived in close proximity to myself, did not have to undergo similar repeated checks because he was a carrier of a 'good passport'.

All those years, I was physically healthy, but still remained under suspicion, and potentially dangerous. I had little power to decide what happened to my body – how many times I was to be X-rayed, poked, pierced with needles, etc. 'Do you want your visa extended, or not?', as if life was that simple. Two years after my arrival, a speech given in parliament defined Australianness as being based on 'Anglo-Celtic-European heritage, Judeo-Christian beliefs, English law and the Westminster parliamentary system'. In the same breath, migrants (especially Asians) were then accused of 'having their own culture and religion', failing to assimilate and forming ghettos. I wondered, 'Can I assimilate into Anglo-Celtic ethnic heritage?' At the same time, pro-multiculturalism Australians, or those that 'promote political correctness', were accused of reverse racism against mainstream Australians, who are forced to fund industries that service 'Aboriginals, multiculturalists and a host of other minority groups'. Like my father, Zoran, years ago, I was now experiencing an intimidating déjà vu.

Around the same time a hairdresser told me there were 'too many Japs at the Gold Coast'. A few years later, during the height of the Children Overboard Affair, a taxi driver let me know that *they* (asylum seekers) were lucky he was not there. No way would he have taken them out of the water after their boat sank. I was later directly warned against speaking my native tongue in public by a 'well-meaning' shop assistant who felt that 'otherwise [we] will never learn to speak properly'. 'Where is your accent from?' 'What is your nationality?' 'How long have you been in Australia?' These questions, asked over and over and over and over again, made one thing very clear to me: when I arrived on that plane in June 1994 the gap between the way I saw myself and the way others saw me increased multifold. Not only had all my systems of social support disappeared overnight, I somehow stopped being me and became 'a foreigner' – a migrant lucky to have been able to come, a Bosnian who escaped the war, a dole-bludger or a job-stealer, a tourist who loved it here so much she decided to stay.

Whether perceived as an exotic other, an interesting other, an inferior other or a threatening other, the fact remained that I was now the *other.* This also meant that, in a matter of days, I even changed my race. 'I can't determine whether the baby has jaundice. His skin colour makes it hard to do so,' said the paediatrician at Brisbane's maternity hospital. Nurses marvelled at his 'lovely olive' skin tone. 'Your son has inherited your olive complexion and your dark hair,' said one of them. When I arrived to Australia I had no idea that my skin was 'olive' and my hair 'dark'. While race was hardly ever explicitly mentioned in former Yugoslavia I kind of believed I was 'white'. I also believed the colour of my hair was, as poetically expressed in Serbo-Croatian, 'chestnut brown'. That being the norm there meant that my race, like the race of white people in general, was invisible. So it came as an utter surprise, even a shock to me, that suddenly, once in Australia, my differences became not only audible but also visible.

Surprisingly, 'local people' at times even knew better than me where I lived or came from. 'Where do you come from?' 'I come from Yugoslavia.' 'But that country no longer exists! Are you a Serb or a Croat?' 'Former Yugoslavia?' 'It is so *funny* that a country is called former!' Not being able to laugh at such funny things made me feel even more alien and isolated. Attending children's parties was at times difficult as the music, the laughter, the cake and candles, the balloons and the girls in pretty lace dresses were in my mind contrasted with images I had just seen on the news, of my hometown being bombed, of my birth-country destroyed. 'Would you like another piece of cake?' was sometimes a decision impossible for me to make as I was somewhat unsure as to which 'reality' was more 'real', the one in front of me or the one at the back of my mind.

For years I worried my 'unpronounceable name' (yet another new identity marker upon arrival to Australia) made it harder for me to find a suitable employment. Finally, in 2007 my suspicion was given some validation by an ANU study that found people with non-Anglo-Saxonsounding names need to send, on average, twice as many applications to be invited for an interview. This validation was quickly undermined by an Australian friend of mine who said, 'Have you perhaps considered that behind your difficulties in getting job interviews may be your personality?' 'If you overdo the impact of a social structure [such as racism or ethnocentrism] at the expense of your own individual agency that could really be extremely disempowering for you,' was the advice of another. 'Leave your past behind, no need for it here,' said a land-of-opportunity enthusiast. 'For centuries Australia has been a place where European rejects have been exported,' shared an Indigenous activist. 'You must be so happy you are in Australia now!' 'We are so lucky here!' 'How do you like it here?' Only one right answer could be given to that last question.

Out: Post-traumatic growth

> Social transformations of violence, like individual ones, are first based on telling the story. This is a consciousness-raising that allows the past to

> become a resource ... and sets the stage for action against repetition of trauma. In all the descriptions of social transformation of trauma ... a common theme is the survivors telling stories that eventually overcome apathy, disbelief, threat, and social systems resistant to change (Tedeschi 1999, p.334).

Hundreds of thousands of people who left the former Yugoslavia since the early 1990s often found themselves 'living peace' in very difficult circumstances. Temporary residence visas, unemployment or underemployment, discrimination, language difficulties, separation from family and many other constrictions and difficulties awaited them in both the neighbouring countries as well as in 'lands of plenty'. Being a temporary or permanent immigrant to a new place is challenging at the best of times. The experience of migration differs depending on the person's circumstances, the length of the migration, how well 'adjusted' to a new life the migrant becomes, attitudes of the locals and whether a new life is perceived as better or worse than life prior to migration. The best-case scenario involves an informed and conscious choice about leaving and the finding of some success after arriving in a desired place, the new life meeting or exceeding the hopeful expectations held prior to departure, and the relatively welcoming attitudes of the locals and the perception by migrants that the new life is offering more than the old. The bestcase scenario also presupposes the ability to exercise a significant degree of personal power over the circumstances of the post-migration experience.

The worst-case scenario involves forceful removal and accidental arrival to a new place, a new life that is worse, overall, than the life prior to departure/war, and an unwelcoming attitude of the locals and the perception/awareness of new arrivals that something bad has happened. It is not uncommon for different members of a family, leaving at the same time and arriving at the same place, to have very different experiences of migration. Different personality types also respond differently to the very same circumstances. Once again, these responses are influenced by a vast range of both external and internal factors, from how a person perceives reality to how others perceive the person.

There is currently a shift away from an earlier focus on pre-migration trauma (Murray et al. 2008) towards an increased focus on resettlement issues, post-migration or post-displacement factors. Research into the psychological wellbeing of refugees resettling in Australia, for example, found that 'post-migration stressors can have a significant impact on settlement outcomes' and may account for a significant amount of PTSD; almost as much as may be accounted for by *pre-migration* trauma exposure (2008, p.8). Worse mental health outcomes were found among those who had experienced loss in resettlement, for example people who were perceived in their home country as having higher levels of education or socio-economic status (2008). Such detrimental changes were also found among those who reported a loss of meaningful social roles and loss of important life projects, and among those who reported lower levels of daily activity, were unemployed or faced economic hardship and/or reported being socially isolated (2008). Compatibility with the host culture and the type of resettlement program also played a role (2008). Several other reports, global in orientation, have confirmed that mental disorders that affect people in all sectors of society disproportionately affect both refugees and migrants (IOM 2003).

The extent to which migration may be a trigger for a potential mental health problem depends on many variables, such as 'the motives for migrating, the duration of stay in the host community, language and cultural barriers, legal status of the migrant, the migrant's family situation, and the migrant's pre-disposition to psychological problems' (2003, p.92). Other studies have concluded that migration in itself does not threaten migrants' mental health (IOM 2006, p.416) and that it can even be beneficial (Stillman et al. 2007). Even more other studies (Furnham & Bochner 1986; Fangen et al. 2010; Sharma et al. 2012, p.65) further confirm that stressors, associated both with the circumstances of migration, and with the post-migration experience, have a greater psychological weight than the (perceived and real) benefits.

In my own case, I was aware that the overall life of most people in Australia, including immigrants, was objectively better than it was in many other places, many other nation-states. Subjectively, however (and many pleasant events and wonderfully supportive people notwithstanding), my own life experience overall felt much worse than the life I had left behind. This could have been due to my relatively low level of exposure to violence, or the fact that I had social support and meaningful work/employment 'for life' (courtesy of surviving elements of socialist ideology and practice) before I migrated. I was also a native speaker in my country of birth, my race was not visible, access to further education and medical services wherein culturally appropriate advice was provided were all givens, and so was my belonging to the local community. Once in Australia, however, most of those systems of social and emotional support disappeared. Furthermore, for the first time in my life I encountered the almost daily practice of what psychologists, in order to describe the everyday actions people take which contribute to someone feeling 'othered', have termed 'micro aggression' (Pierce 1970).

The trouble with the question 'where are you from?' does not lie in the initial question, argues Margo Ford. Rather, it lies with the retort, 'No, where are you *really* from?', when the answer provided is not deemed acceptable (2005, p.72). She calls these conversational practices, common in Australia, instances of 'discrete racism' or of 'subtle forms of interrogation, practised under the guise of polite conversation' (2005, p.77). In effect, these social practices carry 'continuous messages about who is allowed to call themselves Australian and who is not, and can lead to feelings of either belonging or not belonging within the Australian community' (2005). The continuation of a legacy of complex histories of colonisation, the aftermath of two world wars and industrialisation continue to influence some people to believe that nations and nationalities can be ordered hierarchically. There is thus a perception of good migrants, lesser migrants and undesirables, which are always time and place specific. In the Australian context, the initial racism against the Aboriginal people by white settlers and even discrimination against the Catholic Irish (by the Protestant English) continue to be transplanted onto newcomers. In this context, correspondingly, 'speakers of non-dominant languages, accents and dialects often report face-to-face discrimination that appears to rely on linguistic stereotypes rather than [or in addition to the] racial visibility *per se*' (Milojević 2001, p.10). Subtle and not so subtle racism represents: 'an ensemble of social practices and technologies by which dominant classes and groups assert economic, social and interpersonal power over subordinate groups, often on the basis of [both visible as well as] phonotypical appearance' (Luke 2003, p. ix). These practices take many practical forms: 'exclusionary material, physical partitioning of space ... discourse practice, and ... social imaginary and shared cognition' (2003). Discrimination does not occur solely on the basis of race or appearance, rather, 'the "cards" of race, gender, and social class are played out – via linguistic competence, accent and "audibility" as well as through the bodily performance that language always entails' (2003).

Being constructed as a foreigner, by the host of social practices mentioned above, and experiencing isolation, unemployment or underemployment, deterioration of my relative socio-economic status as well as frequent instances of micro-aggression, all carried a particular weight for me. Not only did these experiences pose difficulties in fulfilling certain basic needs (such as wellbeing, identity/belonging, purpose/meaning), they were also insidious reminders of some past traumas. As 'we all know', what happens to foreigners/others – those with a different nationality, ethnicity or dialect – whether they are a minority in somebody else's country, whether they are migrants, refugees or displaced persons and even whether they are seen as the ideological other or the enemy other by the occupying soldiers who came to their native lands from elsewhere is that they:

- are shot dead, as happened to my great-grandfather Mirko
- have to work long(er) hours with immense dedication (and keep quiet) to get semi-accepted in the new society, like my great grandmother Zinka

- are expelled from universities, like my grandmother Mira
- are captured, like my biological grandfather Vasiliy, and have their family taken away and are later punished for surviving
- are sent to working camps, like my grandmother's brother Leon and my grandfather Stanoje
- are murdered in concentration camps, like my grandmother's cousin Danica and her parents
- are tortured, like the civilians Ivan Goran Kovačić wrote a poem about
- require a special permit to walk around their hometown, like Stanoje
- have to run for their lives, like my grandmother Zora and her children
- are murdered in revenge attacks, like my father's cousins
- see their only son taken away and their daughter-in-law nearly beaten to death, like my great-great-grandmother Persa
- see their grandmother nearly beaten to death and have soldiers show them the knives they used to slit other people's throats, like my then eight-year-old father, Zoran
- are taken from trains to be tortured and killed, like those men my uncle Slobodan witnessed

- are attacked with tear gas, armoured cars and batons, like my cousin Mirna are born in barracks without heating at minus 40 degrees, like my mother, Jelena
- are bombed by powerful countries and militaries, like she and all my other family and friends still in the country
- struggle with surviving peace and living trauma, like all of them, millions of others and me as well did and continue to do.

Of course, it was not as if I remembered all these incidents consciously each and every time the ritualised process of othering through 'cordial conversations' took place. Rather, it was as if these incidents were always there, somewhere in the background. Even though I did not think of those events consciously, my body seemed to have remembered them – 1930s and 1940s Russia, the Second World War and the wars in the former Yugoslavia. It felt as if my personal and family biographies finally became ingrained in my own body, in my own biology. In a new and somewhat threatening situation, where for the first time in my life I was the foreigner-other in a place so far away from home, and was constantly reminded of that fact, where I felt incredibly disempowered when trying to materialise my needs and wants within a particular reality, my mind desperately tried to help me to stay safe. And so it became hypervigilant; trying to protect me by reminding me of that other undisputed fact 'we all know': unless you are constantly on the lookout for danger you and your children have very little chance of surviving. In the end, both my emotional as well as my physical health suffered.

And yet, simultaneously, or rather, inseparably, no longer unconscious, my breathing brought me back to that other home, the one that has been within me all along. Breathing connects us to the world around us, writes Ann Gadd. It is both 'the first and the last thing we do when we enter and exit our earthly existence' (2006, p.41). Poets and scientists alike, writes Kabat-Zinn, are aware that our organism, through our breathing, 'pulsates with the rhythms of its ancestry' (2009, p.47). Breathing is one of the rare functions in our body that can be performed consciously or unconsciously and thus this unique function of our breathing has been an 'integral part of many spiritual practices, as a means to make the unconscious known' (Gadd 2006, p.41). The breath itself has played an extremely important role in meditative practices, in developing mindfulness and in healing (Kabat-Zinn 2009, p.48). We cannot *not* breathe, as long as we are alive:

> Even if the air is foul or polluted by our fellow human beings, we are forced to integrate with it, as is every other being. Breathing then mirrors our coexistence. No matter how much we may want to be insular, breathing reminds us that we can't be (Gadd 2006, p.41).

Psycho-spiritual practices of conscious breathing have been used to address specific traumas, generalised anxiety as well as post-traumatic stress disorder. They have also been found to be an 'effective way to restore and accumulate the energy from the spirit in the body when it is disrupted by experiences of racism' (Hunter & Coles 2009, p.213). Together with other interventions at the physical, emotional, behavioural, mental, interpersonal 'whole self' and existential levels (Bourne 2005), these practices of conscious breathing have been proven to minimise living trauma symptomatology. Furthermore, in addition to overcoming or minimising trauma, a broader 'psyche's well-being' and betterment, or *eupsychia* (Maslow 1961), may develop through this process as well. And so, the answer to the question posed earlier in this chapter – Can one go back and function in a normal way after the massive traumas and dislocations that all wars and all situations of life-threatening violence inevitably bring with them? – seems to be no. One can, however, deteriorate, stagnate (stay frozen in time) or alternatively, expand and grow.

Traumatised people, whether traumatised by events that happened to them individually or collectively as members of a particular group, have two basic choices, argues Galtung: one is the way of reliving and recreating trauma, the other, the way of transcendence (2000). Transcendence, writes Galtung, presupposes hope, and hope is located in visions of a positive, constructive future (2004). A similar conclusion was reached by Richard Mollica as a result of his work with traumatised peoples. Survivors of externally created trauma through violence have, he shows, an inherent ability to heal themselves, and in such ways move away from recreating trauma, for themselves and others. The most successful strategies used by survivors to get out of trauma and achieve self-healing involve: Altruism (service to others; an antidote to psychological enclosure); Work (meaningful, purposeful and satisfying) and Spirituality (both as a worldview and a practice) (Mollica 2006). In a violent world, Mollica concludes, these are the best tactics when embarking on a path towards recovery and hope (2006). A broader definition of altruism perhaps also includes cases in which survivors of a trauma (that is, physical, emotional and/or sexual abuse/violence) decide to act as protectors of others (their own or other people's children) and commit not to repeat the same harmful behaviours they experienced once they are in a position of power over others. These too are some common approaches used by survivors during their process of healing. Healing of long-standing injustices involves three steps according to Paulo Freire: denouncing the injustice by defining it; announcing the transformation and making a commitment as to what is one to do about injustice (1998, p.74). Only then is there a possibility of moving beyond it. 'Transformation of the world,' concludes Freire, implies a 'dialectic between the two actions: denouncing the process of dehumanization and announcing the dream of a new society' (1998).

To heal from inter-generational traumas, Yael Danieli further argues, present generations can utilise as significant resources time, the future and hope (1998, 2010b). Given that trauma causes rupture, fixity, a sense of being frozen in time and distorts the normal inter-generational cycle, it is important to recover this via 'bidirectionality of the concept of time' (2010b, p.73). Unresolved trauma results in an absence of closure in the lives of victims/survivors as well as in the lives of their children; this also means that the grief remains timeless (2010b). It is the lack of resolution that ensures the passage of trauma to the next generation – children remember their families' and war history only 'in bits and pieces'. To address this, 'healing of the narrative' – rebridging and filling in the gaps – has been shown to be the 'most integrative and therapeutic' (2010b) method. This means re-interpretation of at least some family experiences as 'positively nurturing', finding strength and stability in family and cultural roots. For example, research by Katharine Baker and Julia Gippenreiter on the long-term impact of family losses because of Stalin's Purges concluded that families who were unable to maintain some sense of connection and continuity with their lost grandparents and were cut off emotionally as well as physically from those grandparents became 'disconnected', less clear about 'who they were or where they were going' (1998, p.423). On the other hand:

> Those who kept a sense of connection with lost family members fared better than those who intentionally or unintentionally let those family members slip into oblivion. Whether the grandparents actually physically survived the Purge was less important than the strength and values passed on to their grandchildren through the knowledge of what had happened to them. Connected grandchildren had a sense of identity firmly rooted in family experience, and many of them continued to enhance their connections through research into their family's past (1998).

Above all, the central element for healing is the bringing of a future dimension into the picture, that is 'the hope and promise enshrined in future generations' (Danieli 2010b, p.73). In this process of re-working the trauma some positive symptoms have been reported by survivors. These include higher achievement motivation in overcoming adversity, increased empathic capacities, personal growth and a newly discovered 'reservoir of spiritual strength'. In that sense, 'trials and suffering may actually serve a positive function in overcoming adversity and lead to personal growth in victims/survivors and their offspring' (2010b).

Similarly, Tedeschi and Calhoun identify at least three broad categories of perceived benefits among survivors of individual and collective traumas. These include 'changes in self-perception, changes in interpersonal relationships, and a changed philosophy of life' (1996, p.456). Perceived changes in self include 'emotional growth', becoming a 'better person', feeling more experienced about life, feeling stronger and more self-assured, as well as potentially stronger, more self-reliant and more confident when dealing with future challenges (1996). Even though some of these perceived changes in the image of self may be 'self-deceptive' or 'self-enhancing illusions' (Taylor & Brown quoted in Tedeschi 1999, p.322), or not confirmed by others and independently verified, they are nonetheless 'the hallmark of mental health' (1999). Changes in interpersonal relationships include 'development of closer family relationships, emotional growth, and an appreciation of how precious these relationships are, and how quickly they can be lost' (Tedeschi & Calhoun 1996, p.456). Further, self-disclosure and the recognition of 'one's vulnerability can lead to more emotional expressiveness, willingness to accept help, and therefore a utilization of social supports that had previously been ignored' (1996). Also, 'part of the positive development of social relationships comes from the greater sensitivity to other people and increased efforts directed at improving relationships' (Tedeschi 1999, p.323).

Lastly, a changed philosophy of life includes 'an increased appreciation for existence, taking life easier and enjoying it more, no longer taking life for granted and living each day to the fullest' (Tedeschi & Calhoun

1996, p.456). While for some, 'spiritual beliefs may be temporarily weakened by tragedy and [still] others may become more cynical and less religious' (1996, p.457), for others trauma may lead to a spiritual quest, a turning to religion as a resource, a strengthening of religious beliefs or to a religious conversion (Tedeschi 1999, p.324). While these new life-worldview schemas may in fact be another example of positive illusions (Tedeschi 1999, p.325), they can nonetheless assist in spiritual development and the development of wisdom, in experiencing emotional relief, regaining some sense of control and intimacy, and, crucially, in finding (new) meaning for both these events as well as life in general.

Based on this and other research within the field of positive psychology, a whole new area of inquiry, studying positive changes following traumatic events of the past, has emerged since the late 1990s. This recent research has indicated 'the possibility of positive impact[s] of negative events' (Tedeschi & Calhoun 1996, p.455), whether these events have impacted individuals or a collective. In the 'frightening and confusing aftermath of trauma, where fundamental assumptions are severely challenged,' write Tedeschi and Calhoun (2004, p.1), such situations can also present 'fertile ground for unexpected outcomes that can be observed in survivors: [a form of] *posttraumatic growth'* (italics added). Tedeschi and Calhoun further define their term as 'positive psychological change experienced as a result of the struggle with highly challenging life circumstances (2004)'. This refers to the 'sets of circumstances that represent significant challenges to the adaptive resources of the individual, and that represent significant challenges to individuals' ways of understanding the world and their place in it' (Janoff-Bulman quoted in 2004, p.1). In other words, it is not the trauma that facilitates growth but rather a conscious and active dealing with it, or *the struggle* with/against highly challenging life events, including whole-life crises.

For all this to take place, recognition and acceptance of the events that have happened is necessary. That is, the popular strategy of denial and moving on without rebuilding cognitive schemas that account for a new and changed reality in the aftermath of trauma(s) is a strategy that can backfire. For post-traumatic growth, trauma/traumas need to be integrated into the expansion of the self (Salick & Aurbach 2006). Social transformation can only happen when survivors tell about 'their experiences and take other actions that enlighten others, obtain justice, and prevent recurrences of similar events' (Tedeschi 1999, p.319). This is part and parcel of giving meaning to trauma 'through social and political action' (1999, p.334). Doing so provides dual benefits: 'The individual transforms the traumatic experience into a basis for a generativity script, and society benefits from the telling of the story' (1999). On the other hand, if higher-order cognitive schemas are not reconstructed to accommodate for traumatic experiences the need for closure may be transferred onwards, and to subsequent generations. Reconstruction of schemas, alternatively, 'produces a view of the world and related behaviour that the survivor perceives as beneficial, not only in managing the trauma, but in living life more fruitfully than it was lived prior to the trauma' (Tedeschi 1999, p.320). It appears, Tedeschi concludes, that it is in 'allowing the trauma to have an impact, rather than avoiding the distressing aspects of it' (1999) which is critical for posttraumatic growth. In summary, it is 'the struggle with the new reality in the aftermath of trauma that is crucial in determining the extent to which posttraumatic growth occurs' (1999, p.321).

Our societies love heroic stories, so there is some danger in the concept of post-traumatic growth, in particular, if people are expected to recover and move on, even grow, too soon. This is unrealistic because neither grief nor trauma recovery follows a predictable line. Both can have periods of progression and/or regression as a response to various internal and external stimuli. Neither process can be forced, even though it can be helped. Post-traumatic growth is not linear; rather it is multidimensional, as persons may report growth experiences in one area while not reporting it in another (1999). Some traumas are more difficult to recover from; for example, victimisation by a trusted person has more negative impact than trauma that results from illness. As well, victims of violence appear to suffer greater traumatic effects than persons who experience other sorts of victimisation (1999, p.325).

One of the few studies that measured post-traumatic growth after war (in Bosnia) found that the overall averages for the post-traumatic growth scale were 'considerably lower than reported in most studies on other kinds of trauma' (Powell et al. 2003, p.71). The study considered it plausible that 'the process of adaptation to terrible events has been hindered in the population studies not only because of the unusual accumulation of traumatic events but also because the individuals themselves as well as the micro-and macrosystems surrounding them have been shaken, changed, or destroyed' (2003, p.82). On the other hand, the former refugees, who spent a considerable amount of time abroad, 'did report significantly more growth than the internally displaced persons' (2003). Once again, the social dimension – improvement, stagnation or deterioration of a society including the social life of an individual – is seen to have a prominent role in the overall wellbeing of people.

This confirms findings in other studies, which report that a good environment and social support do, to an extent, mitigate some of the traumatic effects. A good environment calms down trauma and its consequential symptoms, while good social support can be the most important factor in coping with traumatic stress (Danieli 2010b). A safety network and the reinforcement of trust relationships, which are key characteristics of the communal environment, are also crucial factors in coping with trauma (Tzitoziou et al. 2006). A poor post-trauma environment, on the other hand, can lead to the re-activation of trauma, multiple stressors can further compound trauma, as well as add on traumas of the first generation to later generations (Danieli 2010b). Poor posttrauma environment can lead to second and third traumatic sequences, which could intensify the stress of preceding traumatic events (2010b).

Personal factors and individual coping strategies are equally important. A study on post-traumatic symptoms and growth among Kosovar war refugees confirms that post-traumatic growth is positively correlated with hope and positive cognitive strategies (Aia et al. 2007). 'Hope, religiosity, negative religious coping, and satisfaction with perceived social support' were also positively related to reported post-traumatic growth among traumatised Somali refugees resettled in Hungary (Kroo & Nagy 2011). A study by Hussain and Bhushan found that similar psychological processes, such as 'positive refocusing, refocus on planning, [and] putting into perspective (2011)', partially mediated the relationship between traumatic experiences and post-traumatic growth among Tibetan refugees across two generations. In summary, healing is blocked by a passive, helpless, victim stance, by silences, denials and distractions (Danieli 2010b). Non-acceptance, fighting with a new or old reality, and trying to function as you once did – going back to the past – are also not helpful. It seems that resilience (and growth), on the other hand, are forged through active, collaborative coping efforts, such as remembrance and honouring of stories, displaying of courage, perseverance and mutual support (2010b). Piecemeal and ad-hoc strategies as well, may not be sufficient. Rather, integration of the trauma 'must take place in *all* of life's relevant (ruptured) systems and cannot be accomplished by the individual alone' (Danieli 2006, p.347):

> Rupture repair may be needed in all systems of the survivor, in his or her community and nation, and in their place in the international community. To fulfil the reparative and preventive goals of trauma recovery, perspective and integration through awareness and containment must be established so that one's sense of continuity and belongingness is restored. To be healing and even self-actualizing, the integration of traumatic experiences must be examined from the perspective of the *totality* of the trauma survivors' and family and community member's lives (2006).

Such trauma recovery requires not only recognition that 'personal is political' and 'personal political', but also an ecological understanding of recovery from trauma. Individual differences in post-traumatic response and recovery/growth are 'the result of complex interactions among person, event, and environmental factors' (Harvey 1996, p.3). This approach understands 'violent and traumatic events as ecological threats not only to the adaptive capacities of individuals but also to the ability of human communities to foster health and resiliency among affected community members' (1996, p.5). In that sense, 'racism, sexism and poverty can be thought of as environmental pollutants – i.e. ecological anomalies that foster violence and threaten to overwhelm the health-promoting resources of human communities' (1996). Further, other pollutants and social diseases such as nationalism, imperialism, militarism and androcracy/patriarchy, need to be replaced with the nurturing qualities of peace-promoting worldviews and behaviours, if we are to transcend our individual as well as collective, global, living traumas. In other words, examples of structural, economic, ecological, cultural, epistemological and psychological violence constitute our global pathology, or our 'collective psychopathology' (Koenigsberg 2008). Transcending this global psychosocial pathology, removing pollutants so that we can freely breathe, means replacing pathologies of violence with peace promoting thought patterns/worldviews and social practices. This is a huge task that may need an active engagement by several generations after us. But the sooner we start, the sooner can we hope to bring our living traumas back to health.

Epilogue

> Bibliotherapy ... recognize[s] that no two persons' experiences of an event [or series of events] are identical, or even similar. Therefore, the listener [can benefit from appreciating] both the universal and the unique in the trauma, and what has been gained from it (Tedeschi, 1999, p.334).

To those lucky few who have remained relatively unscathed or not impacted by violence, thank you for listening. To the survivors of various traumas caused by violence, I hope you do not give up. As long as you possibly can, keep on searching for strategies that will bring more health, wellbeing, happiness and peace into your life and into this world.

As for my own journey, after several years of searching I was fortunate enough to come across a GP who listened to me, who understood me and my historical, as well as contemporary social, context. He did not dismiss me as a 'hysterical woman from the Balkans' and my/our condition as 'hopeless'. The trouble with the use of the term 'psycho-somatic' he said, is that people often assume only the impact of the psyche on the body, but the body, as well, significantly impacts on the psyche. This interrelationship is dynamic, ever changing, malleable and significant. Even the brain can physiologically change, and old patterns of acting/re-acting be replaced with the new ones. This plasticity of the brain can be utilised for healing, in a similar way that better social practices can result in better societies. And while I followed his recommendations focused predominantly on the level of the body functioning, I worked on the level of my mind and psyche. Some lifestyle changes were helpful, including dietary changes and adjustments to my physical exercise routines. I tried with good results a number of allopathic and naturopathic treatments my doctor recommended. An underlying physical ailment was identified and finally addressed. New thought patterns were discovered and practised. I feel privileged, thankful and grateful to have had access to all these multiple strategies, even though I actively sought them.

Sadly, the external environment did not change much. The social and political body still needs healing and will continue to do so in the future. We need more citizens to notice the symptoms and understand the underlying causes. We also need more 'doctors' of the world polity to listen to the inter-generational traumas of leaders and states and develop peaceful preventive strategies that move us to transcendence. There is a hope that this is yet to come.

I would like to thank my breathing for settling down, courtesy of a multitude of body-mind-spirit strategies, applied simultaneously and over a significant period of time. At the same time, I would also like to thank my breathing for throwing an initial tantrum, without which, it would have remained unconscious and without which, perhaps, this book would not have been written. A happy ending is still wanting – and yet there is a promise of an alternative beginning.

Endnotes

Introduction

[1] Concepts of attributional bias and the politics of victimhood are discussed and explained in Chapter 2.

[2] *Eutopia* here means a 'better and improved', decidedly not 'perfect society'.

[3] *Eupsychia* here means a 'better and improved self/mind'.

Chapter 1: Communism, utopia

[1] *Pacotopia* – from *paco,* 'peace' in Esperanto (another failed utopian experiment), and *topia,* 'place' – means 'peaceful place'. The purpose of creating Esperanto (which translates as 'one who hopes') was to bring into being an easy-to-learn and politically neutral language that would foster peace and international understanding between people with different regional and/or national languages.

[2] Currently the most promising alternative is the ecological discourse.

[3] The term 'gatherer-hunter' more accurately reflects the main source of nutrition in those

societies. Hunting was mostly supplementary; however, patriarchal and violent societies overemphasised the role of male activity and the organised killing of larger animals at the expense of gathering – 'women's' activity

[4] While the USSR and Russia are more commonly considered 'the motherland' and not the fatherland, in his letter, Vasiliy uses the term Отечество, which is derived from the word father.

[5] Meaning 'hidden', 'secret', from the Greek prefix *kryptō* (κρύπτο).

Chapter 2: War, dystopia

[1] Pronounced Ya'ma.

[2] Poem by Ivan Goran Kovačić (1942–43). Original version in Croatian and translation in English cited at www.ezgeta.com/jama.html.

[3] That is, *Jama* and similar texts should not be studied in primary school, and certainly no such texts in schools should be studied unless there is also emotional support (for example, via teaching emotional literacy) and concrete suggestions regarding actions that prevent violence.

[4] There is a list of 54 countries, but both Yugoslavia as well as six new states that formed after its collapse are listed, and new political

realities demand 'Yugoslavia' be removed from this current list and kept perhaps as a historical data only.

Chapter 3: Feminism, eutopia

[1] After abolishing autonomous status for Kosovo and Vojvodina, two provinces of Serbia were given autonomy in 1974.

[2] That is, disunity of leaders or on ideological grounds between Chetniks and Partisans.

[3] A town in Croatia where mostly Serbs lived.

[4] This combines three other relatively recent indices: The World Economic Forum's *The Global Gender Gap Report,* The Economist Intelligence Unit's *Women's Economic Opportunity Index* and the UNDP's *Gender Related Development Index (GDI)* and *Gender Empowerment Measure (GEM).*

[5] This chapter is a reworking of two texts I previously wrote, Milojević 2010 and 2012.

[6] I use the term hegemonic–androcratic here because in peaceful societies hegemonic masculinity is nonviolent. It is thus only non-peaceful societies that Riane Eisler and others term as androcracy (alternative terms are dominator or patriarchal or warrior-based societies).

Chapter 4: Living trauma, eupsychia

[1] This term is borrowed from the title of Olivera Simić's forthcoming book.

[2] Cited at www.doktor.rs/forum/pulmologija/gusenje-t15984.html.

[3] Cited at www.nezavisne.com/forum/index.php?topic=1339.0.

[4] Cited at ultrazvuk-tarle.hr/dijagnostika/zagreb/kad_pocne_gusiti/.

[5] Cited at www.doktor.rs/forum/neuropsihijatrija/depresija-napad-paniket1686.html.

[6] One notable exception in making this connection is Napoleoni's 2010 book.

[7] Even though Danieli's initial research was predominantly in the context of second-generation Holocaust survivors, her subsequent research as well as research by other scholars seems to confirm that these practices are common across a whole range of traumatised individuals and communities.

[8] Such as the poem *'Jama'* discussed in Chapter 2.

References

Abercrombie N, Hill S et. al. 1984, *Dictionary of Sociology,* Penguin Books, Harmondsworth, Middlesex.

Accad E 2000, 'Violence and Peace: Overview' in C Kramarae & D Spender (eds), *Routledge International Encyclopedia of Women: Global women's issues and knowledge,* vol.4, Routledge, London, pp.1986–91.

Ackerman P & DuVall J 2000, *A Force More Powerful: A century of nonviolent conflict,* St Martin's Press, New York.

Adorno TW, Frenkel-Brunswik E, et. al. 1950, *The Authoritarian Personality,* Harper and Row, New York.

Aia AL, Ticea TN, et. al. 2007, 'Posttraumatic Symptoms and Growth of Kosovar War Refugees: The influence of hope and cognitive coping', *The Journal of Positive Psychology,* vol.2, no.1, pp.55–65.

Alcoff L 1988, 'Culturalism Feminism Versus Poststructuralism: The identity crisis in feminist theory', *Signs,* vol.13, no.3, pp.405–36.

Alexander JC 2001, 'Robust Utopias and Civil Repairs', *International Sociology,* vol.16, no.4, pp.579–91.

Alger CF 1996, 'Reflections on Peace Research Traditions', *The International Journal of Peace Studies,* vol.1, no.1, pp.2–3, cited at www.gmu.edu/programs /icar/ijps/vol1_1/Alger.htm.

Alonso HH 1993, *Peace as a Women's Issue: A history of the US movement for world peace and women's rights (Peace and Conflict Resolution),* Syracuse University Press, New York.

Altwood MA, Bell-Dolan D, et. al. 2002, 'Children's Trauma and Adjustment Reactions to Violent and Nonviolent War Experiences', *Journal of American Academy of Children and Adolescent Psychiatry,* vol.41, pp.450–57.

Amoako KY & Mwaura P 2000, 'Perspectives on Africa's Development: Selected speeches', UN Economic Commission for Africa.

Anderson B 1991, *Imagined Communities: Reflections on the origin and spread of nationalism,* revised edition, Verso, London and New York.

Anderson E 2009, *Inclusive Masculinity: The changing nature of masculinities,* Routledge, London.

Anonymous 2000, 'Letter to the Editor', *Time,* 27 November, p.12.

Another Mother for Peace 2012 cited at www.another mother.org/products-page.

Auerhahn NC & Laub D 1998, 'Intergenerational Memory of the Holocaust' in Y Danieli (ed.), *International Handbook of Multigenerational Legacies of Trauma,* op. cit.

B92 2011, *'Dačić: Ako treba i rat za Kosovo',* 24 November, cited at www.b92.net/info/vesti/index.php?yyyy=2011&mm=11&dd=24&nav_category=640&nav_id=560256.

B92 2012, *'U Srbiji 40% ljudi pije svaki dan', Zdravlje,* 12 February, cited at www.totalportal.rs/zdravlje/313046/u-srbiji-40-ljudi-pije-svaki-dan.

Badiou A 2010, *The Communist Hypothesis,* Verso, London.

Baker KG & Gippenreiter JS 1998, 'Stalin's Purge and Its Impact on Russian Families' in Y Danieli, *International Handbook of Multigenerational Legacies of Trauma,* op. cit.

Bakić-Hayden M 1995, 'Nesting Orientalisms: The case of Former Yugoslavia', *Slavic Review,* vol.54, no.4, pp.917–31.

Barash DP & Webel CP 2002, *Peace and Conflict Studies,* Sage, London.

Barker GT 2005, *Dying to Be Men: Youth, masculinity and social exclusion,* Routledge, London.

Barnaby F 1988 (ed.), *The Gaia Peace Atlas: Survival into the third millennium,* Pan Books, London.

Barry K 2010, *Unmaking War, Remaking Men,* Spinifex Press, North Melbourne.

Bateson G 1958, *Naven: A survey of the problems suggested by a composite picture of the culture of a New Guinea tribe drawn from three points of view,* Stanford University Press, Palo Alto, CA.

Beara V 2011a, 'War Veterans and Family Violence' in DJ Christie (ed.), *The Encyclopedia of Peace Psychology,* Wiley-Blackwell, Oxford.

_____2011b, 'Suicide among War Veterans' in DJ Christie (ed.), *The Encyclopedia of Peace Psychology,* Wiley-Blackwell, Oxford.

Beara V & Miljanović P 2012, *'Gde si to bio sine moj?',* cited at www.veterani.org.rs/index.php?option=com_content&task=view&id=14&Itemid=18.

Beck U 2006, *The Cosmopolitan Vision,* Polity Press, Cambridge, UK.

Beitman BD, Soth AM, et. al. 2005, 'The Futures as an Integrating Force through the Schools of Psychotherapy' in JC Norcross & MR Goldfried (eds), *Handbook of Psychotherapy Integration* (second edition), Oxford University Press, New York.

Belasco A 2009, 'Troop Levels in the Afghan and Iraq Wars, FY 2001–FY 2012: Cost and other issues', Congressional Research Service, Washington, DC.

Bell D 2000, 'Cybercolonization: Introduction' in D Bell & BM Kennedy (eds), *The Cybercultures Reader,* Routledge, London.

Bell P, Bergeret I, et. al, 2000, '*Žene iz bezbjednog skloništa: psihološke i psihijatrijske posljedice ekstremne i prolongirane traume kod žena iz Srebrenice* [Women from the Safe Haven: The psychological and psychiatric consequences of extreme and prolonged trauma on women in Srebrenica]' in E Duraković-Belko & S Powell (eds), *Psihosocijalne posljedice rata, Rezultati empirijskih istraživanja sprovedenih na području bivše Jugoslavije* [The Psychosocial Consequences of War: Results of empirical research from the territory of former Yugoslavia],D O O Otisak, Sarajevo, pp.32–36.

Bennett C 1995, *Yugoslavia's Bloody Collapse: Causes, course and consequences,* New York University Press, New York.

Bennett SH 2003, *Radical Pacifism: The war resisters league and Gandhian nonviolence in America, 1915–1963,* Syracuse University Press, Syracuse, New York.

Berghahn VR 2010, 'Militarism in History' in NJ Young (ed.), *The Oxford International Encyclopedia of Peace,* vol.3, op. cit., pp.27–31.

Bestuzhev-Lada I 1996, 'Communism' in GT Kurian & GTT Molitor (eds), *Encyclopedia of the Future,* Simon & Schuster Macmillan, New York.

Bhabha HK 1994, *Nation and Narration,* Routledge, London.

Bieber F & Daskalovski Z 2003, *Understanding the War in Kosovo,* Frank Cass, London.

Biro M 2011, *'Psihološki aspekti pomirenja: Primer Srba i Albanaca', Interkulturalnost,* vol.1, no.1, pp.294–302.

Blagojević M 1999, 'The Walks in a Gender Perspective' in M Lazić (ed.), *Protest in Belgrade: Winter of discontent,* Central European University Press, Budapest.

Blic online 2009, *'Smanjuje se broj pušača',* 11 October, cited at www.blic.rs/Vesti/Drustvo/114996/Smanjuje-se-broj-pusaca.

Bloch E 1986, *The Principle of Hope,* Basil Blackwell, Oxford.

Bogic M, Ajdukovic, D et al. 2012, 'Factors Associated with Mental Disorders in Longsettled War Refugees:

refugees from the former Yugoslavia in Germany, Italy and the UK', *The British Journal of Psychiatry,* vol.200, pp.216–23, cited at bjp.rcpsych.org/content/200/3/216.full.pdf+html.

Bonta BD 1996, 'Conflict Resolution among Peaceful Societies: The culture of peacefulness', *Journal of Peace Research,* vol.33, no.4, pp.403–20.

Borochov B 1917, '*Poalei Tziyon* Peace Manifesto', cited at www.marxists.org/archive/borochov/1917/stockholm.htm.

Boulding E 1977, *Women in the Twentieth Century World,* Sage, New York.

______1986, 'Utopianism: Problems and issues in planning for a peaceful society', *Alternatives,* vol.xi, no.3, pp.345–66.

______1995, 'Image and Action in Peace Building' in E Boulding & K Boulding (eds), *The Future: Images and processes,* Sage, Thousand Oaks, CA.

______2000, *Cultures of Peace: The hidden side of history,* Syracuse University Press, Syracuse, New York.

______2004, 'Foreword' in G Kemp and DP Fry (eds), *Keeping the Peace,* op. cit.

Boulding E & Forsberg R 1998, *Abolishing War: Cultures and institutions,* Boston Research Center for the 21st Century, Cambridge, MA.

Bourne EJ 2005, *The Anxiety & Phobia Workbook,* New Harbinger Publications, Oakland, CA.

Bowker LH (ed.) 1998, *Masculinities and Violence,* Sage, London.

Brave Heart MYH 2007, 'The Impact of Historical Trauma: The example of the native community' in M Bussey & J Wise (eds), *Transforming Trauma: Empowerment responses,* Columbia University Press, New York.

Breton R 2010, 'Utopias' in NJ Young (ed.), *The Oxford International Encyclopedia of Peace,* vol.4, op. cit., pp.284–86.

Bringa T 2004, 'The Peaceful Death of Tito and the Violent End of Yugoslavia' in J Borneman (ed.), *Death of the Father: An anthropology of the end in political authority,* Berghahn Books, New York, pp.63–103.

Brock-Utne B 2000, 'Peace Education' in C Kramarae & D Spender (eds), *Routledge International Encyclopedia of Women: Global women's issues and knowledge,* vol.3, Routledge, London, pp.1497–99.

_____2010, 'Gender, Socialization, and Militarism' in NJ Young (ed.), *The Oxford International Encyclopedia of Peace,* vol.4, op. cit., pp.207–21.

Brod H & Kaufman M (eds) 1994, *Theorizing Masculinities,* Sage, Thousand Oaks, CA.

Brown A 2003, *The Illusion of Control: Fore and foreign policy in the twenty-first century,* The Brookings Institute, Washington, DC.

Brubaker R 1996, *Nationalism Reframed: Nationhood and the national question in the new Europe,* Cambridge University Press, UK.

Budi Muško 2011, *'Budi Muško – ne budi nasilnik',* Radio Sarajevo, cited at www.budimusko.org/tekstovi; see also pravimuskarac.rs/deklaracija and www.facebook.com/pravimuskarac.rs.

Bulatović L 2006, *Oreol Ili Omča Za Ratka Mladića,* Nikola Pašić, Beograd.

Bunch C 1983, 'Not by Degrees: Feminist theory and education' in C Bunch & S Pollak (eds), *Learning Our Way,* The Crossing Press, Trumansburg, New York.

Burchill S & Linklater A 1996, *Theories of International Relations,* St Martin's Press, New York.

Burke P 2010, 'Communism and Peace Movements', in NJ Young (ed.), *The Oxford International Encyclopedia of Peace,* vol.1, op. cit., pp.374–78.

Butler J 1990, *Gender Trouble: Feminism and the subversion of identity,* Routledge, London.

Butler J 2004, *Undoing Gender,* Routledge, London.

Cady DL 2010, 'Pacifism and Peace Meanings' in NJ Young (ed.), *The Oxford International Encyclopedia of Peace,* vol.3, op. cit., pp.313–16.

Campbell CD & Evans-Campbell T 2011, 'Historical Trauma and Native American Child Development and Mental Health: An overview' in P Spicer, P Farrell, et. al. (eds), *American Indian and Alaska Native Children and Mental Health,* Greenwood, Westport, CT, pp.1–26.

Campbell J 1949, *The Hero with a Thousand Faces,* Pantheon Books, New York.

Carey J (ed.) 1999, *The Faber Book of Utopias,* Faber & Faber, London.

Castleden B & Wareham S 2010, 'War, the Environment, and the Defence White Paper' in MAPW (Medical Association for Prevention of War Australia), *Vision 2030: An alternative approach to Australian security,* Carlton, Vic.

Ćetković, Nadežda, 2003, 'Support for Mothers, Letter to Women's Parliament' in N Ćetković, I Jarić & S Stojanović (eds), *Žene za Žene, SOS telefon za žene i decu žrtve nasilja,* Beograd.

Chitkara MG 1998, *Mother Theresa,* Aph Publishing Corporation, New Delhi.

Cockburn C 2010, 'Militarism and War' in LJ Shepherd (ed.), *Gender Matters in Global Politics: A feminist introduction to international relations,* Routledge, London.

Cohen LJ 2002, *Serpent in the Bosom: The rise and fall of Slobodan Milošević,* Westview Press, Boulder, CO.

Collins English Dictionary 2003, Complete and Unabridged, cited at www.thefreedictionary.com/militarism.

Collins SM & Graham C (eds) 2004, *Globalization, Poverty and Inequality,* The Brookings Institution, Washington, DC.

Čolović I 2002, *The Politics of Symbol in Serbia: Essays in political anthropology,* C Hurst & Co., London.

Connell RW 2002, 'Masculinities, the Reduction of Violence and the Pursuit of Peace' in C Cockburn & D Zarkov (eds), *The Postwar Moment: Militaries, masculinities and international peacekeeping,* Lawrence & Wishart, London.

_____2005, *Masculinities* (second edition), Allen & Unwin, Crows Nest, NSW.

_____2009, *Gender in World Perspective* (second edition), Polity, Cambridge, UK.

Connell RW & Messerschmidt JW 2005, 'Hegemonic Masculinity: Rethinking the concept', *Gender and Society,* vol.19, no.6, pp.829–59.

Connors EA 2007, 'Intergenerational Trauma and Healing' cited at www.acca-aajc.ca/portals/0/2007-winnipegconference/Dr%20Ed%20Connors,%20Revised.pdf.

Cook-Huffman C 2010, 'Gender and Conflict' in NJ Young (ed.), *The Oxford International Encyclopedia of Peace,* vol.2, op. cit., pp.211–15.

Cornis-Pope M 2004, *History of the Literary Cultures of East-Central Europe: Junctures and disjunctures in the 19th and 20th centuries,* John Benjamin Publishing, Amsterdam and Philadelphia PA.

Cortright D 2008, *Peace: A history of movements and ideas,* Cambridge University Press, Cambridge.

Dačić I 2010, quoted in *'SPS proslavio 20 godina od ukidanja Socijalističkog saveza radnog naroda*

Jugoslavije', cited at www.njuz.net/sps-proslavio-20-godina-od-ukidanja-socijalistickogsaveza-radnog-naroda-jugoslavije/#ixzzlsAKXPudH.

Dahl S, Mutapcic A, et. al., 1998, 'Traumatic Events and Predictive Factors for Posttraumatic Symptoms in Displaced Bosnian Women in a War Zone', *Journal of Traumatic Stress,* vol.11, pp.137–45.

Daianu D & Veremēs T 2001, *Balkan Reconstruction,* Routledge, London.

Dakić G & Palić S 2011, *'Udžbenici istorije u Srbiji, BiH i Hrvatskoj vaspitaju decu za nova neprijateljstva',* Blic online, 20 November, cited at www.blic.rs/Vesti/Tema-Dana/290652/Udzbenici-istorije-u-Srbiji-BiH-i-Hrvatskoj-vaspitaju-decu-za-nova-neprijateljstva.

Daly M 1978, *Gyn/Ecology: The metaethics of radical feminism,* Beacon Press, Boston MA.

Danieli Y 1998, *International Handbook of Multigenerational Legacies of Trauma,* Plenum Press, NY and London.

_____2006, 'Essential Elements of Healing After Massive Trauma: Complex needs voiced by victims/survivors' in D Sullivan & L Tifft (eds), *Handbook of Restorative Justice: A global perspective,* Routledge, London and NY.

_____2010a, 'Recovery After Mass Crimes' in NJ Young (ed.), *The Oxford International Encyclopedia of Peace,* vol.3, op. cit., pp.615–18.

2010b, 'Assessinq Trauma Across Cultures from a Multigenerational Perspective' in JP Wilson & CS Tang (eds), *Cross-cultural Assessment of Psychological Trauma and PTSD,* Springer, NY.

Day A, East R, et. al. 2002, *A Political and Economic Dictionary of Eastern Europe,* Europa Publications, London, 2002, p.295.

Deist W, Messerschmidt M, et al. 1990, *Germany and the Second World War: Germany's initial conquests in Europe,* Oxford University Press, UK.

DeKeseredy WS & Schwartz MD 2005, 'Masculinities and Interpersonal Violence' in MS Kimmel, J Hearn & RW Connell (eds), *Handbook of Studies on Men and Masculinities,* op. cit., pp.353–66.

deMause L 1990, 'The Gentle Revolution: Childhood origins of Soviet and east European democratic movements', *The Journal of Psychohistory,* vol.17, no.4, pp.341–52.

Dervin D 2008, 'No Place to Hide: Joseph Stalin's childhood', *The Journal of Psychohistory,* vol.36, no.1, pp.89–93.

Dictionary.die.net. 2012, 'Militarism', cited at dictionary.die.net/militarism.

Djukić S & Dubinsky A 2001, *Milošević and Marković: A lust for power,* McGill-Queen's University Press, Montreal.

Doll B 1995, 'Post-modernism's Utopian Vision' in P McLaren (ed.), *Postmodernism, Postcolonialism and Pedagogy,* James Nicholas Publishers, Albert Park, Vic.

Doroški M 2012, *Intervju. O urušavanju mentalno zdravlja nacije. Strah i stes došli po svoje.* Republished as *Posttraumatski stresni poremećaj,* cited at www.geocities.ws/klubgrbavica/doroski_5.htm.

Drakulić S 1991, *How We Survived Communism and Even Laughed,* Hutchinson, London.

Dudink S, Hagemann K, et. al. (eds) 2007, *Representing Masculinity: Male citizenship in modern western culture,* Palgrave Macmillan, Basingstoke, UK.

Duyvesteyn I & Angstrom J 2005, *Rethinking the Nature of War,* Frank Cass, Abingdon, UK.

Edwards T 2006, *Cultures of Masculinity,* Routledge, London.

Eisler R 1987, *The Chalice and the Blade: Our history, our future,* HarperCollins Publishers, San Francisco, CA.

______ 1997, 'Cultural Shifts and Technological Phase Changes: The patterns of history, the subtext of gender, and the choices for our future' in J Galtung & S Inayatullah (eds), *Macrohistory and Macrohistorians,* Praeger, New York.

______2000, *Tomorrow's Children: A blueprint for partnership education in the 21st Century,* Westview Press, Boulder CO.

______2008, *The Real Wealth of Nations: Creating a caring economics,* Berrett-Koehler Publishers, San Francisco, CA.

Eitinger L 1964, *Concentration Camp Survivors in Norway and Israel,* Universitetsforlaget, Oslo.

Eitinger L & Strøm A 1973, *Mortality and Morbidity after Excessive Stress: A follow-up investigation of Norwegian concentration camp survivors,* Universitetsforlaget, Oslo.

Elshtain JB 1995, *Women and War,* University of Chicago Press, Chicago.

______1996, 'Thinking about Women, Christianity and Rights' in J Witte Jr & JD Van Der Vyver (eds), *Religious Human Rights in Global Perspective:*

Religious perspectives, Martinus Nijhoff Publishers, Leiden, The Netherlands.

Engels F 1877, 'III. Theory of Force (Continuation)' in *Anti-Dühring, Part II: Political economy,* cited at www.marxists.org/archive/marx/works/1877/anti-duhring/ch15.htm.

Enloe C 1990, *Bananas, Beaches and Bases: Making sense of international politics,* University of California Press, Berkeley, CA.

Ervø S & Johansson T (eds) 2003, *Moulding Masculinities,* Ashgate, Aldershot, UK.

Eytan A & Gex-Fabry M 2011, 'Use of Healthcare Services 8 Years After the War in Kosovo: Role of post-traumatic stress disorder and depression', *European Journal of Public Health,* cited at eurpub.oxfordjournals.org/content/early/2011/07/09/eurpub.ckr096.full.pdf_html.

Fangen K, Fossan K, et. al. 2010, *Inclusion and Exclusion of Young Adult Migrants in Europe: Barriers and bridges,* Ashgate, Aldershot, UK.

Farnen RF 2004, *Nationalism, Ethnicity, and Identity: Cross national and comparative perspectives,* Transaction Publishers, New Brunswick, NJ.

Fendler L 1999, 'Making Trouble: Prediction, agency, and critical intellectuals' in TS Popkewitz & L Fendler (eds), *Critical Theories in Education: Changing terrains of knowledge and politics,* Routledge, New York.

Fine C 2010, *Delusions of Gender: The real science behind sex differences,* Icon Books, London.

Fisk R 2005, *The Great War for Civilisation: The conquest of the Middle East,* Vintage, New York.

Fletcher KE 2003, 'Childhood Posttraumtic Stress Disorder' in EJ Mash & RA Barkley, *Child Psychopathology,* The Guildford Press, New York.

Flögel M, Goreta SS, et al. 2010, 'War Stress in the Former Yugoslavia' in G Fink (ed.), *Encyclopedia of Stress,* vol.2, Academic Press, Oxford.

Forcey LR 1999, 'Conflict Transformation' in LR Kurtz and JE Turpin (eds), *Encyclopedia of Violence, Peace and Conflict,* Academic Press, San Diego, CA.

Ford M 2005, 'Imagined Australians in a Culturally Diverse Community' in J Yamanashi & I Milojević (eds), *Researching Identity, Diversity & Education: Surpassing the norm,* Post Pressed, Teneriffe, Qld.

Forum B92 2009, 'Gay Parada', 20 July, cited at forum.b92.net/index.php?s=d295759d6a16db031cc4df2d9380e983&showtopic=50864&st=2085&p=2452190&#entry2452190.

Foucault M 1982, 'Afterword: The subject and power' in HL Dreyfus & P Rabinow (eds), *Michel Foucault: Beyond structuralism and hermeneutic,* University of Chicago Press, Chicago.

_____1984, 'Nietzsche, Genealogy, History' in P Rabinow (ed.), *The Foucault Reader,* Pantheon Books, New York.

_____1986, 'Of Other Spaces', *Diacritics,* vol.16, no.1, pp.22–27.

Frankl V 1946, *Man's Search for Meaning* (revised edition 2004) (originally published as *Trotzdem Jazum Lebensagen: Ein Psychologeerlebt das Konzentrationslager,* and published under a different title in 1959: *From Death-Camp to Existentialism),* Rider, London.

Freire P 1998, *Pedagogy of Freedom: Ethics, democracy, and civic courage,* Rowan & Littlefield Publishers, Lanham ML.

Fromm E 1955, *The Sane Society,* Henry Holt and Company, New York.

Frontal.rs 2012, cited at http://frontal.rs/index.php?option=btg_novosti&idnovost=18538#komentar.

Fry D 2004, 'Conclusion: Learning from peaceful societies' in G Kemp & D Fry (eds), *Keeping the*

Peace: Conflict resolution and peaceful societies around the world, Routledge, London.

Fukuyama F 1992, *The End of History and the Last Man,* Penguin, London.

Furnham A & Bochner S 1986, *Culture Shock: Psychological reactions to unfamiliar environments,* Taylor & Francis, London.

Gadd A 2006, *The Girl Who Bites Her Nails and the Man Who Is Always Late: What our habits reveal about us,* Findhorn Press, Findhorn, Scotland.

Gallagher T 2003, *The Balkans after the Cold War: From tyranny to tragedy,* Routledge, New York.

_____2010, 'Balkan Conflicts' in NJ Young (ed.), *The Oxford International Encyclopedia of Peace,* vol.1, op. cit., pp.168–73.

Gallup G 2003, *The Gallup Poll: Public opinion 2002,* The Gallup Organization, Wilmington, DE.

Galtung J 1996, *Peace by Peaceful Means: Peace and conflict, development and civilisation,* International Peace Research Institute, Oslo.

_____2000, *Searching for Peace: The road to TRANSCEND,* Pluto Press, London.

_____2002, 'Rethinking Conflict: The Cultural Approach', Council of Europe, Strasbourg, cited at www.coe.int/t/dg4/cultureheritage/culture/completed/dialogue/DGIV_CULT_PREV(2002)1_Galtung_E.PDF.

_____2004, *Transcend and Transform: An introduction to conflict work,* Pluto Press, London.

_____2008, *50 Years: 100 peace and conflict perspectives,* Transcend University Press, Bergen, Norway.

_____2009, 'Johan Galtung's View from Europe: Women and men, peace and security', European Commission Speech, 'Making the Difference: Strengthening the capacities to respond to crises and security threats', Brussels, 3 May, cited at http://www.transcend.org/tms/2009/06/women-and-men-peace-and-security-track-1-reinforcing-the-role-ofwomen-in-peace-and-security/.

Galtung J, Jacobsen CG, et. al. 2002, *Searching for Peace: The road to transcend,* Pluto Press, London.

Gareau FH 2004, *State Terrorism and the United States: From counter-insurgency to the war on terrorism,* Clarity Press Inc., Atlanta, GA.

Gavrilović J, Lecic-Tosevski D, et. al. 2002, 'Predictors of Posttraumatic Stress in Civilians 1 Year after Air Attacks: A study of Yugoslavian students', *The Journal of Nervous and Mental Disease,* vol.190, no.4, pp.257–62.

Gilligan J 2001, *Preventing Violence,* Thames and Hudson, New York.

_____2009, 'Shame, Guilt, and Violence', cited at internationalpsychoanalysis.net/wp-content/uploads/2009/02/shamegilligan.pdf.

Glass C 2012, 'Why Men Matter, Part I (The bad news)', 10 January, cited at www.craigglass.org/?p=558.

Glaurdić J 2011, *The Hour of Europe: Western powers and the breakup of Yugoslavia,* Yale University Press New Haven, CT.

Gočanin S 2011, *'Lektira u službi ideologije',* B92.net, 3 October, cited at www.b92.net/kultura/intervjui.php?nav_category=1082&nav_id=546413.

Goldstein JS 2001, *War and Gender: How gender shapes the war system and vice versa,* Cambridge University Press, Cambridge.

Goldstein RD, Wampler NS, et. al. 1997, 'War Experiences and Distress Symptoms of Bosnian Children', *Pediatrics,* vol.100, pp.873–78.

Greenspan M 2004, *Healing through the Dark Emotions: The wisdom of grief, fear, and despair,* Shambhala Publications, Boston MA.

Gregg M & Seigworth GJ (eds) 2010, *The Affect Theory Reader,* Duke University Press, Durham, NC.

Grille R 2005a, *Parenting for a Peaceful World,* Longueville Media, Alexandria, NSW.

_____2005b, 'From Horror to Hope', *Byron Child,* vol.15 (September–November), pp.38–41.

Grosz E 1990, 'Contemporary Theories of Power and Subjectivity' in S Gunew (ed.), *Feminist Knowledge: Critique and construct,* Routledge, London.

Gurvič Z 1965, *Savremeni poziv sociologije,* Veselin Masleša, Sarajevo.

Halberstam D 2003, *War in a Time of Peace: Bush, Clinton and the generals,* Scribner, New York.

Halpern JM & Kideckel DA 2000, *Neighbors at War: Anthropological perspectives on Yugoslav ethnicity, culture and history,* Penn State University Press, University Park, PA.

Haraway D 1988, 'Situated Knowledges: The science question in feminism and the privilege of partial perspective', *Feminist Studies,* vol.14, no.3, pp.575–99.

Harris E 2009, *Nationalism: Theories and cases,* Edinburgh University Press, Edinburgh.

Harris IM & Morrison ME 2003, *Peace Education,* McFarland & Co., Jefferson, NC.

Hart SA 2011, 'Partisans: War in the Balkans 1941–1945', BBC History online, last updated 17 February, cited at www.bbc.co.uk/history/worldwars/wwtwo/partisan_fighters_01.shtml#four.

Harvey MR 1996, 'An Ecological View of Psychological Trauma and Trauma Recovery', *Journal of Traumatic Stress,* vol.9, no.1, pp.3–23.

Haslberger A & Greßler S (eds) 2010, *Epigenetics and Human Health: Linking hereditary, environmental and nutritional aspects,* Wiley-VCH, Wenheim, Germany.

Hatzfeld J 2006 (preface S Sontag, trans. L Coverdale), *Machete Season: The killers in Rwanda speak,* Picador, New York.

Hay LL 1999, *You Can Heal Your Life,* Hay House, Sydney.

Hayden RM 1996, 'Imagined Communities and Real Victims: Self-determination and ethnic cleansing in Yugoslavia', *American Ethnologist,* vol.23, no.4, pp.783–801.

Hearn J 2010, 'Gender and Sexual Scenarios on the Global Scale', *Futura: The Journal of the Finnish Society for Futures Studies,* vol.3, Special Issue on Gender, pp.34–47.

Hegel GWF 2008, *Philosophy of Right* (trans. SW Dyde), Cosimo, New York.

Henderson H 1990, *Building a Win-Win World,* Berrett-Koehler Publishers, San Francisco, CA.

_____1995, *Redefining Wealth and Progress: New ways to measure economic, social, and environmental change; The Caracas report on alternative development indicators,* TOES books, New York.

_____1999, *Beyond Globalization: Shaping a sustainable global economy,* Kumarian Press, West Hartford, CT.

_____2006, *Ethical Markets: Growing the green economy,* Chelsea Green Publishing, White River Junction, VT.

Hershman JD & Lieb J 1994, *A Brotherhood of Tyrants: Manic depression and absolute power,* Prometheus Books, Amherst, MA.

Hertzler JO 1965, *The History of Utopian Thought,* Cooper Square Publishers, New York.

Hicks D & Holden C 1995, *Visions of the Future: Why we need to teach for tomorrow,* Trentham Books, Stoke-on-Trent, UK.

Higate P & Hopton J 2005, 'War, Militarism, and Masculinities' in MS Kimmel, J Hearn, et. al. (eds), *Handbook of Studies on Men and Masculinities,* op. cit., pp.432–47.

Hobbes T 1651, *Leviathan* (Chapter XIII: 'Of the natural condition of mankind as concerning their felicity, and misery'), cited at oll.libertyfund.org/index.php?option=com_staticxt&staticfile=show.php%3Ftitle=585&layout=html#chapter_89842.

Hollis DW 1998, *The ABC–CLIO World History Companion to Utopian Movements,* ABC-CLIO, Santa Barbara, CA.

Hooks B 1991, *Yearning: Race, gender, and cultural politics,* Turnaround, London.

Hourvitz L 2010, 'The March of Folly by Barbara Tuchman', book review, cited at www.stoneschool.com/Reviews/MarchOfFolly.html.

Howell S & Willis RG 1989, *Societies at Peace: Anthropological perspectives,* Taylor & Francis, London.

Hudson W 2003, *The Reform of Utopia,* Ashgate, Burlington, VT.

Hughes R 2000, 'The Phantom of Utopia', *Time,* 26 October, pp.84–85.

Human Security Centre 2005, *Human Security Report 2005: War and peace in the 21st Century,* Oxford University Press, New York.

Humanitarian Law Center 2005, *'Jedanaest godina od otmice u Štrpcima',* 26 February, cited at www.hlc-rdc.org/?cat=235.

Hunter CD & Coles MEL 2009, 'Coping with Racism: A spirit-based psychological perspective' in JL Chin (ed.), *The Psychology of Prejudice and Discrimination, Racism in America,* vol.1, Praeger Perspectives, Westport, CT.

Hussain D & Bhushan B 2011, 'Posttraumatic Stress and Growth Among Tibetan Refugees: The Mediating Role of Cognitive–Emotional Regulation Strategies', *Journal of Clinical Psychology,* vol.67, no.7, pp.720–35.

Hutchinson FP 1996, *Educating Beyond Violent Futures,* Routledge, London.

Ihanus J 2007, 'Stalin's Loss and Shame', *The Journal of Psychohistory,* vol.35, no.1, pp.61–70.

Ikeda D 1995, 'Socialism: Pro and Con' in RL Gage (ed.), *Choose Peace: A dialogue between Johan Galtung and Daisaku Ikeda,* Pluto Press, London.

Inge WR 1949, *The End of an Age: And other essays,* Macmillan Company, London.

IOM (International Organization for Migration) 2003, *World Migration 2003: Managing migration challenges and responses for people on the move,* Geneva.

_____2006, *World Migration 2005: Costs and benefits of international migration,* Geneva.

Jahr C 2010, 'Enemy Images' in NJ Young (ed.), *The Oxford International Encyclopedia of Peace,* vol.2, op. cit., pp.62–63.

Jaramillo DL 2009, *Ugly War, Pretty Package: How CNN and Fox News made the invasion of Iraq high concept,* Indiana University Press, Bloomington, IN.

Jenkins B & Sofos SA (eds) 1996, 'Culture, Politics and Identity in Former Yugoslavia' in *Nation and Identity in Contemporary Europe,* Routledge, Oxford.

Jenkins CJ 2010, 'Ethnic Conflict' in NJ Young (ed.), *The Oxford International Encyclopedia of Peace,* vol.2, op. cit., 2010, pp.95–99.

Jennings LE 1996, 'Dystopias' in G Kurian & GG Molitor (eds), *Encyclopedia of the Future,* Macmillan Library References, New York.

Jones A (ed.) 2006, *Men of the Global South: A reader,* Zed Books, London.

Judah T 2000, *The Serbs: History, myth, and the destruction of Yugoslavia,* Yale University Press, New Haven, CT.

Kabat-Zinn J 2009, *Full Catastrophe Living,* Delta, New York.

Kamenka E 1993, 'Nationalism: Ambiguous legacies and contingent futures', *Political Studies,* vol.41, pp.78–92.

Kanter RM 1972, *Commitment and Community: Communes and utopias in sociological perspective,* Harvard University Press, Cambridge, MA.

Kashmeri SA 2007, *America and Europe after Nine-eleven and Iraq,* Praeger Security International, Westport, CT.

Kaštelan J 2012, cited at www.ezgeta.com/jama.html .

Kaufman M 1994, 'Men, Feminism, and Men's Contradictory Experiences of Power' in H Brod & M Kaufman (eds), *Theorizing Masculinities,* op. cit., pp.142–65.

Kegley CW & Raymond GA 1999, *How Nations Make Peace,* St Martin's/Worth Publishers, New York.

Kelleher WF 2010, 'Peaceful Societies' in NJ Young (ed.), *The Oxford International Encyclopedia of Peace,* vol.3, op. cit., pp.382–84.

Kelly I 2010, 'Nation-States, Causes of Conflict' in NJ Young (ed.), T*he Oxford International Encyclopedia of Peace,* vol.3, op. cit., pp.100–103.

Kemp G 2004, 'The Concept of Peaceful Societies' in G Kemp and DP Fry, *Keeping the Peace,* op. cit., pp.1–10.

Kemp G & Fry DP 2004, *Keeping the Peace: Conflict resolution and peaceful societies around the world,* Routledge, New York.

Kimmel MS 2005, 'Globalization and Its Mal(e)contents: The gendered moral and political economy of terrorism' in MS Kimmel, J Hearn, et. al. (eds), *Handbook of Studies on Men and Masculinities,* op. cit., pp.1–10.

Kimmel M, Hearn J, et. al. (eds) 2004, *Handbook of Studies on Men and Masculinities,* Sage Publications, Thousand Oaks, CA.

Kinder DR & Kam CD 2009, *Us against Them: Ethnocentric foundations of American opinion,* University of Chicago Press, Chicago.

Kiselica MS 2010, 'Promoting Positive Masculinity while Addressing Gender Role Conflict: A balanced theoretical approach to clinical work with boys and men' in C Blazina & DS Shen-Miller (eds), *An International Psychology of Men: Theoretical advances, cases studies, and clinical innovations,* Routledge, London.

Kočić DM 2007, *Istorija: za I razred srednjih stručnih škola (History: For I grade of specialist high schools),* Zavod za udžbenike, Beograd.

Koenigsberg R 2008, 'Political Violence and the Concept of Collective Psychopathology', cited at www.ideologiesofwar.com/old/docs/rk_collective.htm.

Kolakovski L 1980, *Glavni tokovi marksizma,* Tom I-III, BIGZ, Beograd.

Krishnamurti J 1989, *Living in an Insane World,* Krishamurti Foundation of America, Ojai, CA, p.19, cited at thinkexist.com/quotations/violence/.

Kroo A & Nagy H 2011, 'Posttraumatic Growth Among Traumatized Somali Refugees in Hungary', *Journal of Loss and Trauma,* vol.16, pp.440–58.

Kumar K 1987, *Utopia and Anti-Utopia in Modern Times,* Basil Blackwell, Oxford.

Kuzmanović B 2004, *'Intervju: Pucanje po horizontali i vertikali', Dnevnik,* 15 February.

Lafargue P 1883, *The Right To Be Lazy,* Charles Kerr and Co., Chicago, IL, cited at www.marxists.org/archive/lafargue/1883/lazy/.

Lake M 1992, 'Mission Impossible: How men gave birth to the Australian nation – nationalism, gender and other seminal acts', *Gender and History,* vol.4, no.3, pp.305–22.

Lakoff G 2004, *Don't Think of an Elephant: Know your values and frame the debate,* Scribe Publications, Melbourne, Vic.

Lansford T, Watson R, et al. (eds) 2009, *America's War on Terror,* Ashgate, Burlington, VT.

Laufer A & Solomon Z 2006, 'Posttraumatic Symptoms and Posttraumatic Growth Among Israeli Youth Exposed to Terror Incidents', *Journal of Social and Clinical Psychology,* vol.25, no.4, pp.429–47.

Lawlor R 1991, *Voices of the First Day: Awakening in the Aboriginal Dreamtime,* Inner Traditions International, Rochester, VT.

Lawrence BB & Karim A (eds) 2007, *On Violence: A reader,* Duke University Press, Durham, NC.

Lenin V 1917a, 'Can the Bolshevics Retain State Power?', *Prosveschcheniye* 1–2, cited at www.marxists.org/archive/lenin/works/1917/oct/01.htm.

_____1917b, 'What Made the Communards' Attempt Heroic?' in *The State and Revolution,* cited at www.marxists.org/archive/lenin/works/1917/staterev/ch03.htm.

Lev-Wiesel R 2007, 'Intergenerational Transmission of Trauma across Three Generations: A preliminary study', *Qualitative Social Work,* vol.6, no.1, pp.75–94.

Levinson L 2011, 'Recognizing the Multi-generational Trauma of World War II', *Huffpost* 'Healthy Living', 21 May, cited at www.huffingtonpost.com/leila-levinson/war-traumagenerations_b_859547.html.

Levsen S 2010, 'Gender and Militarism in Child Upbringing' in NJ Young (ed),*The Oxford International Encyclopedia of Peace,* vol.2, op. cit., pp.215–18.

Library of Congress 1990, 'Yugoslavia, Socialist Alliance of Workers', *Library of Congress Country Studies,* cited at http://lcweb2.loc.gov/frd/cs/yutoc.html.

Lovrić B 2011, *'Hrvatski ratni veterani umiru barem 20 godina prerano', Vjesnik.hr news portal,* 12 December, cited at http://arhiv.braniteljski-portal.hr/sadrzaj/hrvatska/13487.

Luke A 2003, 'Foreword' in J Miller, *Audible Difference: ESL and social identity in schools,* Multilingual Matters Ltd, Sydney.

Luxemburg R 1911, 'Peace Utopias', *The Labour Monthly,* July 1926, pp.421–28 cited at www.marxists.org/archive/luxemburg/1911/05/11.htm.

Mannheim K 1936, *Ideology and Utopia,* Routledge & Kegan Paul, London.

Maoz I & Eidelson RJ 2010, 'Ethnopolitical Conflict, Psychology of' in NJ Young (ed.), *The Oxford International Encyclopedia of Peace,* vol.2, op. cit., pp.102–105.

Marcuse H 1970, *Five Lectures: Psychoanalysis, politics, and utopia,* Beacon Press, Boston, MA.

Marks MP 2011, *Metaphors in International Relations Theory,* Palgrave Macmillan, Basingstoke, UK.

Martin P 2000, 'The Moral Case for Globalization' in F Lechner & J Boli (eds), *The Globalization Reader,* Blackwell Publishers, Malsden, MA.

Martinović-Vitanović V & Kalafatić V 2009, 'Ecological Impact on the Danube After NATO Air Strikes' in TA Kassim & D Barceló (eds), *Environmental Consequences of War and Aftermath,* Springer, New York.

Marx K 1871, 'The Paris Commune' in *The Civil War in France,* cited at www.marxists.org/archive/marx/works/1871/civil-war-france/ch05.htm.

Maslov A 2001, *Captured Soviet Generals: The fate of Soviet generals captured in combat 1941– 1945,* Routledge, London.

Maslow A 1961, 'Eupsychia – the good society', *Journal of Humanistic Psychology,* vol.1, no.2, pp.1–11.

Mastilović Jasnić I 2011, *'Smrt ćerke bila okidač za brutalnost',* Blic online, 1 June, cited at www.blic.rs/Vesti/Tema-Dana/257271/Smrt-cerke-bila----okidac-za-brutalnost.

McInturff K 2010, 'Gender and Violence' in NJ Young (ed.), *The Oxford International Encyclopedia of Peace,* vol.2, op. cit., pp.222–26.

McKee RG 2008, 'Storytelling for Peace-Building: Toward Sustainable Cultural Diversity', cited at www.gial.edu/GIALens/issues.htm.

McKinley M 2007, *Economic Globalisation as Religious War: Tragic convergence,* Routledge, London.

McPhail K 1999, 'The Threat of Ethical Accountants: An application of Foucault's concept of ethics to accounting education and some thoughts on ethically educating for the other', *Critical Perspectives on Accounting,* vol.10, no.6, pp.833–66.

Messerschmidt JW 2005, 'Men, Masculinities, and Crime' in MS Kimmel, J Hearn, et. al. (eds),

Handbook of Studies on Men and Masculinities, op. cit., pp.196–212.

Mikula M 2008, *Key Concepts in Cultural Studies,* Palgrave MacMillan, New York.

Milburn MA & Conrad SE 1996, *The Politics of Denial,* MIT Press, Cambridge, MA.

Miles R & Brown M 2003, *Racism,* Routledge, London.

Milić A 2011, *'Feministički talasi, orijentacije i pokret u jugoslovenskom i srpskom društvu 20.veka'* in I Milojević & S Markov (eds), *Uvod u Rodne Teorije, Centar za rodne studije,* ACIMSI, Univerzitet u Novom Sadu i Mediterran Publishing, Novi Sad, Serbia.

Milićević AS 2006, 'Joining the War: Masculinity, nationalism and war participation in the Balkans war of secession, 1991–1995', *Nationalities Papers,* vol.3, pp.265–87.

Miller A 1998, 'The Political Consequences of Child Abuse', *The Journal of Psychohistory,* vol.26, no.2, pp.573–85.

Milojević I 2001, 'Poverty-free Futures', *Social Alternatives,* vol.20, no.2, pp.19–24 (revised version published as 'Creating Spaces for Poverty Free Futures', *Development,* vol.44, no.4, pp.98–103).

_____2002, *Futures of Education: Feminist and post-western critiques and visions,* Phd Thesis, School of Education, University of Queensland, Brisbane.

_____2003, 'Gender and the 1999 War In and Around Kosovo', *Social Alternatives,* vol.22, no.2, pp.28–36.

_____2004, 'Analysing Poverty: From abundance and contentment to relative poverty and back' in S Inayatullah (ed.), *The Causal Layered Analysis Reader,* Tamkang University, Taipei, pp.259–66 (previous versions of this article were published in *Social Alternatives* and *Development* journals).

_____2005, *Educational Futures: Dominant and contesting visions,* Routledge, London.

_____2006, 'Hegemonic and Marginalised Educational Utopias' in MA Peters and J Freeman-Moir (eds), *Edutopias: New utopian thinking in education,* Sense Publishers, Rotterdam, The Netherlands.

_____2010, 'From Violent to Peace-oriented Masculinities' in J Johansen & JY Jones (eds), *Experiments with Peace: Celebrating peace at Johan Galtung's 80th Anniversary,* Fahamu Books, Cape Town and Oxford.

_____2012, 'Transforming Violent Masculinities in Serbia and Beyond' in O Simić, Z Volčič, et. al. (eds), *Peace Psychology in the Balkans: Mapping the pathways to peace,* Peace Psychology series, Springer, New York.

Milojević I & Markov S 2008, 'Gender, Militarism and the View of the Future: Students' views on the introduction of the civilian service in Serbia', *Journal of Peace Education,* vol.5, no.2, pp.175–91.

Mirra C 2008, 'Countering Militarism through peace education' in M Bajaj (ed.), *Encyclopedia of Peace Education,* Information Age Publishing, Charlotte, NC.

Mišković I 2010, *'Prošle godine izdato 10 miliona kutija sedativa',* Blic online, 18 March, cited at www.blic.rs /Vesti/Drustvo/181292/Prosle-godine-izdato-10-milion a-kutija-sedativa.

Mollica R 2006, *Healing Invisible Wounds: Paths to hope and recovery in a violent world,* Houghton Mifflin Harcourt, Boston, MA.

Morgan DHJ 1994, 'Theater of War: Combat, the military, and masculinities' in H Brod & M Kaufman (eds), *Theorizing Masculinities,* op. cit., pp.166–83.

Mosse GL 1996, *The Image of Man: The creation of modern masculinity,* Oxford University Press, New York.

Mueller J 2010, 'War: Aversion to War' in NJ Young (ed,), *The Oxford International Encyclopedia of Peace,* vol.4, op. cit., pp.327–30.

Murawska-Muthesius K 2006, 'On Small Nations and Bullied Children: Mr Punch draws Eastern Europe', *The Slavonic and East European Review,* vol.84, no.2, pp.279–305.

Murray KE, Davidson GR, et. al. 2008, *Psychological Wellbeing of Refugees Resettling in Australia,* The Australian Psychological Society, Melbourne.

Nagata DK 1998, 'Intergenerational Effects of the Japanese American Internment' in Y Danieli (ed), *International Handbook of Multigenerational Legacies of Trauma,* op. cit., pp.125–39.

Nagel J 2005, 'Nation' in MS Kimmel, J Hearn, et. al. (eds), *Handbook of Studies on Men and Masculinities,* op. cit., pp.397–413.

Nakosteen MK 1965, *The History and Philosophy of Education,* The Ronald Press Company, New York.

Nandy A 1987, *Traditions, Tyranny, and Utopias: Essays in the politics of awareness,* Oxford University Press, New York.

Napoleoni L 2010, *Terrorism and the Economy: How the war on terror is bankrupting the world,* Seven Stories Press, New York.

Nathanson S 1993, *Patriotism, Morality, and Peace,* Rowan & Littlefield Publishers, Lanham, ML.

Naumović S & Jovanović M 2004, *Childhood in South East Europe: Historical perspectives on growing up in the 19th and 20th century,* Lit Verlag, Münster, Germany.

Neile C 2010, 'Storytelling for Peace', International Story Telling Center, cited at www.storytellingcenter.net/resources/articles/neile1.htm. (retrieved January 2010)

Niens Ulrike 2010, 'Direct Violence, Psychology of' in NJ Young (ed), *The Oxford International Encyclopedia of Peace,* vol.2, op. cit., pp.591–94.

Nietzsche F 1977, *A Nietzsche Reader* (ed. and trans. RJ Hollingdale), Penguin Books, New York.

Nisbet R 1982, *Prejudices: A philosophical dictionary,* Harvard University Press, Cambridge, MA.

Norris D 2008, *Belgrade: A Cultural History,* Oxford Universtiy Press, New York.

Oberg J 1999, 'Bombings – Incompatible with humanitarian concerns', Transnational Foundation for Peace and Future Research (TFF), *The Free Press Info* #60, 24 March, cited at www.math.yorku.ca/sfp/newsl/sfp21.

______2001, Transnational Foundation for Peace and Future Research (TFF) Peace Browser bulletin, 18 November.

Oberschall A 2007, *Conflict and Peace Building in Divided Societies: Responses to ethnic violence,* Routledge, London.

Orwell S & Angus I (eds) 1968, *The Collected Essays, Journalism and Letters of George Orwell,* Penguin, Harmondsworth, UK.

Oxford Dictionary online 2012, 'Militarism', cited at oxforddictionaries.com/definition/militarism.

Ozmon H 1969, *Utopias and Education,* Burgess Publishing Company, Minneapolis, MN.

Paige GD 2009, *Nonkilling Global Political Science,* Center for Global Nonkilling, Honolulu, HI.

Papić Z 1994, 'Nationalism, Patriarchy and War in Ex-Yugoslavia', *Women's History Review,* vol.1, pp.115–17.

Paris R 2004, *At War's End: Building Peace after Civil Conflict,* University of Colorado, Boulder, CO.

Parpart JL & Zalewski M (eds) 2008, *Rethinking the Man Question: Sex, gender and violence in international relations,* Zed Books, London.

Pavković A 2000, *The Fragmentation of Yugoslavia: Nationalism and war in the Balkans,* Macmillan Press, Hampshire, UK.

Pavković M 2012, *'Svakim danom nas je sve manje',* cited at www.radiosamobor.hr/novosti.php/2012/02/28/Prva-knjiga-o-suicidima-hrvatskih-branitelja.html.

Pearson L 1972, 'Victor Gollancz Humanity Award Acceptance Speech', cited at www.unac.org/en/link_learn/canada/pearson/part_iv.asp.

Pešić V 1994, 'Bellicose Virtues in Elementary School Readers' in R Rosandić & V Pešić (eds), *Warfare, Patriotism, Patriarchy: The analysis of elementary school textbooks,* Centre for Anti-War Action Association MOST, Belgrade.

Pettman I 1996, *Worlding Women: A feminist international politics,* Allen & Unwin, Sydney.

Phillips S 2000, *Stalinist Russia,* Heinemann Education Publishers, Oxford.

Pierce CM 1970, 'Offensive Mechanisms: The vehicle for micro-aggression' in F Barbour (ed.), *The Black 70s,* Sargent, Boston, MA.

Pilgrim P 1992, *Peace Pilgrim: Her life and work in her own words,* Friends of Peace Pilgrim and Ocean Tree Books, Shelton, CT.

Pivac N, Kozarić-Kovačić D, et al. 2007, 'Neurobiology of Posttraumatic Stress Disorder' in S Begec (ed.), *The Integration and Management of Traumatized People after Terrorist Attacks,* IOS Press, Amsterdam.

Polak F 1973 *The Image of the Future,* Elsevier Scientific Publishing Company, Amsterdam.

Politika 2008, *'Simbol Kruševca od izuzetnog značaja',* naslovi.net, 5 July, cited at www.naslovi.net/2008-07-05/politika/simbol-krusevca-od-izuzetnog-znacaja/731363.

Polk K 1994, *When Men Kill: Scenarios of masculine violence,* Cambridge University Press, Cambridge, UK.

Popović P 2009, *'Australijski Knindža', Elektronske Novine,* 5 February, cited at www.e-novine.com/index.php?news=22204.

Popović P & Davidov-Kesar D 2011, *'Srbija razgovara: mora li se kod psihijatra zbog sedativa', Politika,* 3 October, cited at www.politika.rs/rubrike/Drustvo/Srbija-razgovara-mora-li-sekod-psihijatra-zbog-sedativa.lt.html.

Postman N 1993, *Technopoly: The surrender of culture to technology,* Vintage Books, New York.

Powell S, Rosner R, et. al. 2003, 'Posttraumatic Growth After War: A study with former refugees and displaced people in Sarajevo', *Journal of Clinical Psychology,* vol.59, no.1, pp.71–83.

Priebe S, Bogic M, et al. 2010, 'Mental Disorders Following War in the Balkans: A study in 5 countries',

Archives of General Psychiatry, vol.67, no.5, pp.518–28.

Radivojević B 2006, *'Sedativ svakom Srbinu!', Večernje Novosti,* 20 March, cited at www.novosti.rs/vesti/naslovna/aktuelno.69.html:181147-Sedativ-svakom-Srbinu.

Ramet SP 2005, *Thinking About Yugoslavia: Scholarly debates about the Yugoslav breakup and the wars in Bosnia and Kosovo,* Cambridge University Press, Cambridge, UK.

Raphael B, Swan P, et. al. 1998, 'Intergenerational aspects of trauma for Australian Aboriginal people' in Y Danieli (ed.), *International Handbook of Multigenerational Legacies of Trauma,* op. cit., p.336.

Reardon B 1993, *Women and Peace: Feminist visions of global security,* State University of New York Press, Albany, New York.

______2000, 'Sexism and the War system' in DP Barash (ed.), *Approaches to Peace: A reader in peace studies,* Oxford University Press, New York.

Redžić E 2005, *Bosnia and Herzegovina in the Second World War,* Frank Cass, New York.

Reeser TW 2010, *Masculinities in Theory: An introduction,* Wiley Blackwell, Oxford.

Reus-Smit C 2004, *The Politics of International Law,* Cambridge University Press, Cambridge, UK.

Reyes G, Elhai JD, et. al. (eds) 2008, *The Encyclopedia of Psychological Trauma,* Wiley, Hoboken NJ.

Rigby A 2010, 'Communitarian Peace Experiments' in NJ Young (ed.), *The Oxford International Encyclopedia of Peace,* vol.1, op. cit., pp.378–80.

Rivett K 2004, *After Defensive War,* Australian Scholarly Publishing, Melbourne.

Roberts DW 2008, *Human Insecurity: Global structures of violence,* Zed Books, London.

Roeder PG & Rothchild D (eds) 2005, *Sustainable Peace: Power and democracy after civil wars,* Cornell University Press, Ithaca, New York.

Rogel C 2004, *The Breakup of Yugoslavia and the War in Bosnia,* Greenwood Press, Westport, CT.

Rosandić R 1994, 'Patriotic Education' in R Rosandić & V Pešić (eds), *Warfare, Patriotism, Patriarchy,* op. cit., pp.41–57.

Rosandić R & Pešić V 1994, *Warfare, Patriotism, Patriarchy: The analysis of elementary school textbooks,* Centre for Anti-War Action Association MOST, Belgrade.

Roy A 2003, 'Confronting Empire', cited at www.ratical.org/ratville/CAH/AR012703.html.

Ruddick S 2004, 'Maternal Thinking as a Feminist Standpoint' in SG Harding (ed.), *The Feminist Standpoint Theory Reader: Intellectual and political controversies,* Routledge, New York.

Sabes-Figuera R, McCrone P, et. al. 2012, 'Long-Term Impact of War on Healthcare Costs: An eight-country study', cited at www.plosone.org/article/info%3Adoi%2F10.1371%2Fjournal.pone.0029603

Salick EC & Auerbach CF 2006, 'From Devastation to Integration: Adjusting to and growing from medical trauma', *Qualitative Health Research,* vol.16, no.8, pp.1021–37.

Šarić P 1990, *'Alternativa nasilju',* Duga, 18 August, pp.67–69.

Savković B (ed.) 1998, *Serbia, Who Is That?,* Alternativa, Belgrade.

Seidler VJ 2005, *Transforming Masculinities: Men, cultures, bodies, power, sex, and love,* Routledge, London.

Senehi J 2002, 'Constructive Storytelling: A peace process', *Peace and Conflict Studies,* vol.9, no.2, pp.41–63.

_____2010, 'Storytelling and Peace' in NJ Young (ed), *The Oxford International Encyclopedia of Peace,* vol.4, op. cit., pp.111–13.

Shakhireva S 2007, 'Swaddled Nation: Modern Mother Russia and a psychohistorical reassessment of Stalin', *The Journal of Psychohistory,* vol.35, no.1, pp.34–60.

Sharma M, Atri A, et. al. 2012, *Foundations of Mental Health Promotion,* Jones & Bartlett Learning, Burlington, MA.

Shechter H & Salomon G 2005, 'Does Vicarious Experience of Suffering Affect Empathy for an Adversary? The effects of Israeli's visits to Auschwitz on their empathy for Palestinians', *Journal of Peace Education,* vol.2, no.2, pp.125–38.

Shiva V 1993, 'Monocultures of the Mind', *Trumpeter,* vol.10, no.4, cited at www.trabal.org/ad_ict4d_reader/shivamono1993.pdf.

Siebers T (ed.) 1994, *Heterotopia: Postmodern utopia and the body politics,* The University of Michigan Press, Ann Arbor, MI.

Simić O 2011, 'Speaking the Unspeakable, Remembering the Wished to Be Forgotten', *International Feminist Journal of Politics,* vol.13, no.2, pp.248–55.

Simon B 1983, 'The History of Education' in P Hirst (ed.), *Educational Theory and its Foundation Disciplines,* Routledge & Kegan Paul, London.

Simon WF 1980, *Time for Truth,* Berkley, New York.

SIPRI (Stockholm International Peace Research Institute) 2011, 'World military spending reached $1.6 trillion in 2010, biggest increase in South America, fall in Europe according to new SIPRI data', Press Release, 11 April, cited at www.sipri.org/media/press releases/milex.

Sklevicky L 1996, *Konji, žene, ratovi,* Druga & Ženska infoteka, Zagreb.

Slaughter R 1998, 'The Knowledge Base of Futures Studies' in D Hicks & R Slaughter (eds), *Futures Education: World yearbook of education 1998,* Kogan Page, London.

Smith P, Perrin S, et al. 2002, 'War Exposure among Children from Bosnia-Hercegovina: Psychological adjustment in a community sample', *Journal of Traumatic Stress,* vol.15, pp.147–56.

Spencer M (ed.) 2000, *The Lessons of Yugoslavia,* Elsevier Science, Amsterdam.

Špirić Z 2008, *Ratna psihotrauma srpskih veterana. Udruženje boraca rata Republike Srbije od* 1990.god., Beograd.

Staub E 2000, 'Genocide and Mass Killing: Origins, prevention, healing, and reconciliation', *Political Psychology,* vol.21, no.2, pp.367–82.

_____2003, *The Psychology of Good and Evil: Why children, adults, and groups help and harm others,* Cambridge University Press, Cambridge, UK.

Stenton M 2000, *Radio London and Resistance in Occupied Europe: British political warfare 1939–1943,* Oxford University Press, New York.

Stephenson CM 2009, 'Gender Equality and the Culture of Peace' in J De Rivera (ed.), *Handbook on Building Cultures of Peace,* Springer, New York.

Stevens A 2010, 'Attractions of War' in NJ Young (ed.), *The Oxford International Encyclopedia of Peace,* vol.4, op. cit., pp.325–27.

Stillman S, McKenzie D, et. al. 2007, 'Migration and Mental Health: Evidence from a natural experiment', Department of Economics Working Paper, University of Waikato, New Zealand.

Stojaković G 2011, *'Prilog za istoriju ženskog pokreta u Vojvodini i Srbiji u 19. i 20. veku'* in I Milojević & S Markov (eds), *Uvod u RodneTeorije, Centar za rodne studije,* ACIMSI, Univerzitet u Novom Sadu i Mediterran Publishing, Novi Sad, Serbia.

Stokes G 1997, 'Review of Maria Todorova. Imagining the Balkans', H-Net Reviews, September, cited at w ww.ess.uwe.ac.uk/genocide/reviewy3.htm.

Strauss O 1918, in *The Independent*, Independent Publications, University of Michigan, Ann Arbor, MI.

Sullivan D & Tifft L (eds) 2006 *Handbook of Restorative Justice: A global perspective*, Routledge, London and New York.

Sullivan S 2002, *Marx for a Postcommunist Era: On poverty, corruption, and banalit* y, Routledge, London.

Suvin D 2000, 'Of the utopias that have been conceived...', 'Utopia: The search for the ideal society in the western world' exhibition, The New York Public Library, cited at utopia.nypl.org/I_meta_3.html.

Sveaass N 2012, 'Trauma – from an Individual and a Group Perspective' in DJ Christie (ed.), *The Encyclopedia of Peace Psychology*, vol.1, Wiley-VCH, Germany.

Svoboda D 2004, 'Living in a Communist Country', *Education Forum*, cited at educationforum.ipbhost.co m/index.php?showtopic=1743.

Swain J 2005, 'Masculinities in Education' in MS Kimmel, J Hearn, et. al. (eds), *Handbook of Studies on Men and Masculinities*, op. cit., pp.213–29.

Tagore R 1916, 'Nationalism' in *Four Chapters,* Macmillan, London, 1976.

Tanaka G 2005, 'Storytelling and Peace Education', *Journal of Peace Education,* vol.2, no.1, pp.93–97.

Tanjug 2012, '19 years since massacre in Štrpci', cited at http://www.b92.net/eng/news/crimesarticle.php?yyyy=2012&mm=02&dd=27&nav_id=78996.

Tedeschi RG 1999, 'Violence Transformed: Posttraumatic growth in survivors and their societies', *Aggression and Violent Behavior,* vol.4, no.3, pp.319–41.

Tedeschi RG & Calhoun LG 1996, 'The Posttraumatic Growth Inventory: Measuring the positive legacy of trauma', *Journal of Traumatic Stress,* vol.9, no.3, 1pp. 455–71.

______2004, 'Posttraumatic Growth: Conceptual foundations and empirical evidence', *Psychological Inquiry,* vol.15, no.1, pp 1–18.

TFF (Transnational Foundation for Peace and Future Research) 1992, 'Preventing War in Kosovo', cited at www.transnational.org.

Thomson M 2012, 'U.S. Military Suicides in 2012: 155 days, 154 dead', cited at battleland. blogs.time.com/2012/06/08/lagging-indicator/.

Tickner JA 2002, 'Feminist Perspectives on International Relations' in W Carlsnaes, T Risse-Kappen, et. al. (eds) *Handbook of International Relations,* Sage, London.

Todorova MN 1994, 'The Balkans: From discovery to invention', *Slavic Review,* vol.53, no.2, pp.453–82.

______1997, *Imagining the Balkans,* Oxford University Press, New York.

______1999, 'Bones of Contention', cited at www.clas.ufl.edu/events/news/articles/199911_todorova.html.

Trifunović D 1998, KNJIŽEVNOST, 3 January 2011, cited at riznicasrpska.net/knjizevnost/index.php?topic=405.0.

Tziotziou A, Livas D, et al. 2006, 'Coping with Traumatic Experiences in a Communal Setting: Therapeutic communities', *International Journal for Therapeutic and Supportive Organizations,* vol.27, no.4, pp.589–99.

UN (United Nations) 2012, 'Women in Peacekeeping', cited at www.un.org/en/peacekeeping/issues/women/womeninpk.shtml.

UNAC (UN Association of Canada) 2010, 'Cultures of Peace' factsheet, cited at www.unac.org/en/projects/peace/role.asp.

UNECE (UN Economic Commission for Europe) 2012, Statistical database, Gender statistics, Crime and Violence, cited at w3.unece.org/pxweb/database/STAT/30-GE/07-CV/?lang=1.

UNHCR (UN High Commissioner for Refugees) 2009; 2010, both cited at www.unhcr.org/statistics.

UNICTY (UN International Criminal Tribunal for the former Yugoslavia), cited at www.un.org/icty/transe54/060125ED.htm.

Utopian Dreamer 2012, 'Paxtopia', cited at www.utopiandreamer.com/paxtopia.htm.

Veblen T 2009, *Absentee Ownership: Business enterprise in recent times, the case of America* (first edition 1923), Transaction, New Brunswick, NJ.

Vissing Y & Moore-Vissing Q 2010, 'Warless Societies' in NJ Young (ed.), *The Oxford International Encyclopedia of Peace,* vol.4, op. cit., pp.342–45.

Vladisavljević N 2008, *Serbia's Antibureaucratic Revolution: Milošević, the fall of communism and nationalist mobilization,* Palgrave Macmillan, London.

Vlahović V 1981, *Španski građanski rat, Sabrani radovi I,* Izdavački Centar Komunist, Belgrade.

Vlajković J, Srna J, et. al, 2000, *Psihologija izbeglištva,* Željko Albulj, Belgrade.

Vojna enciklopedija 1974 (knjiga osma), Beograd, Vojnoizdavački zavod.

Vojska Srbije 2012, cited at www.vs.rs/index.php?news_article=47ad6a7c-2d27-102f-8d2f-000c29270931.

Voros J 2008, Listserv post cited at www.wfsf.org.

Wachtel A 1988, *Making a Nation, Breaking a Nation: Literature and cultural politics in Yugoslavia,* Stanford University Press, Palo Alto, CA.

Walklate S 2004, *Gender, Crime, and Criminal Justice* (second edition), Willan Publishing, London.

Warren KJ & Cady DL 1994, 'Feminism and Peace: Seeing connections', *Hypatia,* vol.9, no.2, pp.4–21.

Warters W 2010, 'Male Violence, Unlearning of' in NJ Young (ed.), *The Oxford international Encyclopedia of Peace,* vol 2., op. cit., pp.659–62.

Weber A 2006, 'Feminist Peace and Conflict Theory' in *Encyclopaedia on Peace and Conflict Theory,* Routledge, London, cited at www.uibk.ac.at/peacestudies/downloads/peacelibrary/feministpeace.pdf.

Weber T 2008, *Our Friend 'the Enemy': Elite education in Britain and Germany before World War I,* Stanford University Press, Palo Alto, CA.

Weir S 2008, *History's Worst Decisions and the People Who Made Them,* Murdoch Books, Sydney.

White Ribbon 2012, 'Australia's campaign to stop violence against women', cited at www.whiteribbon.org.au/myoath.

Whitehead SM & Barrett FJ (eds) 2001, *The Masculinities Reader,* Polity Press, Stafford BC, Qld.

WHO (World Health Organization) 2005, *Mental Health Atlas,* Department of Mental Health and Substance Abuse, Geneva.

Wikipedia 2010, 'Otpor', cited at en.wikipedia.org/wiki/Otpor!

______2012, 'Anti-bureaucratic revolution', cited at en.wikipedia.org/wiki/Anti-bureaucratic_revolution.

Wilson JP & Tang CT (eds) 2010, *Cross-cultural Assessment of Psychological Trauma and PTSD,* Springer, New York.

Woito R 2010, 'Pacifism, Critical' in NJ Young (ed.), *The Oxford International Encyclopedia of Peace,* vol.3, op. cit., pp.308–13.

Wolf N 1991, *The Beauty Myth: How images of beauty are used against women,* Anchor Books, New York.

Woodword S 2008, 'The Security Council and the Wars in the Former Yugoslavia' in A Vaughan Lowe, A Roberts, et. al. (eds), *The United Nations Security Council and War: The evolution of thought and Ppractice since 1945*, Oxford University Press, Oxford.

Wright EO 2010, 'The Real Utopias Project: A general overview', cited at www.ssc.wisc.edu/~wright/OVERVIEW.html.

York S 2002, *Bringing Down a Dictator* (movie), cited at www.aforcemorepowerful.org/films/bdd/.

Young JE & Klosko JS 1994, *Reinventing Your Life: How to break free from negative life patterns and feel good again,* Plume Books, New York.

Young NJ (ed.) 2010a, *The Oxford International Encyclopedia of Peace,* vols 1 to 4, Oxford University Press, New York.

______2010b, 'Socialist Internationalism and Peace Movements' in NJ Young (ed.), *The Oxford International Encyclopedia of Peace,* vol.4, op. cit., pp.58–60.

Zaharijević A 2008, *Neko je rekao feminizam? Kako je feminizam uticao na žene XXI veka,* Heinrich Böll Stiftung, Beograd.

Zajović S (ed.) 2009, *Antimilitarizam i žene,* Žene u Crnom, Beograd.

Zajović S, Perković M, et. al. (eds) 2007, Žene za mir, Žene u Crnom, Beograd.

Zalewski M 2007, 'Do We Understand Each Other Yet? Troubling Feminist Encounters With(in) International Relations', *The British Journal of Politics & International Relations,* vol.9, no.2, pp.302–12.

Zimmerman ME 1994, *Contesting Earth's Future: Radical ecology and postmodernity,* University of California Press, Berkeley, CA.

Žižek S 1999, 'Human Rights and Its Discontents', Presentation to the European Graduate School, 16 November, cited at www.egs.edu/faculty/slavoj-zizek /articles/humanrights-and-its-discontents/.

Back Cover Material

Breathing: Violence In, Peace Out investigates the long term impact of transgenerational trauma and of personal and collective experiences with war and other acts of collective violence. It also looks at the possibilities for the emergence of more peaceful futures, including the individual and social practices necessary to bring them about. It explores the links between personal histories and world events and helps us to understand life's dualities: violence and peace, self and other, safety and threat, stability and change, oppressing and freeing, past and future.

The text moves between two voices, as Milojević journeys between the personal ('breathing in'), which describes her family's experience with violence, while the second academic voice ('breathing out') tries to make sense of it. The rhythm created in the text by inhaling and exhaling is used as a device to reflect not only what we take from the world but also what we give back to it. Milojević asks: Can we go back and function in a 'normal way' after the massive trauma that all wars and situations of life-threatening violence inevitably bring with them? And what happens to the people who are impacted by them, once these events are over?

Breathing: Violence In, Peace Out is an inquiry into alternative futures as Milojević explores a range of possibilities, both for each of us personally, and for the world.

A

B

T

U

V

Z

Printed in Dunstable, United Kingdom

91343448R00281